Caring for Our Children

Caring for Our Children

*The History of Nursing
Royal Children's Hospital, Melbourne*

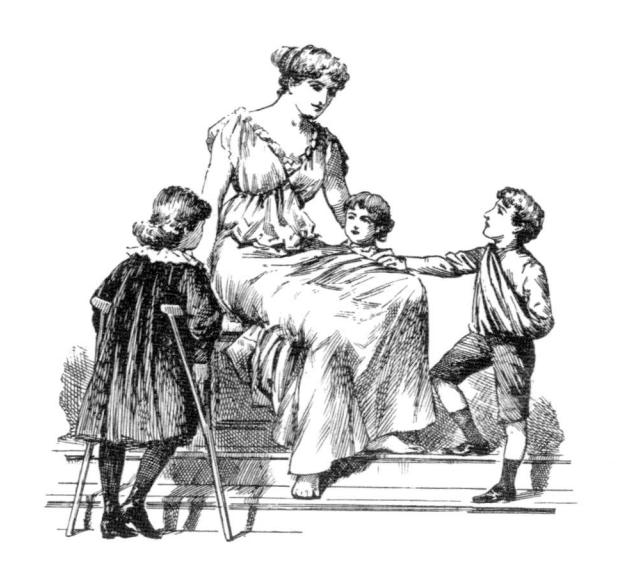

Margaret McInnes

AUSTRALIAN SCHOLARLY PUBLISHING
MELBOURNE

© Margaret Elizabeth McInnes 2006
First published 2006 by
Australian Scholarly Publishing Pty Ltd
Suite 102, 282 Collins Street, Melbourne 3000
PO Box 299 Kew, Victoria 3101
tel (03) 9654 0250   fax (03) 9663 0161
www.scholarly.info
aspic@ozemail.com.au

A National Library of Australia
cataloguing-in-publication entry
for this title is available.
ISBN 1 74097 119 1

Printed by BPA Print Group.

Designed by Green Poles Design.

Contents

Foreword	vii
Royal Children's Hospital Nurses' Code	viii
Introduction	ix
Acknowledgements	xi

PART 1 *1870–1900*

1	Foundation of a Children's Hospital	3
2	The Dawn of Professionalism	21
3	A Growing Workforce	45

PART 2 *1900–1924*

4	The Years of Miss Player	65
5	The War Years	79
6	War Nurses Return	93

PART 3 *1924–1947*

7	Between the Wars	111
8	Nursing Disabled Children	133
9	The Years of World War Two	153

PART 4 *1947–1962*

10	A New Era	185

PART 5 *1963–1987*

11	A New Hospital	227
12	Intensive Care and Theatre Nursing	253
13	Transition to Tertiary Education	273
14	Special Nursing	291

Epilogue	312
Notes	315
Appendix 1 Prize winners	334
Appendix 2 Graduates of the RCH School of Nursing 1890–1987	340
Select Bibliography	372
Index	375

Appreciable care has been taken in writing Caring for Our Children. Former staff members of the Hospital have been interviewed, and their views and recollections have been incorporated into this History. Care has also been taken to ensure that where those views might be thought contentious, they are clearly shown to be the views of individuals at the time. The author is indebted to the many who in one way or another participated in this project, and who generously offered her their views and comments.

Foreword

The history of nursing at the Royal Children's Hospital is absolutely fascinating, having commenced in 1870 when the Hospital for Sick Children was first established by a group of philanthropic men and women.

From the very beginning good nursing was essential, and all through this remarkable story shines the inspirational devotion and dedication of the nurses.

For many years, their workload was almost unbearable, their living conditions primitive and their pay, more often than not, non-existent, but their tender loving care for the patients was magnificent.

Gradually over the years evolution towards professionalism and tertiary education went ahead, and now paediatric nurses are well-educated and able to cope with the ever-increasing technology which is needed in modern nursing.

I would like to congratulate Mrs McInnes most warmly on having covered every aspect of nursing. Her book is compulsive reading for all those interested in the history of nursing at the Royal Children's Hospital.

DAME ELISABETH MURDOCH, AC DBE CBE

Royal Children's Hospital Nurses' Code

As graduates, we acknowledge that the education we have completed has prepared us to be responsible members of Society, particularly in the care of sick children.

We intend to use the skills we possess for the benefit of our future patients and to further develop our nursing knowledge for the good of all.

We will recognise the individual rights of the sick person, including cultural beliefs, privacy and confidentiality.

We will continue to be intelligent, caring and concerned citizens.

We will unite with other members of the health team and ancillary professions in meeting the emotional, physical and social needs of our patients, so contributing to the welfare of the community.

Introduction

The Royal Children's Hospital nurses occupy a unique place in the growth of the nursing profession with their contribution to child health and welfare in Australia. The first certificated children's nurses date from 1889.

The first part of this story marks the beginning of formal children's nursing at the Hospital for Sick Children in the 1870s under the guidance of Sarah Anne Bishop, herself an uncertified but very experienced nurse from the Ballarat goldfields hospital, and Dr William Snowball, Australia's first paediatrician. The work was dangerous, with infections rampant, the death of children a daily occurrence and the nurses' own health severely compromised.

In common with charity hospitals founded in Australia, general nursing adhered to principles adapted from the Nightingale School of St Thomas' Hospital in London. Melbourne was influenced by the nineteenth-century development of hospitals for children in England and Europe, particularly Great Ormond Street Hospital for Children in London. Physician Dr Charles West's book *How to Nurse Sick Children* (London, 1854) predates Florence Nightingale's writing.

From small beginnings the Children's Hospital branched into diverse locations providing convalescence, rehabilitation, and specialist in-patient and out-patient care. The gentle enclosed world of nineteenth-century children's nursing had to adapt to growing specialties and received general registration. By the mid-twentieth century, several hundred nurses were employed in a hospital with annexes of some 400 beds.

From the 1950s developments in clinical paediatrics were so pronounced that children's nursing was challenged by the disappearance of many childhood illnesses; the widespread use of antibiotics and immunisation made long-term nursing of children in hospital unnecessary. Increasing specialisation in paediatrics called for more sophisticated approaches, while modern theories of child development showed a growing transformation in the relationship between hospitals, staff, children and their parents.

In the final part of the story, we see a transition to tertiary education and a fading of the hundred-year-old apprenticeship system. Nursing at the Royal Children's Hospital underwent transformation to unit management and orientation. The last Nursing School ended in 1987. The Hospital is affiliated with Melbourne

University as a centre for postgraduate training in paediatric nursing for Victoria, Tasmania and the Territories.

For some years, the League of Former Trainees of the Royal Children's Hospital have been collecting memorabilia, photographs and research material in order to preserve their history. This book cannot possibly tell the whole story and it is hoped that others may be inspired to carry on.

Acknowledgements

In the course of researching and writing this book, I have been generously assisted by hundreds of people in Australia and around the world who gave their time, recollections and hospitality. It is not possible to acknowledge each individual, but for those who began the process in this journey, I reserve special thanks. Most will find their names in the text and notes.

A special thank you goes to Sandra Willis, who designed the questionnaire without which I could not have traced the wide range of former nurses. Miss Rae Anstee AM, President of the League of Former Trainees, offered support and encouragement at all times, while the editorial sub-committee showed special dedication: Audrey Grant (Chair), Adele Brain OAM, Nance Gooderham and Heather Telfer. Dr Peter Yule gave me enormous encouragement with his attendance at committee meetings, reading chapters and offering invaluable advice.

The History would not have been possible without the Archival Records collected over many years by nurses themselves and the support and work of Bronwyn Hewitt, the Royal Children's Hospital Archivist.

I would like to acknowledge the kind hospitality of Mr Nicholas Baldwin, Archivist of Great Ormond Street Hospital for Children in London, when I visited that institution in search of records of the Melbourne nurses who received training there. He allowed me access to Dr Charles West's 1854 handbook for nurses, *How to Nurse Sick Children*, a most precious archival possession. Ms Cheryl Norris of the School of Nursing at the University of Tasmania assisted me with advice in my search for answers to the puzzle of the origin of the early Children's Hospital Nightingale nurses.

My grateful thanks go to Ms Elizabeth Kennedy, Corporate Counsel for Women's and Children's Hospitals, who generously and willingly helped me with her timely advice.

Last, but not least, I owe it all to my husband, Dr Laurie McInnes, for his unfailing support and advice.

MARGARET MCINNES
February 2006

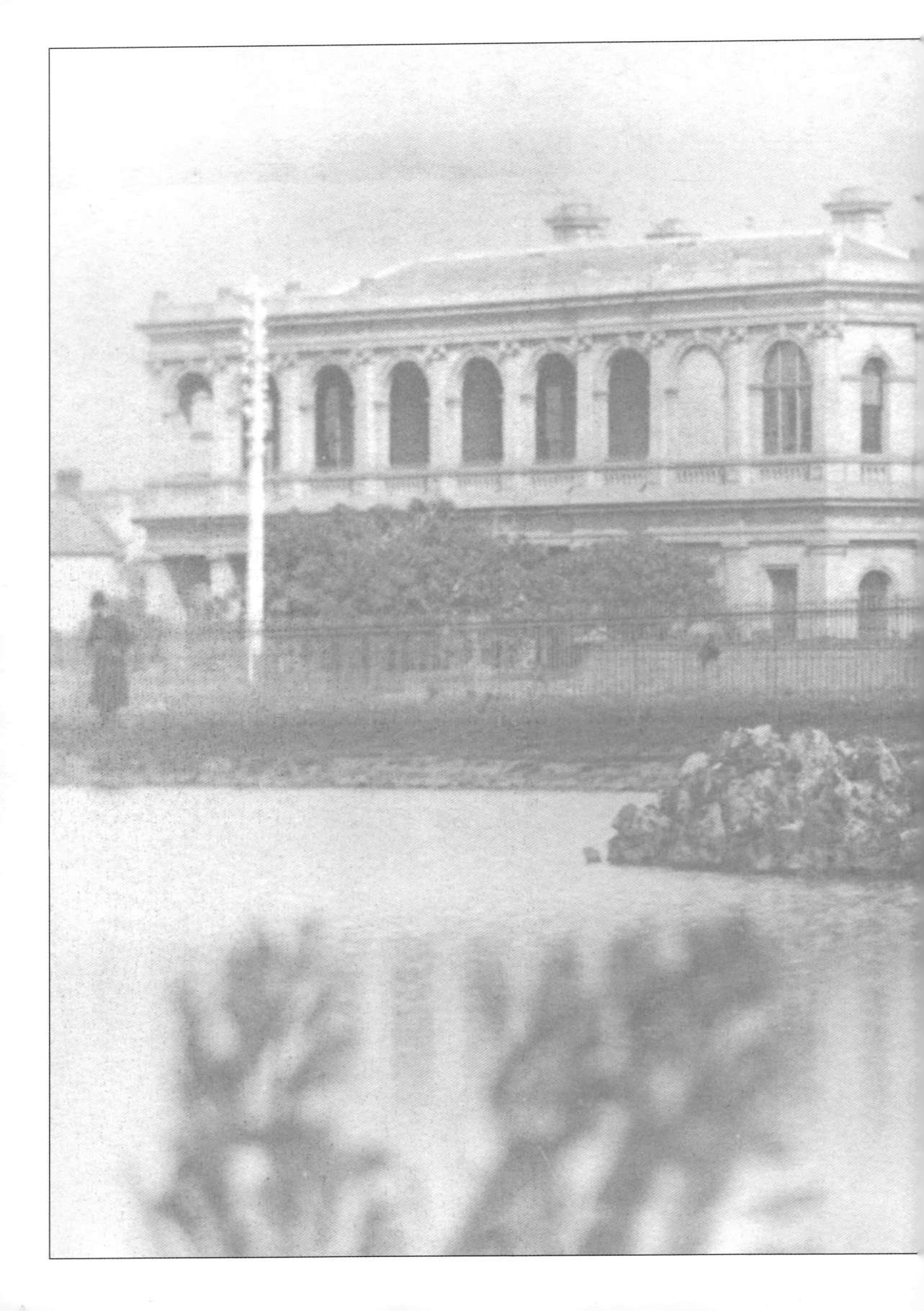

Part 1

1870–1900

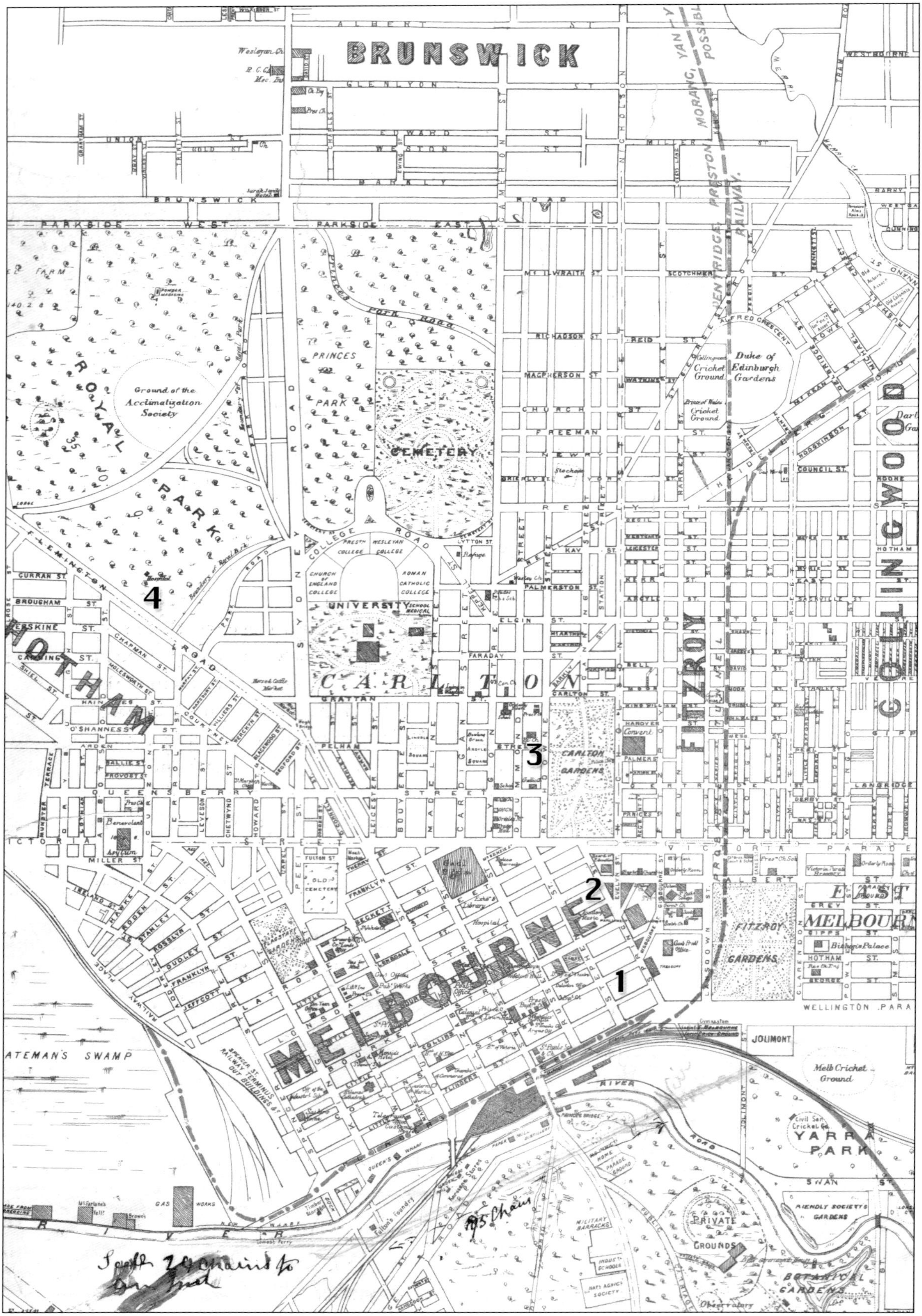
BRUNSWICK
ALBERT ST
GLENLYON ST
EDWARD ST
WESTON ST
BARKLY ST
BRUNSWICK ROAD
PARKSIDE WEST
PARKSIDE EAST
ROYAL PARK
Ground of the Acclimatization Society
PRINCES PARK
CEMETERY
UNIVERSITY
CARLTON
FITZROY
COLLINGWOOD
HOTHAM
MELBOURNE
EAST MELBOURNE
Duke of Edinburgh Gardens
CARLTON GARDENS
FITZROY GARDENS
FLAGSTAFF GARDENS
OLD CEMETERY
JOLIMONT
Melb Cricket Ground
YARRA PARK
FRIENDLY SOCIETYS GARDENS
PRIVATE GROUNDS
BOTANICAL GARDENS
BATEMAN'S SWAMP
GAS WORKS
RIVER
MILITARY BARRACKS
SPENCER ST RAILWAY TERMINUS & GOODS SHEDS
QUEENSBERRY STREET
VICTORIA STREET
VICTORIA PARADE
WELLINGTON PARADE
FLEMINGTON ROAD
SYDNEY ROAD
COLLEGE ROAD
GRATTAN ST
ELGIN ST
FARADAY
PELHAM
MORANG, YAN-YEAN, PRESTON, HEIDELBERG RAILWAY POSSIBLE
1
2
3
4

CHAPTER 1

Foundation of a Children's Hospital

the 1870s

The hospital is a little world, in which experience only teaches wisdom. There are a thousand small matters to learn that the novice only grasps by patience and observation, details which come under the head of hospital etiquette, as rigorous as any code of law.[1]

Grace Jennings Carmichael, one of the Children's Hospital's first trained nurses and noted nineteenth-century literary writer, was the author of these words. As fresh today as when she penned them in the 1880s, the words convey the very first insight we have of the life and closed world of the Children's Hospital nurses. A healthy, bright-eyed country girl from Orbost in the Snowy River country of East Gippsland, Grace conjured up scenes of hospital life within 'the windowed walls, in the dim-lit wards with the rows of beds, the faces of the sick children and the cheerfulness of the womanly figures in caps and aprons moving noiselessly amongst them'.[2]

The Hospital for Sick Children in Nurse Grace's day in the late 1880s was away up the slight hill from the sounds and the noise and the bustle of the city, in the more salubrious streets near the Carlton Gardens. This first permanent hospital was a splendid building on the corner of Rathdowne and Pelham streets with beds for sixty

---

Map of Melbourne, 1877.
1   First Hospital for Sick Children, Stephen Street, 1870–73.
2   Spring Street, 1873–75.
3   Corner of Rathdowne and Pelham streets, Carlton, 1875–1963.
4   Parkville, 1963.

Map Collection, State Library of Victoria.

children. On fine days, children were seen on small cane couches on the long, broad balconies, their books and toys about them. The chattering and laughing in the fresh air and sunshine belied the reality of those with medical conditions where the 'typhoid fiend reigned supreme'.[3]

The nurse's responsibility and vigilance were infinitely important; she became observant, wise and intuitive. When there were only two or three nurses for the night, they did their rounds with a quick stealthy turn through the dim-lit wards, tucking in a bed here, moving an uncomfortable child there. Now and then a moan from a corner, or the typical shrill night scream of a hip disease patient, pierced the silence 'with startling intensity'.[4]

Our story begins some years earlier on a fine spring day on Friday 9 September 1870 when the Free Hospital for Sick Children began. At the behest of Robert Williams Pohlman, a County Court Judge, a group of people from Melbourne's elite society, touched by the sense of misery and sorrow in many poor households, met at the Parsonage at the old St James' Cathedral in William Street, to establish a Free Hospital for Sick Children.[5] These well-intentioned, like-minded people with a strong tradition of philanthropy and charity were Mrs Chambers, Mrs Clark, Mrs Stafford, Mrs Jennings, Mrs McPherson, Mrs Moline, Mrs Puckle and Mrs Rintel, upper-class wives of men representative of the medical, business and legal professions of Melbourne.

The idea was initially the inspiration of Dr John Singleton and Dr William Smith, both of whom had a special interest in the diseases of children. Singleton, a medical doctor and crusader against vice in the dark lanes and alleys of the city, saw a great need for a hospital for children. For a few months in 1870, Smith, a recent immigrant and medical practitioner, conducted a practice in the dubious precinct of Romeo Lane (Crossley Street) and Juliet Terrace (Liverpool Street), off Bourke Street, between Spring Street and Stephen Street (Exhibition Street). This area was known by police for its disorderly and immoral associations. Together, the two doctors decided to take the matter in hand.[6]

At the inaugural meeting of the founding Committee, Singleton's free dispensary, a small two-storey, six-room cottage at 39 Stephen Street, with a frontage of eighty-eight feet and a door directly onto the busy street, was chosen as the site of the first Free Hospital for Sick Children.[7]

DR JOHN SINGLETON was born in Dublin in 1801. After serving an apprenticeship with an apothecary, he studied medicine at Dublin University and gained his MD from the University of Glasgow in 1838. An Anglican, he became a temperance advocate and an evangelist at a young age. He moved to Victoria in 1850 with his family and set up practice in Collins Street. In 1860 he went to Warrnambool, where he was instrumental in setting up the Framlingham Aboriginal Settlement.

On his return to Melbourne in 1867, Singleton resumed medical practice and with Bishop Charles Perry and other people of influence, including Judge William Pohlman and Sir William Stawell, founded the Society for the Promotion of Morality. Of all the organisations supported by the society, the ones Singleton had the most to do with were the Model Lodging House for Men in King Street, the 'Retreat for Friendless and Fallen Women' in Islington Street in Collingwood and the Collingwood Dispensary with links to Melbourne City Mission. He saw the Children's Hospital as combining free medical care and Christian mission, but soon left it because of religious differences with the Committee.

A competent physician and vocal advocate of public health, Singleton highlighted the high infant mortality and the scourges of typhoid and tuberculosis. He was against the widespread use of alcohol in the practice of medicine. He died in 1891, a famous figure among the poor and downtrodden. Some of the institutions he founded bear his name today.[8]

DR WILLIAM SMITH came to Melbourne in 1870 and in that year was appointed the first curator of pathology at the Melbourne Hospital and lecturer in anatomy at the Melbourne Medical School. Associated with Dr John Singleton in the establishment of the first Children's Hospital, he was appointed Honorary Surgeon. He retired from the Hospital within a year and took up practice in Casterton, returning to England in 1875 to become a lecturer at Oxford.[9]

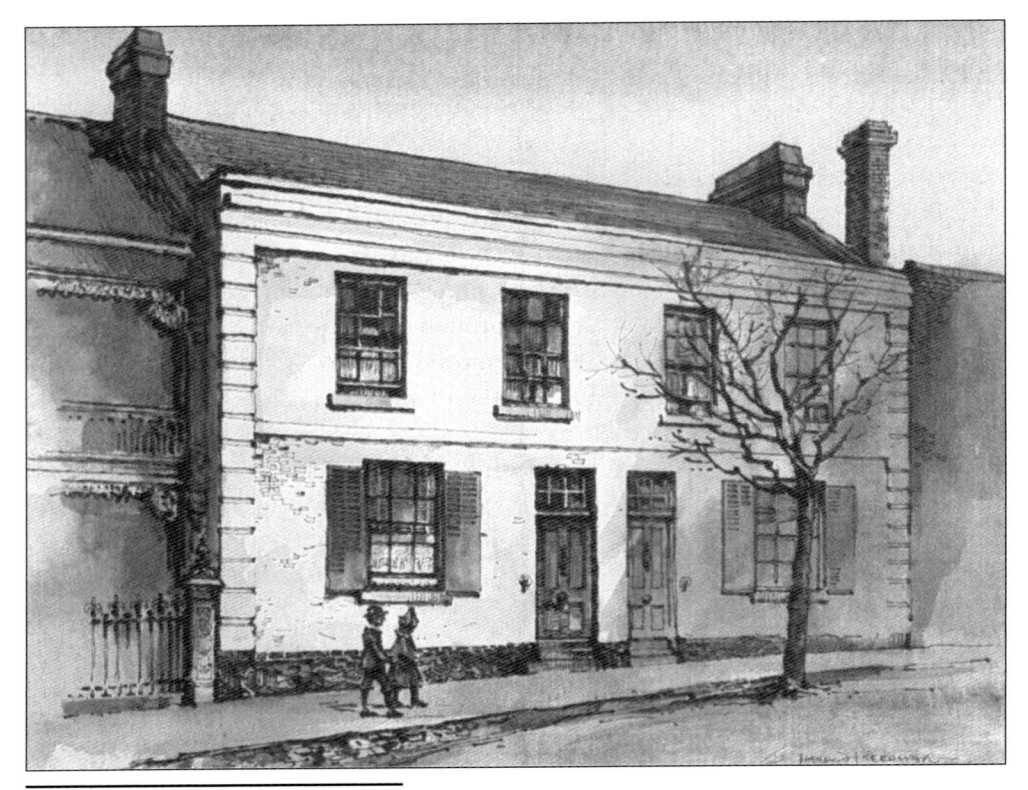

Free Hospital for Sick Children, 39 Stephen Street, Melbourne, 1870.
Sketch by Harold Freedman.

Melbourne in the 1870s

It is not difficult to imagine Melbourne as it was in the heady days following the gold rushes. To the observer and visitor, the city was visually beautiful with graceful buildings and a vibrant youthful population. Victoria had grown at a staggering rate; by 1870 there were half a million people, half of those in Melbourne. The high birth rates of the late 1850s and 1860s created an extraordinarily large number of young people, and the profile of inner Melbourne changed with a significant influx of dependent women seeking accommodation and a future for their children.[10]

Wealth generated from the goldfields created optimism; business enterprises flourished with well-developed communications networks, the railways and the telegraph. Exports from the Victorian hinterland were shipped through the busiest port in the southern hemisphere, while imports flooded Melbourne with all the good things money could buy. Fine buildings dominated the skyline. By night the city had a Bohemian air; flickering gas lamps lit the streets for people seeking excitement in the theatres and other attractions. Decorative terraces and suburban villas appeared in miraculous time. Streets became the playgrounds for children in the crowded city and in the new suburbs pushing out to the north and south: Richmond, Brunswick, Collingwood, North Melbourne, Fitzroy and Carlton. South of Melbourne's Yarra River, the merchant middle classes built mansions away from the city to enjoy leafy streets and an outlook of botanical gardens and boulevards.

But there was another side to the city; Melbourne was rough and dirty. The city council proved unable to provide adequate services where immigration and a mobile population added to crowding, disease and filth. Reticulated water was piped into Melbourne in 1857 but there was no underground sewerage. Following legislation of 1869 outlawing cesspits, human waste was removed by the 'night man' to be delivered into depots such as Royal Park, dumped conveniently on the side of the road or in the river from the Johnston Street Bridge in Abbotsford. Liquid refuse, chamber slops, ablution water, drainage from urinals, stables, cowsheds and noxious trades flowed through open bluestone gutters down the length of city streets to the ultimate destination of the Yarra and Port Phillip Bay.

Child health and mortality

In colonial times Australian children were particularly vulnerable to unhygienic living conditions. The new country of wide spaces, sunlight, fresh air and freedom to roam was initially beneficial to the growth and development of children. By the 1850s and 1860s, however, the medical profession expressed concern with childhood mortality as many children were 'living in a state highly incompatible with infantile life'.[11] The chances of infants surviving decreased in the overcrowded and insanitary industrial inner-suburbs, where people lived in appalling conditions and knowledge of nutrition and hygiene was poor. Babies had a slim chance of survival when food and milk was delivered in open carts by horses leaving steaming, stinking heaps of manure and urine, while poor waste disposal services ensured rubbish, offal, dead animals and filth piled up outside every front door and in every backyard.

In one quarter of 1853, 37 per cent of deaths in the general population in Melbourne occurred in children under five years, but 50 per cent of these were under one year. In the years 1854–57, infant mortality was 20 per cent of births.[12] By the 1880s, of every 100 children born, 90 might survive to the age of one year, 82 to five years and only 78 to adulthood. Lack of fresh, suitable food and clean milk led to a high summer mortality. The disorders of babies and young children in colonial times were vague: atrophy, marasmus, debility and inanition (in modern terms, failure to thrive) were often caused by lack of nourishing food. The transmission of gastroenteritis, a major cause of the large numbers of deaths of babies in the first year of life, was poorly understood. In 1876, the Annual Report of the Hospital for Sick Children noted that 'the mortality of children in this colony is altogether the consequence of causes of a social nature'.[13]

We only have to look around the old graveyards in Victoria to understand the ravages of infectious diseases. Largely absent in the first few years of settlement, whooping cough, measles, diphtheria and scarlet fever caused intermittent epidemics with catastrophic results in the second half of the nineteenth century. The actual morbidity is difficult to assess as interpretation of diagnosis among diseases such as typhoid, typhus fever, gastroenteritis, dysentery and intestinal disorders is confusing. The most frightening, diphtheria, was sometimes confused with scarlet fever, croup, angina, sore throat or laryngitis. Diphtheria first appeared in Victoria in 1858 but declined between 1892 and 1895 with the introduction of diphtheria antitoxin. It challenged nurses who witnessed toxaemia and suffocative deaths; the Children's nurses were closely involved with Hospital doctors as tracheostomy and, after 1891, intubation were introduced. Pulmonary tuberculosis, tubercular bone disease, rheumatic fever and osteomyelitis left children disabled, or to die after years of suffering.

Accidents were common. A contributing factor was the huge volume of heavy horse-drawn vehicular traffic. Contemporary photographs show 'slum' children playing in the streets, rarely wearing shoes; poor children were visible at the kerbside and in the lanes of the inner suburbs. Amputation injuries were common. In the decade 1860 to 1870, there were literally hundreds of reports of 'suspicious' cases of death, and in the *Medical Journal* of 1863 it was noted that at inquest about 25 per cent of deaths of children under three could be attributed to infanticide, neglect, ignorance and maltreatment.[14] Many undetected cases of illness leading to death were reported in the *Argus*. On Monday 18 October 1870, the City Coroner, Dr Youl, held an inquest on the body of William Andrew Risby, aged three years. William was playing in the yard at his mother's house in Carlton. He was found dead. The cause of death was said to be convulsions, and a verdict was returned to that effect.

The need for a children's hospital

Thirty-five years after the foundation of Melbourne there was only one general hospital for the poor of the city. Built in 1846, it was unable to meet the needs of the vastly changing and growing population. The conditions and overcrowding in adult wards caused great distress and the majority of inmates were suffering from accidents, tertiary syphilis and the lunacy of delirium brought about by the 'demon drink'. A hospital was planned for the south of the Yarra, the Alfred, but it did not provide care of the children of the poor. The Melbourne Lying-in Hospital and Infirmary for Diseases of Women and Children (Women's Hospital), founded in 1856, took children in a very limited way until 1868.[15]

Two main services were developed for children of the poor in Melbourne in the latter half of the nineteenth century. The first was the provision of orphanages, church welfare services, refuges and industrial schools. The earliest of these, the

Emerald Hill Protestant Orphan Asylum, was established in 1850. Refuges took children at times of severe distress; for example, the Carlton Women's Refuge, founded in 1854 by Dr Charles Perry, the Anglican Archbishop of Melbourne, became a haven for women and children during the depression of the 1890s.

There were also a few, scattered shopfront children's dispensaries where mothers could receive advice and a bottle of medicine; the most notable of these were the Collingwood and Richmond dispensaries run by Dr Singleton. These dispensaries, and later the Children's Hospital, were for children of the poor. The infants and children of middle and upper-class families, also susceptible to the diseases of the period, were nursed at home and attended by doctors who were paid their fee. Thus, in the early life of the Hospital it was a charitable institution for the poor, and only later, as medicine and nursing became more sophisticated, did it cater for sick children of all classes.

The idea of separate hospitals for children was growing throughout the civilised world. The Hôpital des Enfants Malades in Paris, the first Children's Hospital in Europe, was founded in 1802 and pre-dated the first special facility in Britain, Dr John Bunnell Davis' Universal Dispensary for Children, an out-patient clinic, opened in 1816. The most influential and first children's hospital of major importance in the world was the Great Ormond Street Hospital for Sick Children, founded in London in 1852, from which the Melbourne Children's, the first in the British colonies, is reputed to have taken the lead.

There were doubters. Children's hospitals engaged the attention of Florence Nightingale, regarded as an authority on nursing and influential in matters of sanitary reform. Her shrewd remarks about hospitals for children were far-reaching and ambivalent. While acknowledging the greater susceptibility of children than grown people to all noxious influences, 'the want of fresh air, of proper warmth, want of cleanliness in house, clothing, or body…and careless dieting…and by want of management in charge of them,' she was concerned that the child was better off with the mother. She recognised the life duration of babies as 'the most delicate test of sanitary conditions, [but] the remedies were certainly not the establishment of a Child's Hospital'.[16]

In 1868, the first Nightingale nurses arrived with Lucy Osburn in Sydney at the invitation of the Colonial Secretary Henry Parkes. There was a new awareness and confidence that much could be achieved in Australia towards a more unified and organised health care.

Some members of Melbourne's medical establishment became outspokenly critical of the need for a children's hospital. Dr Guy Fetherston, the President of the Medical Society, said:

> That social conditions did not justify it…that the classes which supply patients for such a hospital here, are in very different circumstances from

those in the old country. There, the poor classes were so very poor, their habitations so wretched, their surroundings so miserable, their food so scanty, that the term home means only suffering and misery.

The notion was that the poor could help themselves; their trouble was of their own doing. 'None but the intemperate, the unthrifty and incapable can be excluded from the prevalent rule of prosperity.'[17] It was suspected that some doctors were afraid of losing income with the establishment of a 'Free Hospital' but this was hardly justified when many poor families could not find a sixpence compared with the doctor's fee of half a guinea.

Diseases of children were little understood in Australia until the Melbourne Children's Hospital began in 1870. With a few early exceptions, medical interest had focussed on childbirth and child rearing. In the 1860s, enlightened attitudes towards the meaning and importance of childhood and changing perceptions of children as the source of future progress in a colonial society, paralleled scientific and medical developments in Europe and England. Alongside educational theorists came the germ theory of disease described by Pasteur and in 1867 Joseph Lister found a connection between airborne bacteria and wound infections. Carbolic sprays and steam sterilisation aided the development of surgery, ushering in a new and more progressive era in the study of medicine. Improvement in the application of anaesthesia, first developed in 1849, widened the scope of surgery with some success.

But it was the transformation of nursing by Florence Nightingale that made possible a new era in the care of hospital patients. While antiseptics and anaesthetics widened the horizons of surgery, hospitals were needed to house the patients. Nursing, previously thought to consist of the administration of medicines and the application of poultices, was suddenly thought of as the key to good organisation in three areas: the care of the patients, the war against infection and the moral tone of the hospital. The nurse could do more good than the physician and surgeon. It took several years before the principles of asepsis and antisepsis came into widespread use, but without good nursing there could not be a children's hospital.

Women and nursing

In the early days of settlement employment options for women were limited. Many found work in domestic service as maids, cooks or washerwomen while there were some opportunities for the better educated as private school teachers, and governesses. With the growth of the manufacturing industries and commerce, women were increasingly absorbed in factory work, in clothing, footwear and food processing. Shop counter work, as well as the less common government and professional services gradually expanded and became more available to women.[18]

Nursing had a history of extremely low status in Australia, not only because of the historical use of convict labour and the depiction of the nurse by Charles Dickens in his literary work,[19] but also as a result of the multicultural makeup of the population. For example, in the large Catholic Irish population in Australia, nursing was connected with the Religious Orders working with the poorest of the poor, the homeless, the drunkards and vagrants, orphans and incurables—the hidden and untouchable elements of the community.

Most nursing took place in homes as an extension of domestic life and involved bathing, feeding and the cooking of bland invalid food. Nursing outside the home gradually became an option with the proliferation of the Victorian country goldfield hospitals and with the growth of the charity network. As there were few employment openings outside a woman's social class, her bid for independence and freedom as well as her need to earn a living were inextricably bound with her finding a safe place to live. Hospital nursing with live-in conditions provided that security.

As Florence Nightingale's vision began to spread—with its focus on character, moral superiority, fortitude, courage, purity, unselfishness, perseverance and obedience—nursing became more respectable and one of the few occupations outside the home for 'women of breeding'. Family approval of nursing grew as their daughters began to live in hospital nurses' homes with home sisters and nursing superintendents. Importantly, the care of children provided the opportunity to work in a gentle motherly role, away from the potential moral contamination of male adult wards in general hospitals.

Nursing rapidly moved outside the home into hospitals as the idea of service and duty based on doing 'good works' became popular in the minds of the middle and upper classes. This was particularly so among members of Ladies' Guilds and church groups. As rudimentary nursing schemes began, remuneration was exceedingly low in return for board; the reward for selfless sacrifice was the expectation of a certificate of competency at the conclusion of the period of training. Not only were the wages low but the hours worked were incompatible with continuing good health; the nurse's work was hard, dangerous and—before technological innovations such as steam laundries, gas-fired hot water and cooking stoves, piped water and manual washing machines—extremely dirty. The duties and pay were sometimes less than those for domestic service. The causes and treatment of diseases were unknown. Hospitals were more often than not life threatening from infectious diseases for which there was no known prevention or cure.

The Hospital Committee

The role of the first Committee of the Children's Hospital at Stephen Street was very different to that of the other hospitals in Melbourne at that time. Usually at the Melbourne Hospital the subscribers, the Honorary Medical Officers and the Hospital Secretary had a right to vote. At the Hospital for Sick Children, ladies had tight control and outnumbered men on the Committee; caring for children was regarded as a task best left to the women. At the seventh meeting in November 1870, a resolution was passed that 'the Committee [is] to consist of 24 members and with Mrs Frances Perry, the Anglican Bishop's wife to be president of the Ladies Committee'. Mrs Patterson and Mrs Ettershank, ladies known for their 'good works', were among those invited to join the Committee.[20]

For many years there was no constitution. Instead, the members, social equals, made up their own rules, nominating those known to them and ruling all matters domestic and financial, as well as those involving staffing and the eligibility criteria of patients for admission. A Gentlemen's Committee consisted of lawyers, accountants and businessmen but, apart from financial dealings and lobbying, the men had no direct influence in the day-to-day running of the affairs of the Hospital, being frequently over-ruled by the ladies.

Initially, the twelve rules of the Hospital concerned management of the institution with protocols about subscriptions, eligibility for child admission, privileges for clergymen, the selection of the most urgent cases and the empowerment of medical officers to exclude or dismiss cases they saw as unfit for treatment. 'Ineligibility' for admission affected those whose parents were financially viable and therefore able to seek private care; it also affected those cases regarded as medically incurable. Victorian ladies of the upper class administered charity relief with a code distinguishing the 'deserving' poor and the 'undeserving' others. The former, perceived to have fallen down on their luck through no fault of their own, led respectable lives; the lifestyles of the latter involved abuse, gambling, drinking, swearing and general immorality. Remarkably, the only infectious disease barred from admission was smallpox.

The Committee members were determined to remain free of influence of one religion or sect. The attendance at meetings of Mrs Perry, the Bishop's wife, became sporadic and, on 2 October 1871, her resignation was accepted without comment. The reasons we can speculate upon, and unhappily, Dr Singleton resigned also one month later. In his memoirs Singleton stated, 'I could not feel that where God was not acknowledged I had proper place or business'.[21] Both Mrs Perry and Dr Singleton had requested prayers to commence each meeting, but this had been refused. Overtures by the clergyman Dr Bromby, Principal of Melbourne Grammar School and the husband of a Committee member, to conduct a fundraiser with a public talk on *The Origin of the Species*, was likewise refused. His daughter, Miss Eliza Bromby, an experienced nursing graduate of King's College Hospital in London, offered to assist with the training of the children's nurses. Although there is evidence that she spent some time as a Committee member, no record exists of her offer ever being taken up.

Consolidating an image in status-conscious Melbourne was important to gain trust and support in the charity network. Some Committee members in the early days of the Hospital were connected to many of the great squatting and pastoral families: the Clarkes, Chirnsides and the Austins. Lady Janet Clarke joined the Committee three times but attended meetings infrequently due to regular overseas visits and other charity obligations. The Chirnside family was represented by Annie, the wife of the landowner George, and Isabella, the wife of Robert. Catherine Austin (née Mack) of Berrybank married her cousin Albert Austin, owner of 200,000 acres in the Western District. The family of eleven children moved to Toorak in the 1870s and Catherine became a Children's Hospital Committee member for nearly twenty years, being President from 1899 to 1903.

The Children's Hospital was founded to provide assistance to children of the poor working class of the inner streets and industrial suburbs of Melbourne. The Committee never wavered in their care for the needy, although it took some time for their actions to catch the public imagination. It was undesirable, they felt, that children should be exposed to the sounds and moral evil associated with the great wards of the Melbourne General Hospital. It had been shown that institutions that specialised in services for children offered the greatest hope for their recovery. Some years later, when the Hospital had moved to Carlton, the Committee took this one step further. In the minutes of November 1880, the Vice-President Mrs Elizabeth Testar, by then sixty-one years old, mentioned 'that there were boys and girls in the same ward'. She moved a resolution 'that this should not be allowed and that no boys or girls over five years should be together'.

The Cottage Hospitals

The Hospital for Sick Children initially opened as an out-patient dispensary but it soon became evident that numbers of sick poor children would need overnight admission. The Providing Committee (the forerunner of the House Committee, in modern terms) prepared a simple inventory of requirements. By purchase or goodwill they obtained: six beds or cots, one bedstead for a nurse, mattresses, mackintoshes, sheets, soap, quilts, pillows and cases, a hip bath, a water can, pails, washing tubs, a fountain tray, chairs, a stair broom, a boiler for washing and a table. The first two children were admitted to 39 Stephen Street (re-named Exhibition Street) on 22 December 1870.

The Committee can be admired for opening a special hospital for children; there was no precedent in Australia. The Committee was very aware that there was a need to train nurses. They came to rely on the medical expertise and advice of the appointed consultants, Professor Halford of Melbourne University and Dr Motherwell, a renowned physician.

We know nothing about the personal characteristics of the first staff members, but the nursing and housework were first divided between a Mrs Bail and another person, with Mrs Bail taking precedence and receiving board and wages at the rate of £26 per annum from 1 November 1870. An increase of five shillings was promised from the 14th of the month, presumably after her passing the test of competency. A Mrs Sheldon was appointed for a fortnight with board and wages of seven shillings a week. As an example of the uncertain prospects, both appointments were terminable at a week's notice.[22] Enormous faith was invested in the character of the housekeeper and other domestic helpers.

Historical research has shown that in the city streets of Melbourne, the small cottages like the first Children's Hospital had no running water, taps, toilet facilities or bath. Water was delivered by cart or collected from a street pump at a large drinking fountain in the street.[23] It was then stored in the house fountain, a portable receptacle with a tap, kept near the wood-fired stove for convenience. The other source was a rain tank. Lavatories had a pan system with a trapdoor at the back lane for emptying. Some had dirt closets. The bathing of a child was carried out by sponging in bed or, if they were well enough, in the hip bath kept near the stove for warmth. Emptying was hard work; the housekeeper carried jugs up and down stairs, as the upper rooms were typically accessed by a steep narrow staircase. A rule required the patients to bring with them a change of linen, and the washing was done at the expense of the charity only in the case of those who resided at a great distance from the hospital. Bed mattresses became a problem, not only from soiling but also from bed bugs. A request for straw mattresses was rebuffed. This matter came up constantly, but the Secretary was directed to ask the Doctor's opinion on the matter. The begrudged cost of fumigation and destruction of mattresses was an early example of the frugality practised by the Committee.[24]

Stephen Street was never considered a permanent location. General nuisances, noise and hopelessly small premises caused the Committee to seek another house whilst waiting for a permanent home on land allocated at Parkville. In October 1873 children were moved to a new location, a narrow three-storey house on the hill in Spring Street facing the peaceful vista of the Treasury Gardens. A few doors from Flinders Street, this house was almost back to back in the same city block as the previous location but away from the crowds and dust of Stephen Street.

Community interest grew in the activities at the little Hospital. In September 1874, the Collingwood Gas Company offered to supply a meter free of charge, provided that the Committee agreed to take gas from them every alternate month. The Providing Committee did buy a gas stove served with Collingwood gas, a great innovation. This eastern facing house, although slightly larger and quite elegant, with pretty verandas open to fresh air and the morning sun, was not all it seemed. When the new Homeopathic Hospital took over the building after the Children's Hospital moved in 1875, it was found that the wooden bed frames and mattresses were full of bugs and had to be taken to the tip.[25]

Little is known about the first children admitted to the Hospital, but the case study published by Dr William Smith in the *Australian Medical Journal*, 'On

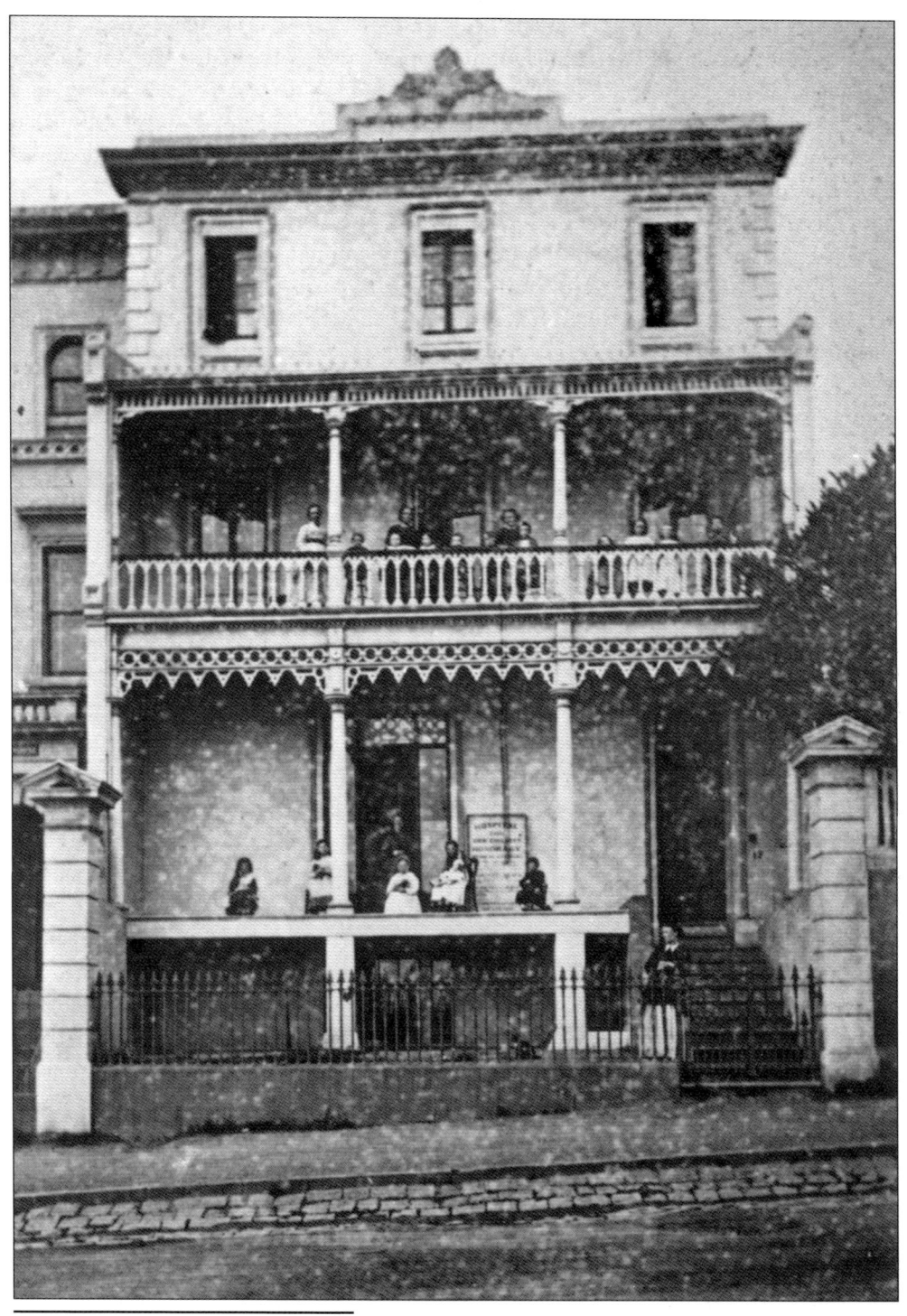

Children's Hospital, Spring Street, 1873–75.

Syphiloma' in January 1871, told the story of 'Clara, aged 5, who had caries of the frontal bone [of the skull] with bulbous eruptions on the palms from birth. She exhibited nervous symptoms, congestion of the brain and became unconscious and paralysed. The diagnosis was syphilis.'[26] Dr Charles Hunter's Annual Report for 1876 is the first definitive list of diseases treated. By far the most prevalent were typhoid and infantile fever, with paralysis, hip joint disease, atrophy and debility, bronchitis, scrofula (tuberculous abscesses), talipes, necrosis, syphilis, heart disease, fractures and dysentery being common also.

The nurses

Victoria had no organised general nurse training in 1870. The first specialist training was a three-month course in midwifery at the Lying-in Hospital (Women's Hospital), which began in 1862. Families preferred to be attended at home where most people were born, lived and died; hired nurses had varied reputations and it was accepted that the mother and members of the family, or a trusted domestic nurse, would assume responsibility for sick children. When hospitals needed nurses, the simple way was to advertise in the daily papers. Nursing was considered no more than a domestic or housekeeper job, the prerequisite being trustworthiness and respectability. Unfortunately, there are no Children's Hospital records to tell us how these nurses carried out the actual work or procedures in the early days.

The Hospital was run as a domestic establishment with kind neighbourhood women and trustworthy housekeepers handy in the sickroom who fed, bathed and comforted the living and laid out the dead. The very nature of caring for dangerously ill children demanded devotion to the job and a certain empathy. The nurse's responsibility and vigilance were infinitely important; she became observant, wise and intuitive. Practical bedside nursing skills were handed down from one nurse to another. It does seem that a great deal of the nurses' time was devoted to dusting, scrubbing, fetching and carrying water and other heavy tasks. Water was carried in china basins, with the nurse navigating a narrow staircase while wearing a full heavy twill dress. The nurse also had to provide adequate food and medicines, toileting, sponging, bathing and clean up messes.

Marian Harvey was appointed as the first Matron in September 1873 at a salary of £60 per annum. Her staff at Spring Street consisted of a cook, a helper and a general servant. Selected from thirty-two applicants, Miss Harvey was one of three educated sisters who came to Australia in 1859. She lived at Ballarat for some years and was said to be quite experienced for her role. Unfortunately, no personal records survived of her life but all three sisters followed nursing careers; Sarah and Emily both became matrons of the Women's Lying-in Hospital, and Sarah married one of the Medical Officers, Dr Guy Fetherston.[27] None of the sisters trained in a formal sense but all were the epitome of the 'lady nurse' of the Nightingale image. Marian's appointment was controversial: certain members of the community hinting at favouritism. On 13 September 1873, the *Argus* published a letter from Samuel Mullen, the Melbourne bookseller and sometime Hospital auditor, with an accusation that an influential member of the Committee pledged a majority of votes in advance. It was a first hint that the Children's Hospital was gaining notoriety as an elitist organisation. The Committee denied any impropriety.

With Miss Harvey's appointment the staff was arranged into a more orderly system. A general servant, Clara Huxley, was soon replaced by Sarah Murphy at a salary of eight shillings a week. Mrs Bail, having fulfilled the role of housekeeper and nurse since the Hospital began, assumed the title of Head Nurse, the first such position, and Anna Ford was engaged as the assistant nurse. A small hierarchy was established.

The nurse's day began at 6 am and, except for meal breaks, she was on duty continuously as a companion to the children until ten in the evening. The first hospital had room for only six beds; the work was intensive. Hospital rules precluded the admittance of young babies; there was no accommodation for nursing mothers. The move to Spring Street did provide more room and the Matron or her assistant slept overnight. In May 1874, the minutes record that the Committee directed Miss Harvey to employ a night nurse to sleep in the ward for the time John Ashton was a patient in the Hospital. And Dr Wigg was asked not to admit such young children again. He responded with a request 'that in cases where the medical men think it necessary to admit very young children to the Hospital they be empowered to do so and to forward a certificate of such cases to the Committee'. The Committee was convinced. Miss Harvey arranged for a nurse to sleep in the ward with the children.

Marian Harvey resigned in March 1875 to care for her sister Sarah's children following Sarah's death in childbirth. Nothing is known about her from that date. Unfortunately, no photographs survived. She died in Sale in the 1880s.

The doctors

With the resignation of Dr Singleton and Dr Smith in 1871, a succession of Medical Officers gained experience by attending the Out-patients Room. Drs William a'Beckett, Joseph Black and Henry Wigg were the new Honorary Consultants; suburban general practitioners, they were well-respected in the profession. But the most influential in the foundation and reputation of the nursing school was William Snowball.

A young graduate of the Melbourne Medical School, Dr Snowball had recently returned from Europe and England where he devoted much attention to the study of diseases of children at the Great Ormond Street Hospital for Sick Children in London. Appointed Resident Medical Officer at the Melbourne Children's Hospital in 1878 and Honorary Consultant in 1882, he became the major influence in the foundation and progress of the discipline of paediatrics in Australia as well as the driving force in the establishment of nurse training at the Children's Hospital. As an advocate of home nursing and domestic science, he introduced external classes in invalid cookery for nurses. He also assisted in the drafting of *Notes for Nurses*, loosely adapted from the book *How to Nurse Sick Children* written in 1854 by one of the most famous paediatricians of the century, Dr Charles West of Great Ormond Street Hospital. He further developed the first Hospital Pharmacopeia.[28]

Dr Snowball became known far and wide, receiving testimonies from the parents of children who travelled from the west coast of Tasmania, then a hazardous journey for such ill children. Lady Janet Clarke, a Committee member and friend, deeply admired his skills and sent letters of thanks preserved in the archives; as the consultant to the Clarke children, his visits to the family mansion 'Cliveden' in Clarendon Street, East Melbourne, were frequent.

Carlton

The Committee had been looking for permanent premises and, in 1875, the offer came to buy the elegant villa mansion of Justice Sir Redmond Barry on an acre of ground at the corner of Rathdowne and Pelham streets in Carlton. It was a building large enough for thirty children. In 1876, the Carlton address became the first permanent home of the Children's Hospital.

Sarah Anne Bishop, an experienced Matron from Ballarat, was chosen to replace Marian Harvey and reorganisation of staff began. A Miss Garson, 'having given her services to the Hospital for some time it was decided to engage her at £1 a month to make herself useful and be trained as a nurse'. The following year the Committee decided that 'it was desirable to engage nurses at low wages in consideration of the training they would receive'. Unfortunately time lapsed without a competent Head Nurse to train the young and inexperienced staff.

Despite this, the Annual Report of 1880 announced once again that 'classes have been arranged for the proper training of nurses employed in the hospital and have already have been productive of great benefit'. Matron Bishop and Dr Snowball were thanked as those 'whose great zeal and energy have greatly contributed to the success of the Hospital'. In a decade, the Hospital for Sick Children had become established from small beginnings to a solid foundation. But it would be almost another ten turbulent years before nursing would become a professional career.

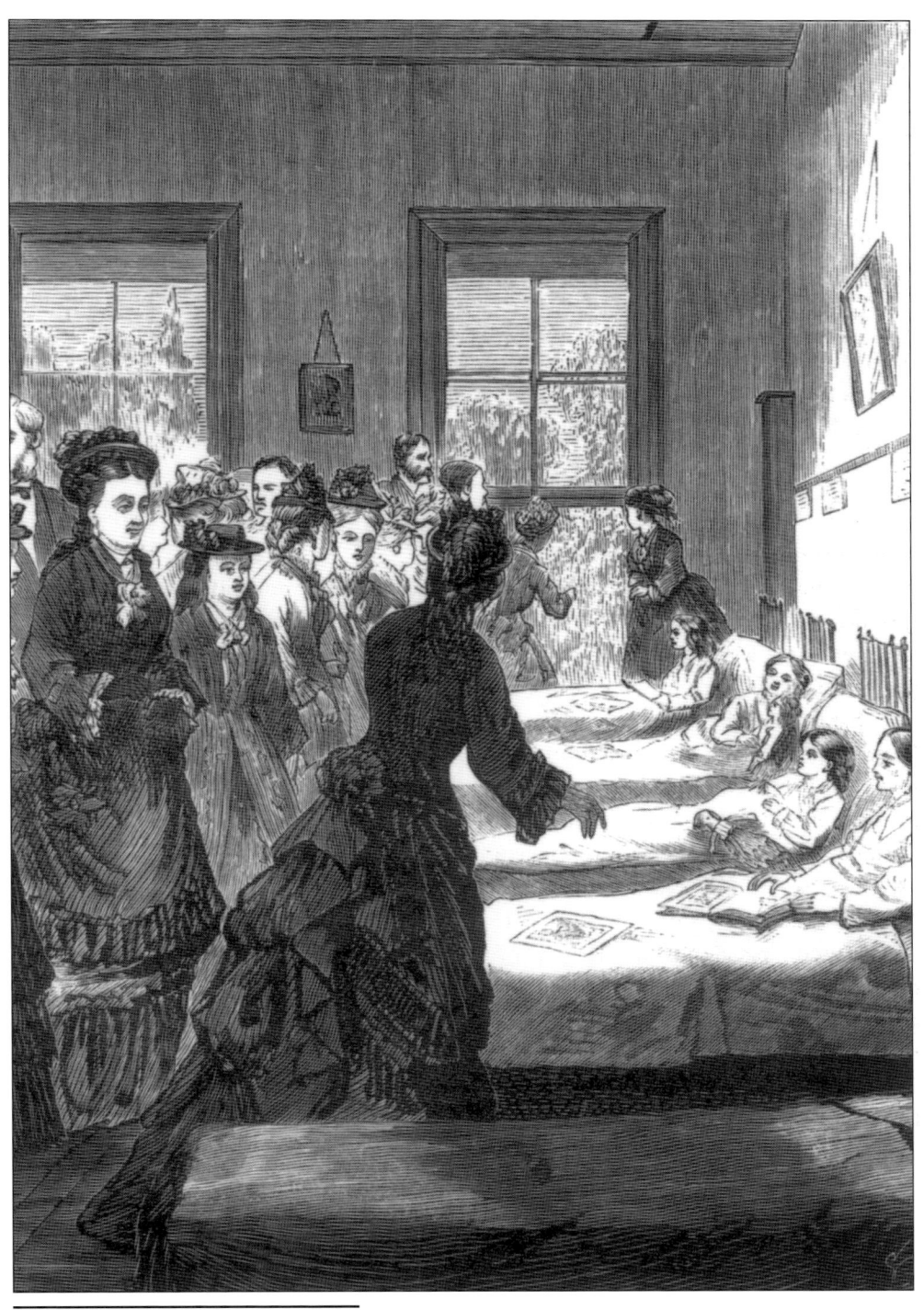

Opening of the new Hospital for Sick Children, Melbourne. Lady Bowen Ward.
Print: Wood Engraving, Samuel Calvert, 1876. La Trobe Collection, State Library of Victoria.

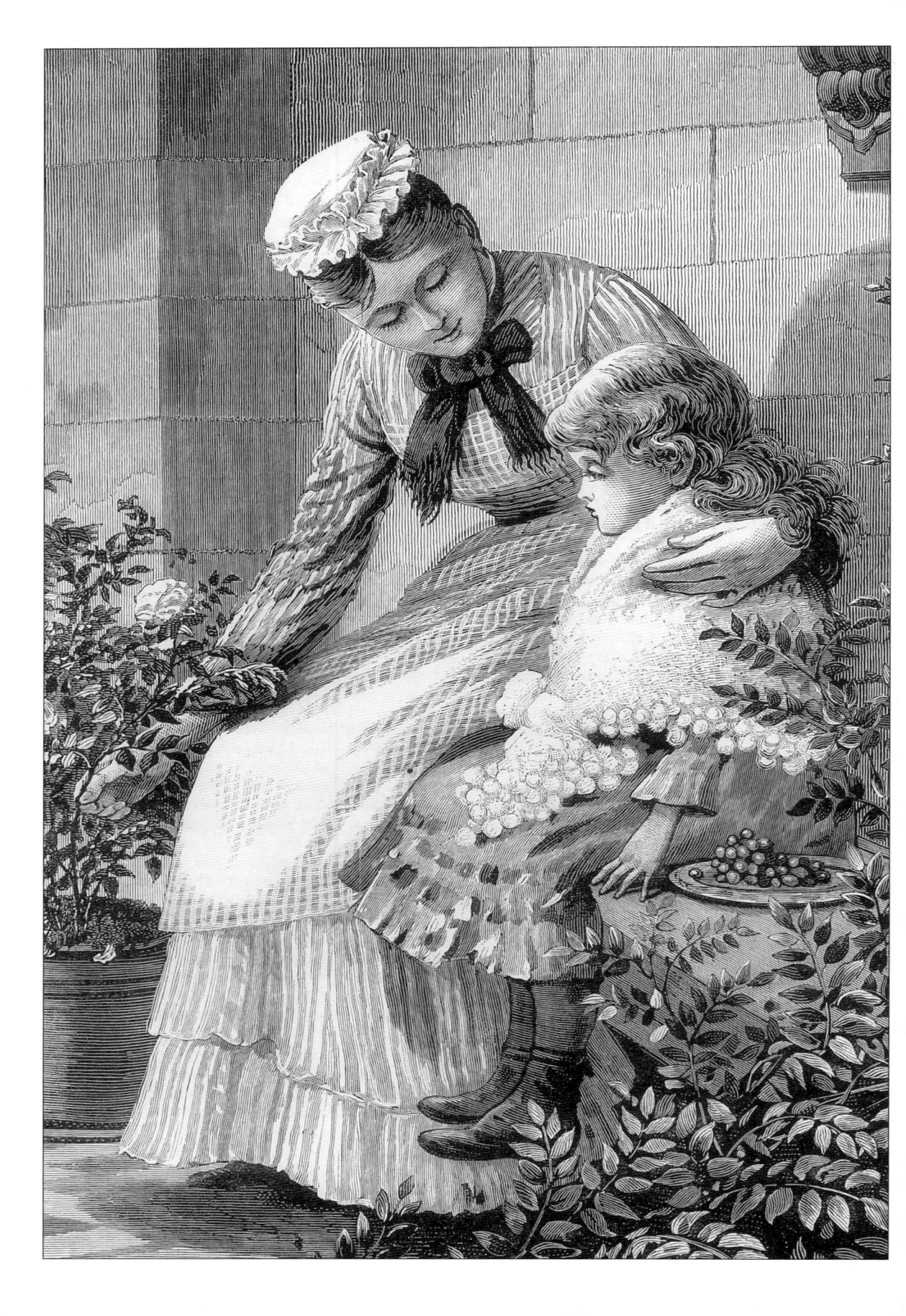

CHAPTER 2

The Dawn of Professionalism
the 1880s

*W*e know very little about the early nurses at the Children's Hospital. Their feelings, aspirations, experiences and disappointments were not revealed in their enclosed world. They left no memoirs, diaries or letters, personal working records or possessions. A few photographs from the 1880s reveal young ladies posing in the garden of the stately mansion in Carlton, appearing rather slighter in stature than their modern counterparts. Their clothes are feminine in the fashion of the Victorian era: long, finely striped dresses with puffed-up sleeves, stiff collars, white aprons, black button-up boots and nursery maid caps. There is little to distinguish them from the domestic servants of the day. We wonder about their discomfort in such cumbersome clothing during the onslaught of the hot north winds on a Melbourne summer day.

The evidence of the nurses' actual day-to-day work is sketchy until the 1880s. Nurse Rose Vaughan's handwritten 'Notes on Nursing', dated 1886, details the Nightingale influence in Australia by then. Nurses were expected to have personal qualities of fortitude, courage and perseverance, and, above all, obedience: 'One of the first duties of a nurse is to obey the instructions from the medical man'.[1]

A significant amount of the nurses' time was spent learning observation techniques and carrying out medical orders. The observations and records of the patient's symptoms, so critical in the care of children, enabled the doctor to make a

---

Getting Better. A scene at the Children's Hospital.
Print: wood engraving. George Rossi Ashton, 1881. La Trobe Collection State Library of Victoria.

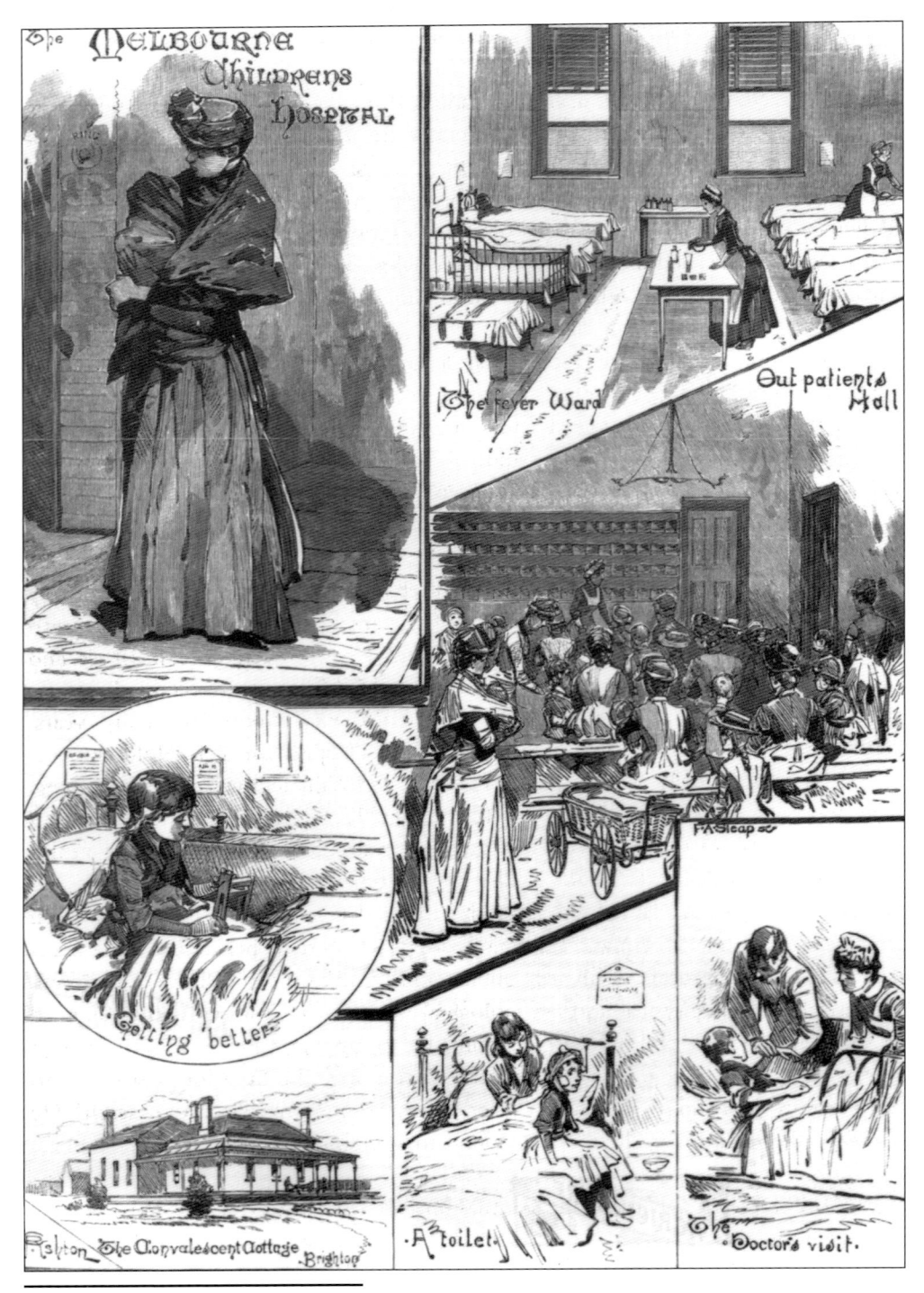

Scenes at the Children's Hospital.
Print: Wood Engraving, George Rossi Ashton 1887. La Trobe Collection, State Library of Victoria.

diagnosis. In no other profession was a relationship so marked by mutual dependency as that between doctor and nurse.

The doctor was accepted as the leading spirit of the institution, and much happiness and stability in hospital life depended on his interest and endorsement of nurses and nursing. But without competent nursing, the ability to soothe the child and (sometimes) the parents, to provide orderliness and cleanliness, to administer medicines and take observations, the Children's Hospital could not exist. When the doctor visited the bedside, the nurse hailed his visit with relief. Nurse Grace Carmichael described this relationship eloquently:

> ...I know of no more intellectual fellowship than that which exists between a cultivated man and woman, in the relationship of doctor and nurse, where the professional intercourse is honourably observed and the good work is carried on in the mutual helpfulness which will always link together two utterly different, yet inseparable arts namely, doctoring and nursing of the sick.[2]

From the beginning, the Ladies' Committee depended on a group of Honorary Medical Officers, all prominent members of the medical profession in nineteenth century Melbourne. Doctors William a'Beckett, Henry Wigg, Joseph Black and Edwin James, consultant surgeon Professor George Halford, and consultant physicians James Neild and James Motherwell, continued their support for many years, contributing to the reputation and goodwill of the Hospital for Sick Children.

But it was not until doctors Charles Hunter and William Snowball were successively appointed as Resident Medical Officers in 1877–78, that the Committee paid serious attention to the instruction of nurses. Dr Hunter advocated public health education. He made observations of the degradation caused by poor housing and crowded insanitary living conditions and witnessed thousands of poverty stricken parents trudging up Pelham and Nicholson streets to present their child at the Outpatients Hall. This prompted his first publications dealing specifically with children. He described their physical and psychological needs in institutions, and their need for stimulation: 'Each child will get less nursing, petting, and joyous exercise than a baby at home. Dancing, jumping, and fondling stimulate the liver, lungs, stomach to keep healthy—but in a sick baby, a sudden movement might cause death.' He described the need for fresh air and hygiene, for example:

> A fire is useful and promotes ventilation, but it is dangerous to shut the windows and doors and other inlets. It [the fire] sucks the air through the walls but most soils are more open than the walls and as the air is sucked through the soil below the house, so surely, will it bring with it foul and deadly odours from the drainage water with which our bad surface drains

soak the soil...for twenty feet on each side...with the worst of their filth. Who can tell what diseases may be below their houses ready to enter once the fire is lighted...[3]

The Children's Hospital Committee printed one thousand of Dr Hunter's pamphlets.

Following the first rush of enthusiasm, nurse training waned. Ward hygiene, hospital administration and Listerian method infection control lagged for want of instruction.

In August 1882, Drs a'Beckett and Snowball, by now elected to honorary positions, met to devise ways to bring a more scientific approach to the training of nurses. Post-operative nursing care was critical to the recovery of sick children, therefore necessary to the reputation of the surgeon. Their first resolution was to hire a competent person to begin the process.

WILLIAM SNOWBALL was born in 1853 in Sydney. His father, a Yorkshire stonemason and builder, moved the family to Melbourne shortly after William's birth. He was educated at Melbourne Grammar School and studied medicine at Melbourne University. The faculty consisted of seven students. After graduation he sat for the FRCS in Edinburgh and became a Licentiate of the College of Apothecaries in London.

As a young doctor, Dr Snowball paid attention to the study of diseases of children at Great Ormond Street Hospital in London and in the children's hospitals of Europe. Returning to Melbourne in 1877, he practised as a physician and surgeon in Carlton; first as a Resident Medical Officer to the Hospital for Sick Children from 1876 to 1882, and then, as Honorary Medical Officer from 1882 to 1901. His private practice was conducted from his home, 'Frosterley', on the corner of Drummond and Victoria streets, Carlton. Much of the Hospital's medical and nursing development was planned from this address.

William Snowball was best known as a kindly physician with a sympathetic 'bedside manner'. Many upper-class Melbourne women, including Lady Janet Clarke, solicited his advice and treatment for their sick children. His reputation spread as far as Rosebery, on the West Coast of Tasmania, from where a child was sent on the perilous journey to be treated successfully by him.

William Snowball was influential in the establishment of the Children's Hospital Nursing School in the late 1870s, and developed curriculum in anatomy, physiology and *materia medica*: the basis for nurses' lectures for generations. Ahead of his time, his vision extended beyond the hospital to the home. Children's Hospital nurses learned to negotiate and conduct themselves in private employment, to advocate hygiene and cleanliness, to prevent illness and accidents, and improve child nutrition. In the 1890s, through his connection with the philanthropist Sir William McPherson, William Snowball established a course in invalid cookery for Children's Hospital Nurses. In the twentieth century this facility became the Emily McPherson College of Domestic Science.[4]

Head Nurses

The key to nurse teaching in nineteenth-century hospitals was the appointment of an experienced Head Nurse, in modern terms a Charge Nurse. Ward Sisters had not yet been designated because very few women were trained for that position in Australia and the term was not used until the twentieth century. The Head Nurse would allow the Matron to attend exclusively to household and administrative matters. The first appointment at the Children's proved to be less than satisfactory. She left the Hospital without any notice on a Sunday 'not being in a condition to attend to her duties'. It seems that she was drunk. Her successor, Miss MacFarlane, was employed at a salary of £40 to be raised to £50 at the beginning of the year 'if she fulfilled the duties required of her to the satisfaction of the committee'.[5]

But many nurses, even those with experience, had little idea what to expect in a children's hospital. If they did not have the personal attributes, that is, the stoic qualities of faithfulness and courage to withstand the long hours and heartbreak of tending sick and dying children, they did not last very long. Four months after Miss McFarlane began, she sent a letter saying that 'as she found herself a little deficient in the surgical part of her work she thought it right not to have a salary raise, but that she was willing to stay'. However, she left in a matter of weeks.

The Committee widened the net by advertising in Sydney, Adelaide and Hobart. In April 1879, a Mrs Bellaine, of the Hobart Hospital, was appointed to assist Matron Bishop. None of Mrs Bellaine's records of interview survive but she was described in the Hospital's Annual Report as a 'Nightingale Nurse'.[6] This can be explained by the fact that a few nurses from the Hobart Hospital, which was established in 1875, had voluntarily at their own expense travelled from that hospital to Sydney to spend time at Lucy Osburn's training school.[7] Over time, the Nightingale nursing principles were absorbed throughout the public hospitals in the cities and regions of Victoria. Mrs Bellaine's appointment marked a period of stabilisation in the nursing staff. There was now one night nurse, an out-patients' nurse and seven assistant nurses. The assistants were engaged at £15 per annum for the first year, to £30 in the third year then progressing towards a certificate of competency after one year to the satisfaction of the Committee.

Despite the appointment of a worthy Head Nurse, things did not go altogether smoothly. Ellen Healy left in October 1881, complaining 'she could get no instruction from the Head Nurse who promptly assured the Ladies' Committee she had instructed Ellen in every way she could'.[8] Some nurses simply wanted to go home. They were tired of working sixteen hours a day, seven days a week with two afternoon hours off and one day off every second week. This was detrimental to good health, and probationers were not prepared for a career little better than domestic service where half a year was spent in the rough manual labour of scrubbing, waxing, polishing and cleaning fireplaces. The low pay caused hardship to many. Wages increased very little in ten years. In the 1870s a night nurse was awarded £35 per annum when the cook received £36, but the Committee rationalised this by the offset of free board, food and instruction. In the 1890s depression, salary reductions affected night nurses severely. Their pay was reduced from £35 to £30, and that of first-year trainees from £20 to £15 per annum.

Hospital nursing

Although anaesthetics and antiseptics expanded the procedures that doctors performed, pathology and X-rays were still unknown. Bacteriology was in its infancy and specialties had not developed. Treatment was primitive by today's standards. Many procedures were positively dangerous to patient and nurse if they were not followed correctly. Time-consuming fomentations were prepared by taking a large piece of flannel dipped in boiling water and sometimes infused with marshmallow, camomile flower or poppy seed, then wringing it out tightly with two sticks, or rolling it in a towel. The foment was placed on the patient 'with a mackintosh above to prevent dampness arising'. A common turpentine, 'stupe', was applied as hot as could be borne, covered with a larger piece of wool and bandaged securely. Salicylate foments were prepared every four hours for children suffering with rheumatic fever.

Painful festering sores, carbuncles and boils, commonly suffered by children, were treated with poultices prepared with linseed meal stirred in boiling water, until a 'soft mess was secured and spread on a cloth an inch thick'. Mustard and linseed, one to ten parts stirred in hot water, was placed on muslin on the skin until 'well reddened but not blistered'. Commonly, household poultices were made of stale breadcrumbs softened in very hot water. Variations were charcoal, bran, kaolin, boracic acid, thymol and peppermint oil. To prevent bedsores, the nurse 'sponged the parts with brandy or spirits of wine, alum and water followed by a sprinkle of violet powder or powdered rice'.

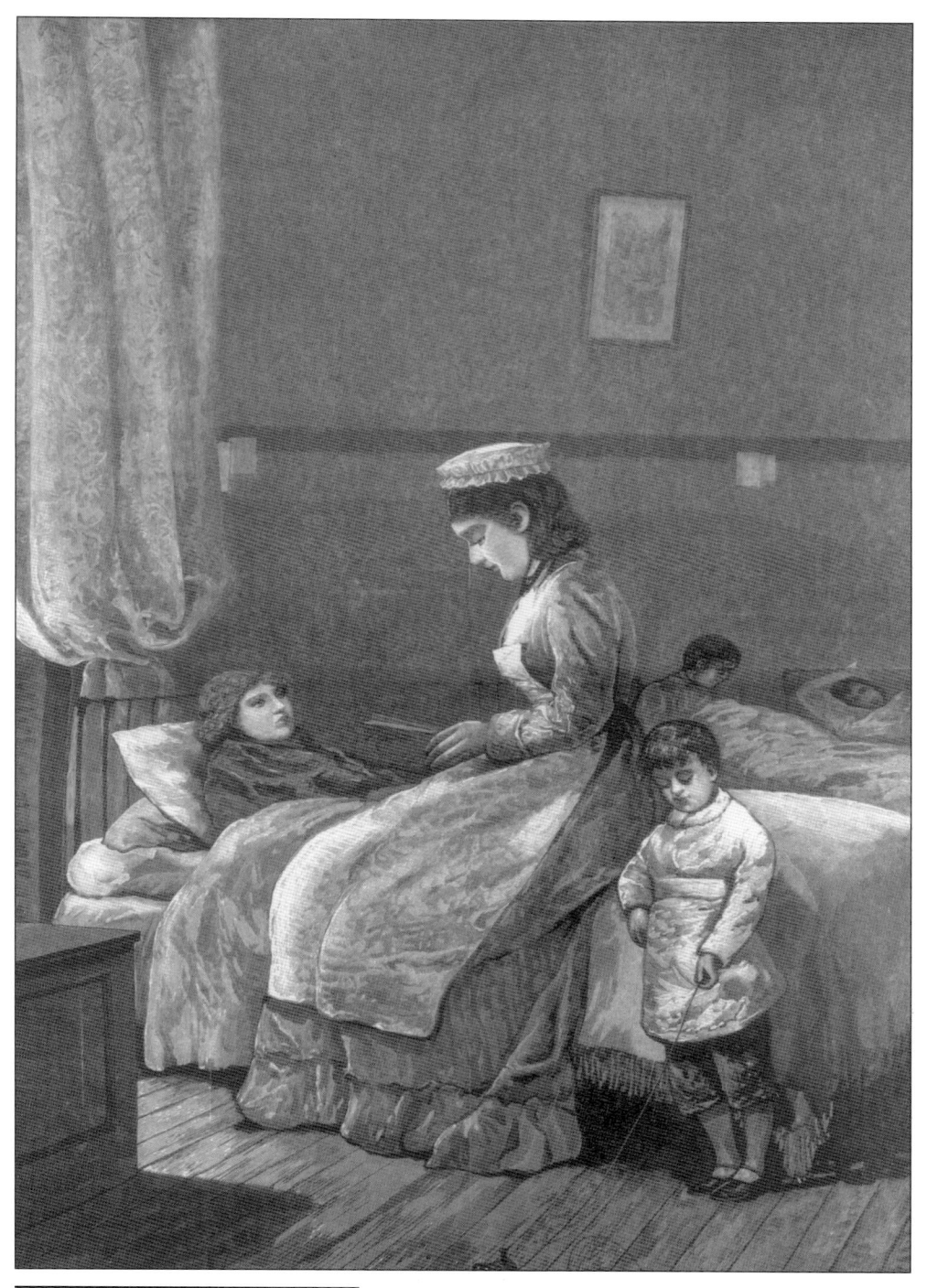

Convalescent. A sketch at the Children's Hospital.
Print: Wood Engraving, George Rossi Ashton, 1881. La Trobe Collection, State Library of Victoria.

Simple tasks were time consuming; for example: 'to take a temperature, if the arm has been exposed, and is cold, place it [the arm] under the bedclothes for quarter of an hour before…It should be taken before the patient is washed in the morning and again in the evening'.

From the main building there was much fetching and carrying of meals from the kitchen and wood for the fires. In a rush at 'about seven in the morning, nearly a dozen nurses might be seen scampering across the yard, and congregating in the laundry, waiting for the advent of the hard-working laundress, who looked upon the nurses as her natural enemies'.[9]

Poor appetites were coaxed with tiny spoons of tonic: water and brandy. Preparation of beef tea, a standard of the 'sick diet', fell to the nurse's lot: a half-pound of meat was minced, pounded and mixed with one pint of water, twenty grams of bicarbonate of soda and four drams of 'pancreatic', then boiled, stirred and strained. Several hours later, the unfortunate child was subjected to drinking the liquid.

Nurses were expected to know about the application of bloodsucking leeches. It was very important to check and count them at the end of the procedure to ensure none was lost. Curious methods were used to entice the creatures to 'latch on', such as salt and sugary water. The nurse administered emetics, purges and opiates in complicated mixtures of bottled medicine to rid the body of worms and hydatids, constipation and fevers. The prescribed medicines, bitter and nauseating, were followed by a slice of lemon rubbed around the mouth.

The patient could be dosed with inhalations and potions, passed down from colonial folklore: one tablespoon of Old Woman's Cough Mixture contained aniseed, laudanum, paregoric and peppermint, each to cover a threepenny piece, then mixed with one cup of honey and dissolved in a quart of boiling water, with spirit added to 'keep it good'.

Particular emphasis was placed on the observation, care and state of the mouth and tongue—'sometimes a diagnostic sign…to be observed most carefully for paralysis—or if jerking, St Vitus Dance or Trembling Fever'. Various afflictions could be diagnosed by the colour of the tongue: black in the case of typhoid, and bright scarlet and strawberry for fever.

Infectious diseases nursing

Drills were to be learned off by heart: incubation and quarantine periods for typhoid, scarlet fever, diphtheria and smallpox. Unfortunately, infectious diseases broke out in the wards all too frequently and a nurse could be assigned without notice to the small, two-roomed, detached isolation pavilion at the end of the garden—a lonely twenty-four-hour vigil. A child dangerously ill with diphtheria was nursed in a steam fog from the kettles, as well as carbolic and eucalyptus sprays. Grace Carmichael described the long days:

From the windows we had views of the orchard encircled with red brick walls. The vines were dying gorgeously, though a few late clusters of grapes might reward a search through the crimson and yellow leaves. The nearest building was the mortuary, not the liveliest of prospects when time hangs heavily on the hands. At night that little house would sometimes be brilliant with light, and the voices of the doctors could be heard, creating a sense of companionship, in spite of the grim suggestiveness of their being there.[10]

Supplies left at the door by the handyman, food and wood to keep the fire going, broke the monotony. If she was lucky, 'nurse' was provided with relief for an hour or two to step into the fresh air in the garden, to the sights and sounds of the outside world. Should the patient succumb, as too often happened, there was the gentle preparation and the last rites. The child, dressed in a delicate shroud, was carried by the nurse just a few steps down the path, past the vines and the orange trees, to the mortuary in the cool of the evening dusk.

The remaining important task upon returning to the pavilion concerned disinfection of the sick room. First she rolled the bedding for removal to the fumigation room, then liberally sprinkled and washed the walls and floors with carbolic acid by spraying. Finally, the room was filled with choking sulphur: one teaspoonful of black oxide of manganese mixed with two teaspoons of common salt poured on sulphuric acid—one or two drops. Sulphur was burned, one or two

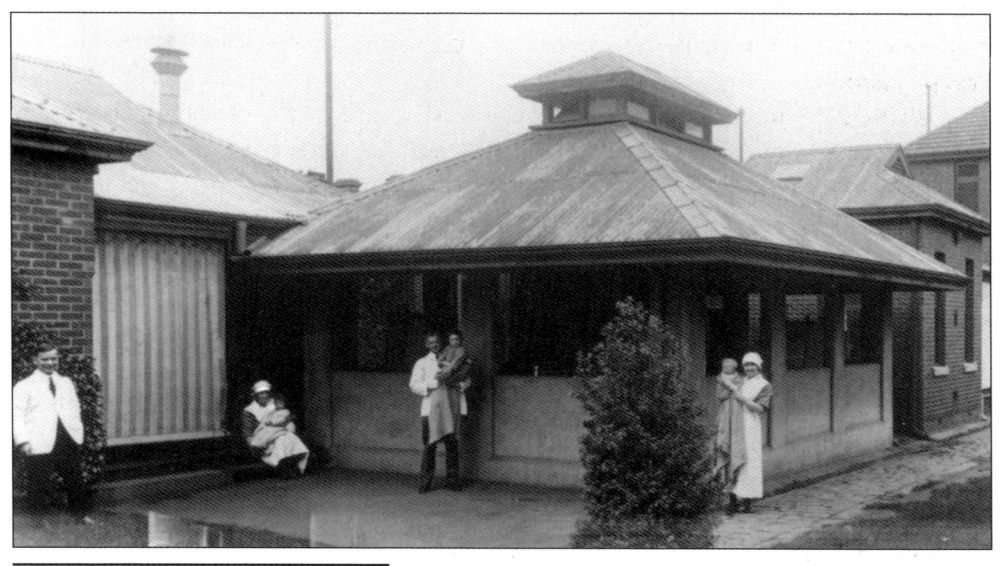

Infectious Diseases Pavilion, 1918. At rear, Pathology Department facing Drummond Street.

tablespoons to 1,000 cubic feet. Barely had the nurse completed her work when she heard the urgent and ominous sounds: the chatter of voices as another child was carried hurriedly into the pavilion.

A great deal depended on the nurses' observations. The acutely ill patient became totally dependent on the devotion of the nurse, as this case study shows,

> 'Annie', aged eight years, from an inner suburb of Melbourne, was admitted in March 1885, rather emaciated and pale, with a hectic flush on both cheeks, slightly delirious. Pulse very weak, 120, respirations hurried and shallow, temperature 103°F. Sonorous rhonchi over both lungs and bases dull. Her tongue was covered in 'sordes'. Annie had been very ill for a fortnight before admission suffering with headaches, vomiting and general malaise, a slight cough, no appetite and slight diarrhoea with light coloured motions.
>
> She was nursed in her bed with cool sponges of vinegar and water, ice-packs to her head, frequent starch enemas, and frequent 'draughts'. For restless nights…sips of Potassium Bromide and Chloral Hydrate, Quinine Sulphate, and tincture of Bella Donna were given. Laudanum foments were applied to the abdomen. Delirious and moaning though conscious at intervals, Annie slept on average for two hours. Her 'stepladder' temperature see-sawed: approximately 104°F in the evening to 98.4°F in the morning, her pulse was very quick and weak. She passed two or three light coloured motions a day, sometimes more, of undigested milk. She took some nourishment. Over many days, Annie's tongue was clean and shiny, dry and glazed. Frequent cleansing with Liq. Ferri Perchlor with glycerine gave temporary relief.
>
> **9 April** Tongue quite clean—she looks puffy about the eyes and hand. Perhaps she had been lying on her hand. Very low. Heart, second sounds, clearly audible. Still moans if touched but is not so touchy as usual. One motion, hands trembling.
> **10 April** Tongue clean but v. dry. Moaning a good deal.
> **11 April** (27th day in Hospital). Very restless and moaning. 'Draught' given in the night. Tongue very dry and glazed looking.
>   6 pm. (Dr) called in to see patient and found her in a state of collapse. Hot bottles were put to her feet and sides, draughts of whiskey and water given.
> **12 April** At 9 am, 5 mins after the second dose of whiskey, despite all good endeavours, the patient died without a struggle.
>   Diagnosis—typhoid and broncho-pneumonia.
>   Annie lived 42 days [from the onset of this condition].[11]

During Annie's illness, the nurses administered purges and enemas, bed baths and sponges, sips of water and brandy, ice-packs and packing sheets. Lowering the temperature was a complicated business. First, a mackintosh was placed on the bed, then three single blankets. A sheet was dipped in icy cold water. The nurse manually wrung out the sheet and, after placing it folded on the bed, brought it up to the neck, winding under and over the arms. The patient was then wrapped and tucked up like a parcel with three blankets overlapping, but 'not for longer than 5 minutes, according to the instructions'. The feet were left clear, presumably to test body temperature and observe the colour.

The Hospital

Less than six years after the acquisition of Redmond Barry's house, the two wards—ante-rooms accommodating thirty-four children off a central hall—were cramped. In August 1886, Dr Snowball came before the Committee* representing the Honorary Medical Staff to request the enlarging of the Hospital. Thirty extra beds were necessary for urgent cases being refused every day. An Operating Ward was required, an additional Honorary Medical Officer, an Honorary Pathologist and two Resident Surgeons. Two years later, the matter of accommodation was becoming urgent when Dr Snowball reported the Outpatients Room and the mortuary were too small. At that point, the Ladies gave up the board room for the doctors' use. Plans were drawn up for a new board room, an enlarged 'dead house', and drying and fumigation rooms. With the expected increase in the number of patients, additional accommodation was required for more nurses, but the Committee in its forward planning only found it necessary to provide accommodation for four additional nurses.

Many modifications occurred: mains water and a gas cooking range, cisterns, dirt toilets and a suitable bath for children. A pedalled, gas-fired, manual washing machine was donated by Mr J. B. Were in 1876.[12] A steam boiler provided hot water to the kitchens, laundry and bath. The once beautiful garden became crowded with a conglomeration of small buildings: an isolation pavilion and mortuary, converted stables, laundry and wood shed. The spacious garden tended so carefully in Redmond Barry's day, the orchard, vines, exotic trees and vegetable plots, disappeared. The gardener's cottage, although condemned as being not fit for habitation, was repaired and whitewashed.

There was very little room for extensions and the drainage was suspect. Underfloor flooding was blamed for outbreaks of diphtheria. In May 1888, a communication was received by the Town Clerk of Melbourne City Council that 'complaints had been made of an offensive smell in the street channels supposed to be from the use of sulphur baths at the Children's Hospital. The practice was to be discontinued.' The Hospital Secretary replied, 'measures would be taken to abate the nuisance as much as possible'.[13]

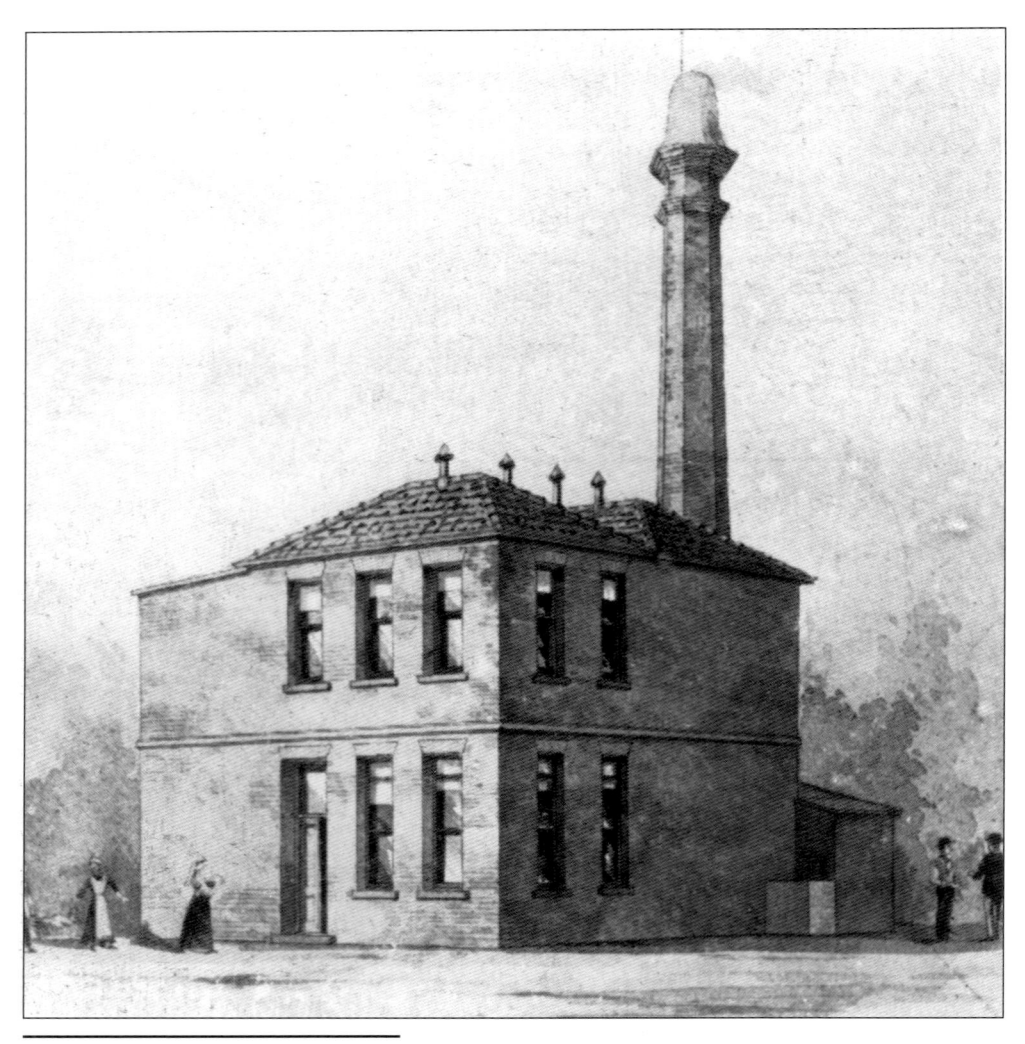

The steam laundry, 1890.

Lord and Lady Loch officially opened the extension, a second storey with a colonnaded balcony, on 7 December 1887. The floors were divided into departments: Surgical upstairs, the Elizabeth Ward (boys), Centre Ward, Sumner Ward (girls) and Medical below with Centre Hall and the Lady Bowen Ward. The balcony faced the Carlton Gardens and the new Exhibition Building. The 'house' now provided accommodation for sixty children.

The terrazzo-floored operating theatre facing Pelham Street was flooded with the northern light by day through large skylights and tall narrow windows. By night, emergency surgery was performed in gaslight. Carbolic acid permeated the building, mingling with the nauseous vapours of chloroform and open ether. The operating

The Dawn of Professionalism

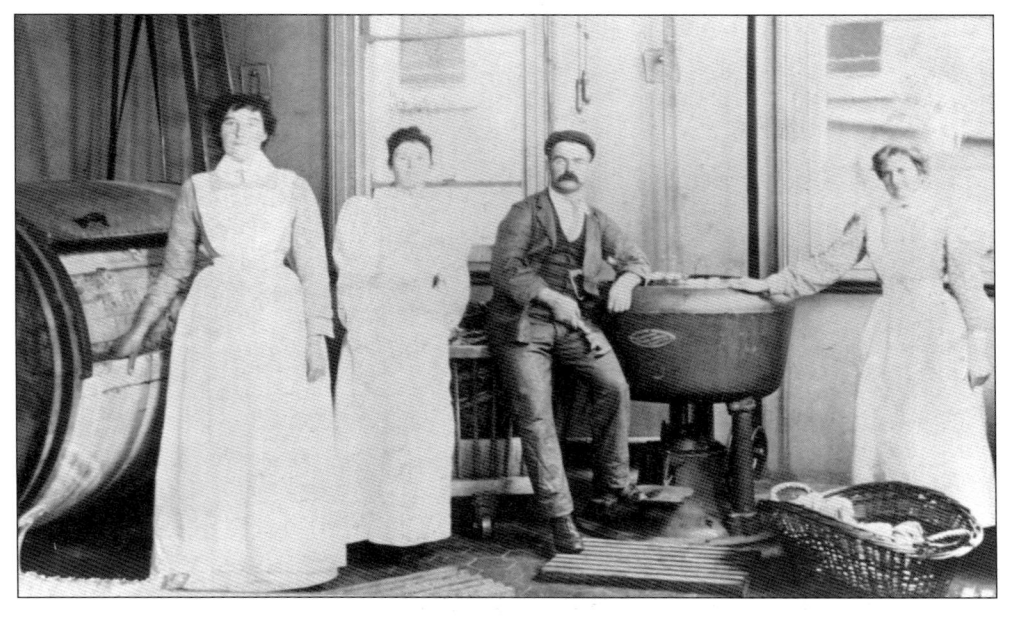

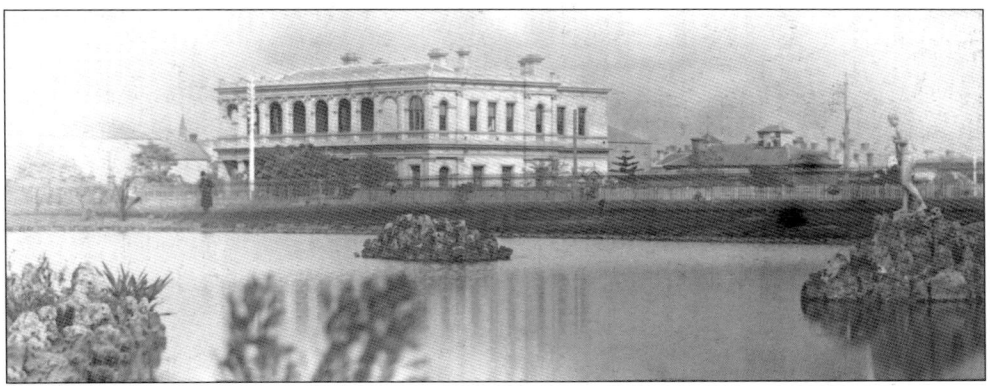

Top: Gas-fired, pedal washing machine, 1890.
Bottom: Redmond Barry's house, 'Carlton Gardens', at the corner of Rathdowne and Pelham streets, converted in 1876 to the Children's Hospital.

theatre, well furnished with operating table, stands and hand basins, was sterilised by Listerian methods, both saviour and curse—infection was dramatically reduced but the toll on nurses' well-being was considerable. Before the advent of surgical gloves, hands were washed and dipped in large basins of carbolic. Nurses complained of chronic skin irritations, tired legs, sore feet and general debility. Steam sterilisation of instruments was yet to come.

The number of in-patients doubled. Despite boom times in Melbourne, for the very poor of the inner suburbs, the Children's Charity Hospital became a haven.

Patients arrived on wooden wheels or the cast-off tyre of an old-fashioned perambulator. The better-off came in buggies and carts or cabs. Grace Carmichael observed: 'up and down this street—not the most aristocratic of localities—there is always a string of characteristic-looking folks, hospital bent'.[14] But the great majority travelled by cable tramway to Pelham Street or Victoria Street. The cable network circled the inner suburbs. For a penny, mothers and children could alight at Nicholson or Lygon streets, take a short walk through the Carlton Gardens, and crowd around the front door and inside the Hall to join the bedlam. Hospital rules dictated that no babies were to be admitted; there was scarce accommodation and none for nursing mothers. Children with known infectious disease were issued with a red ticket or, more commonly, told to go home.

The Committee soon planned a new Out-patients Department but that was in the future. By 1890, attendances increased to 27,879. In 1893, Maria Thomas was appointed Out-patients Nurse-in-Charge and she remained in that position for twenty-five years, overseeing the growth and development of an increasingly busy and complex department.

MARIA THOMAS, Out-patients nurse, later Sister-in-Charge from 1894, began her training in 1888, receiving her certificate in 1891. She held this position until retirement in 1922. Described as a 'martinet', she was a formidable character with a mountain of knowledge, striking terror into generations of doctors and nurses. She never trusted doctors, particularly the anaesthetists, and was known not to allow surgery to commence until (unknown to the doctor) she was quite satisfied the child was asleep—by surreptitiously pinching the patient on the thigh under the sheet. Maria decided to end her career following the appointment of Grace Wilson as the Matron. The Committee gave Maria six months' leave on full pay in recognition of her long and devoted service.

Matron Sarah Bishop and the nurses

Sarah Anne Bishop was appointed Matron in 1875 and for twenty-four years the ladies of the Committee were content with her role as administrator and housekeeper. This was confirmed when she requested a salary increase: the Committee unanimously decided that 'in consideration of Mrs Bishop's long and fruitful service her salary should be raised to £150 per annum'. Major administrative changes envisaged by the Nightingale system, to 'lady superintendent' or 'director of nursing', did not interest the Committee. The title, in fact, was not implemented until the twentieth century. Most importantly, Matron was required to be trustworthy, loyal and dedicated, to maintain competent and stable staff, and provide weekly reports to the Committee. Her domain was 'the house', where she had charge of the nursing staff and trainees, the maids, the cook, the laundrywoman, handyman, gardener and errand boy.

Mrs Bishop was extremely kind. Over the years she brought about a range of improvements to ensure that life was a little more comfortable for her nurses, domestics and the doctors. Dr Arthur Jeffreys Wood claimed 'she made the doctors the most comfortable in Melbourne'.

Her thoughtfulness was illustrated many times; for example, when she appeared to give evidence before the Royal Commission on Charitable Institutions in 1892, she firmly recommended that nurses have a sitting room.[15] She campaigned with the Committee for incremental improvements in living conditions: the cold flag stones in the maids' room were covered with wooden floors and, some years later, with carpet. She had overhead gas lamps installed over the night nurses' personal pantry cupboard on the back porch. When Nurse Eliza Booth died of typhoid fever in the nurses' quarters, Mrs Bishop pleaded with the Committee: 'her [Eliza's] friends are in very poor circumstances'. The Committee agreed to pay £5 towards her burial.[16]

Her kindness extended to 'a woman whose baby was born in the street outside the Children's Hospital'. She reported: 'the small ward was opened on Sunday to accommodate the poor woman' who was later transported to the Women's Hospital.[17] During the economic distress and severe weather of June 1892, Mrs Bishop sought, and was given permission, to distribute a limited supply of tram tickets to the 'most necessitous cases'.

Mrs Bishop's kindly personality and quiet authority were particularly useful in handling the first generation of nurses, some of whom were working-class daughters of inner-suburban families, with little education. Some subsequently became well-regarded, practical nurses. In all of the twenty-four years of Mrs Bishop's tenure, only one slip was recorded for which she was severely reprimanded: in the early days of her employment, she inadvertently opened a bank letter by mistake. Her main ally was the President, Mrs Elizabeth Testar, a down-to-earth, quiet, unpretentious lady who was appointed to the Committee in 1871.

Mrs Testar undoubtedly followed the development of the Alfred Hospital in the 1870s. The Melbourne public was entertained in the daily press about the antics and goings-on of the 'clever and haughty' Edinburgh-trained Nightingale Nurse, Miss Haldane Turriff, recruited to the Alfred from Lucy Osburn's team at the Sydney Hospital. Miss Turriff was found to be, among other things, 'uncivil to the medical staff' and she failed to implement a nurses' training school. There was certainly no such impropriety at the Children's.

SARAH ANNA BISHOP (née Gove) was born in 1835, but like many thousands of people who arrived in Ballarat in the 1850s, her origins are obscure. The only clues to her personal details have been found on her son's death certificate of 1916. Her name has been found on a shipping list from Britain in 1857. She was appointed to the Ballarat Hospital in 1864 when her son Tom was four years old. Highly regarded, she contributed significantly to administrative stability at that institution where formerly there was 'strife and confusion'.[18] Nothing is known of her husband and it is assumed she was a widow.[19]

Mrs Bishop was chosen from twenty-eight applicants for the position of Matron at the Children's Hospital in 1875. None of the records of her appointment have survived. Sarah Bishop served the Hospital from 1875 to 1899, with responsibilities for the nursing and domestic staff. She retired as the Hospital was embarking on a major rebuilding programme in 1899.

Little is known about the circumstances of her death, which occurred on 20 May 1904. No burial or death certificates can be traced in Victoria.

The frequent turnover of nursing staff could be partly explained by the three years required to train; a great length of time to give up a personal life for what amounted to live-in domestic service. One nurse explained 'that she was leaving as she found she was learning nothing about nursing which had been her motive for entering the institution'.[20] Instruction of a more intellectual nature was not available. Some probationers came before the Committee for 'misbehaviour', a cover for discontent, cheekiness and failure to comply with the rules. Overcrowding and long hours caused feelings to run high. In December 1886, Nurse Stewart resigned as a Head Nurse—she was leaving 'on account of a misunderstanding with Dr Snowball'. In June 1887, Matron Bishop dismissed Nurse Blackburn for her disobedience to orders. There were often tensions between nurses and doctors over orders for treatment and treatments given.

Matron Bishop introduced nurses' uniforms for practical reasons, one of which was to demarcate nurses from domestics. The Committee thought it desirable to have one pattern of print dresses while on duty. In 1878, Mr Mars Buckley, whose wife was a member of the Ladies' Committee, offered to obtain the print from the

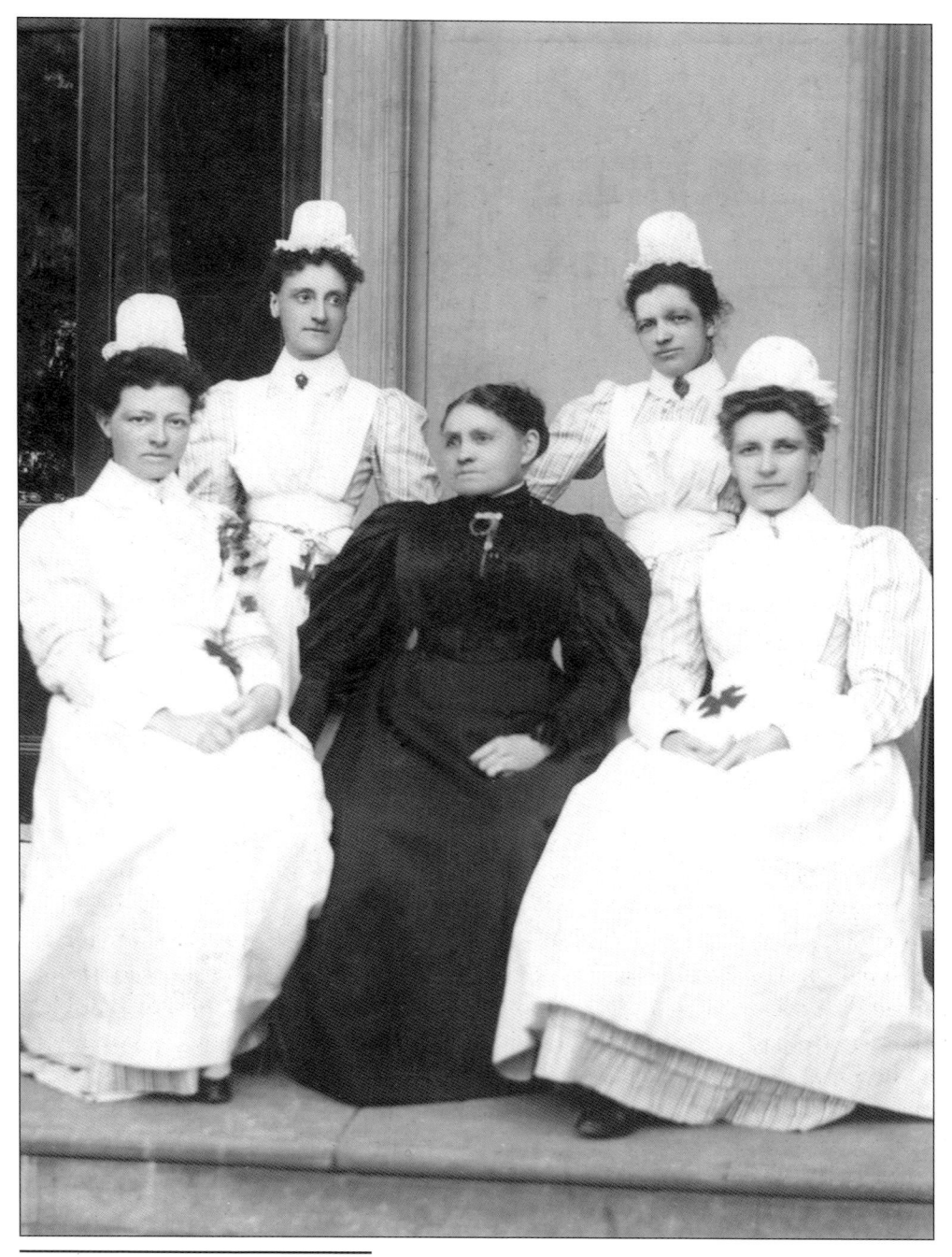

Mrs Bishop and her nurses, 1895. *Back right*: Nurse Ida Bevan.
RCHA/Bevan Collection.

manufacturers through his partners.[21] But there was little else to adequately define these young women as trained nurses. As an incentive to stay the distance, a certificate of competence was little compensation for the risk of infection, as Grace Carmichael explained: 'the first dread of the new probationer...the bodily strain of long hours and heavy labour, from which no nurse can escape, if she enters any important hospital with the object of thorough training'.[22]

When the Hospital was extended with a second floor in 1886, the night duty nurses had double the number of patients—sometimes more than sixty. Bed-making began as early as 4 am, with every child lifted, at least twenty from bed to bed in heavy splints. Each mattress was turned.

Food and supplies came via lifts and hatches raised and lowered by a series of ropes and pulleys. During the typhoid epidemic of the late 1880s, questions were raised by a Committee member about the amount of work expected of one nurse in charge of eighty patients, many with typhoid. The Matron and Head Nurse stated that 'there were only two night nurses, one up and one down-stairs, but if they required assistance it was to be given'.[25]

ELIZABETH TESTAR was born in 1819 in England, but nothing else is known about her early life. In 1850 she married Thomas Testar, and soon after came to Australia. He became a clerk and accountant for the Denominational Board and, in 1862, the Secretary and Accountant for the Board of Education. Mr Testar lost his job in 1878 but Elizabeth continued to be heavily involved in the affairs of the Hospital for Sick Children.

A childless woman, she joined the Committee in 1871 and was appointed to the original Providing Committee. In 1871, she was elected Vice-President, and in 1885 President, an office she retained until 1899. She took a leading part in the design of the Brighton Convalescent Cottage in 1885, the alterations to Redmond Barry's house in 1886, and the planning of new Hospital buildings up to 1900. She retired at the age of eighty and died at her home in St Kilda in 1908. A ward in the upper storey extensions at Carlton was named the Elizabeth Ward after Elizabeth Testar and Lady Elizabeth Loch.

The Dawn of Professionalism

GRACE JENNINGS CARMICHAEL was twenty-one years old when she began her training as a nurse at the Hospital for Sick Children and was one of the first four graduates in 1889–90. By then she was a published poet in the *Australasian*.

Born in Ballarat on 24 February 1867, Grace was the daughter of a Scottish gold miner, Archibald Carmichael, and Margaret Jennings, née Clark. Her father died when she was three. The family moved to Melbourne and in 1875 her mother married Charles Naylor Henderson. In 1879, Henderson became manager of Orbost Station, one of the vast properties of W. J. T. Clarke in remote Gippsland where Grace's romantic vision of the Australian bush was formed. At the age of eighteen, seeking employment, she lived as a lady's secretary and companion before beginning her training as a nurse.

Her book, *Hospital Children*, the most well known of her literary output, published by George Robertson in 1891, is a synthesis of her experiences and the most graphic account ever produced of the inside of the old Hospital at Carlton. Her entry to the Hospital coincided with one of the worst typhoid epidemics Melbourne had experienced, and she contracted the illness. Near death, she left the Hospital but her strong and healthy constitution carried her through. Eventually she returned to the Hospital to sit the final exam, passing with credit, one of the first nurses to gain the certificate. At the conclusion of her training she moved away from the Hospital forever, to nurse a boy, the subject of one of her most famous poems *The Wooden Legs,* at Barunah Downs Station near Geelong.

Grace married the English architect Francis Henry Mullis in 1895, at the age of twenty-eight. He was thirty-five. They moved to South Australia where their first son Geoffrey was born, and then to England where Grace had four more children, two of whom died in infancy, one a baby girl. Following her husband's imprisonment for embezzlement, Grace fell into dire poverty and died of pneumonia in the Leyton workhouse on 9 February 1904, at the age of thirty-seven, far away from her beloved Gippsland. Her surviving children, three boys, aged seven, four and one, were left destitute and taken to the Northampton workhouse until a public appeal in 1910 raised money to bring them back to Australia.[23]

The people of Orbost Historical Society commissioned a sensory garden and relief sculpture in Grace's memory on the 'Old Forest Road', the site of the old cattle station where she grew up. The artist has depicted

Grace in the nurse's uniform of the Children's Hospital. She was buried in a pauper's grave at Wood Grange Park Cemetery in London. Twenty-three years after her death, in 1927, a headstone was erected—a white marble book with the words 'A Wattle Day Tribute to the Memory of Jennings Carmichael, an Australian Poetess', opposite a spray of wattle and words from her own verse:

'*Ah, little flower I loved of old,*
Dear little downy heads of gold.'[24]

Another memorial can be found at Ballarat.

A duty of care

Emphasis was placed on simple tasks well done: the wards were to be kept clean and aired, children were to be properly nourished and, if a nurse was not able to make a child happy, she was dismissed; to be unkind was unacceptable. A tradition developed that Children's Hospital nurses were required to have qualities of loving, caring motherliness, intuitiveness, sympathy and an extraordinary amount of patience. The Committee took the welfare of the children very seriously.

Nevertheless, in April 1889 a scandal occurred when Nurse Alma came before the Committee and acknowledged she had given a child a slap but she said she 'was sorry for having done so and promised it should never happen again'. In October 1886, a report of another incident caused severe distress to the Hospital management: a nurse had been unkind to a child, the 'statement being fully confirmed by the Head Nurse and acknowledged by herself. The nurse was dismissed by the Committee.'[26]

The most serious breach of the nineteenth century at the Children's concerned Nurse Maud Barlow. A mother complained that, as she was leaving the Hospital on Sunday 1 December 1889, she heard her child 'suddenly stop crying and going back to the ward found that a pillow had been thrown over the child's face'. Nurse Barlow admitted to the act and stated that it was not done in ill temper or unkindness. 'The child was a fine fat boy and showed no marks of unkindness'. Nurse Barlow was dismissed.

This incident caused uproar amongst nursing and medical staff. The Head Nurse, Alice Martelli, and Nurse Barlow appeared before the Committee and, after an exhaustive investigation, Nurse Barlow remained dismissed. Matron Bishop was instructed to 'suspend any nurses in any serious complaint and to read the nurses' rules weekly. Alice Martelli's anger that her authority had been usurped by the Committee prompted her letter of resignation:

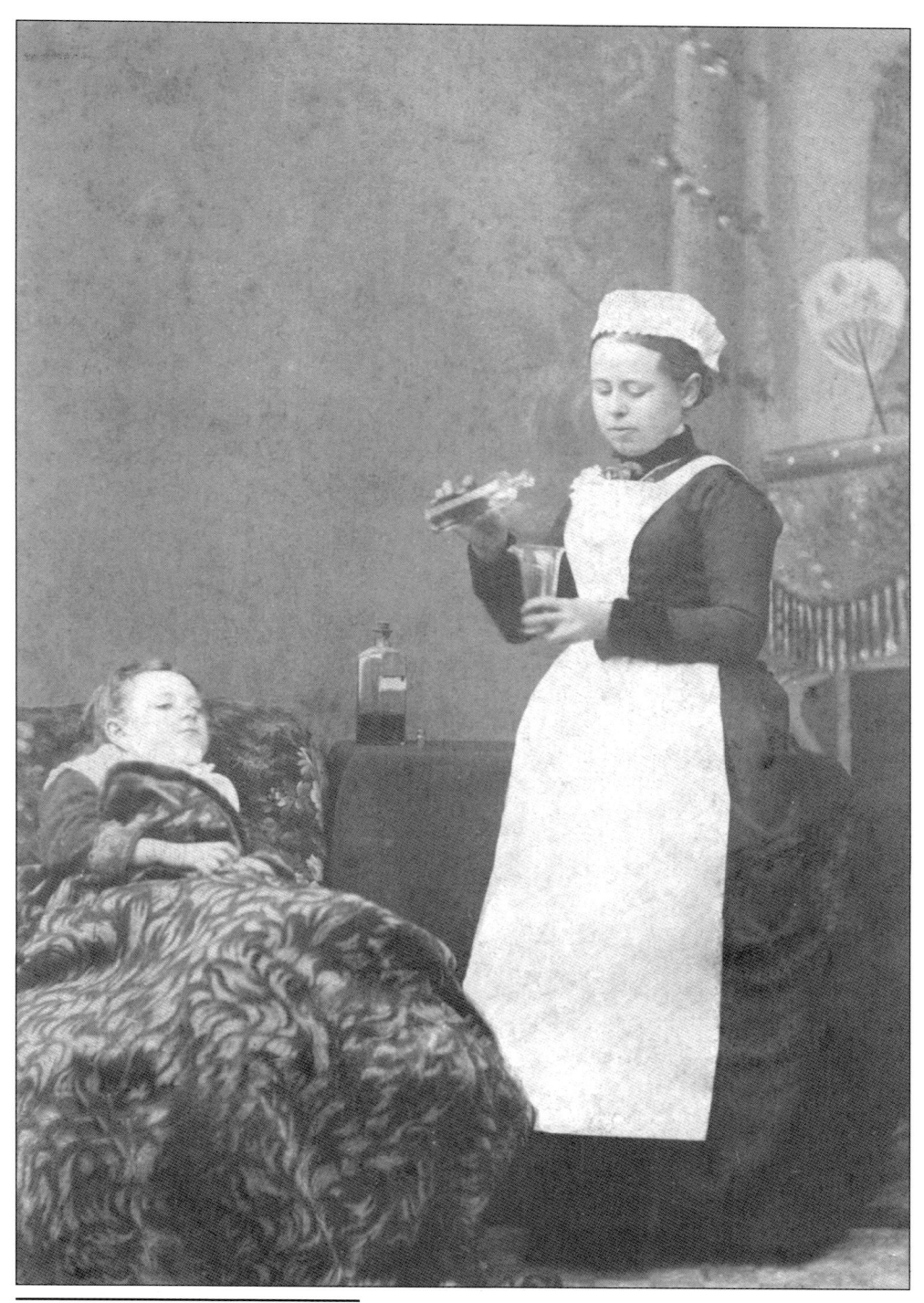

Nurse Lillias Sharpe Fraser at the Hospital for Sick Children, 1880s.
RCHA/Cuddy Collection.

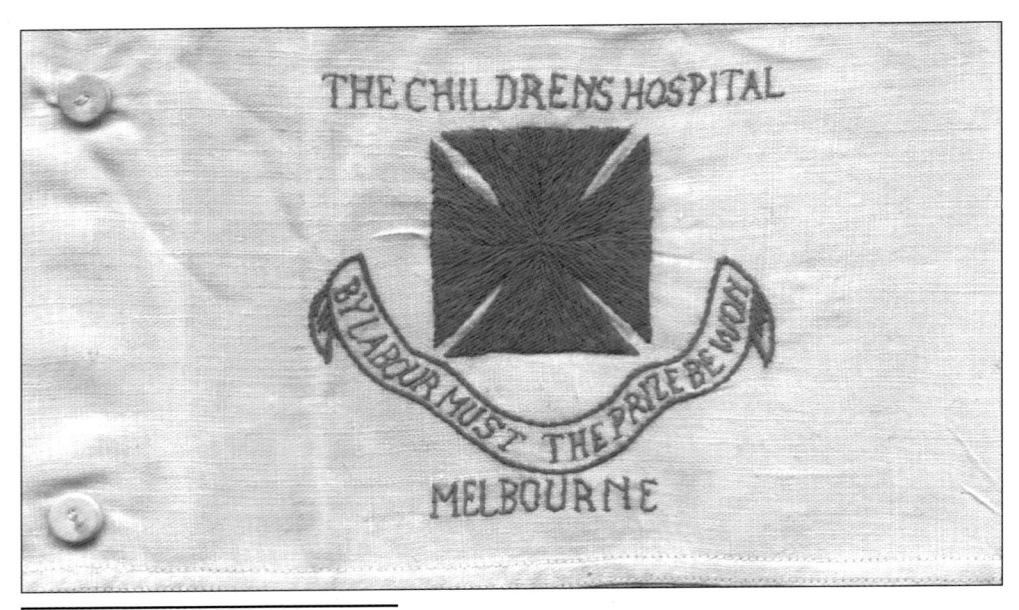

Hand-embroidered armband with the Knights of St John Cross: 'By Labour Must the Prize be Won'.
RCHA/Grace Collins Collection.

>I have the honor to place in your hands my resignation of the post of Head Nurse to this Hospital. It is with the utmost regret I take this step which I feel has been forced on me…Your total disregard for my humbly expressed wishes, as evidenced by your recent action in dismissing a nurse well trusted by me, and with whom I respectfully and most earnestly asked you to deal leniently, amounts in effect to a vote of want of confidence…I would like to place before you the case of the nurses generally—women mostly now of gentle breeding, who cheerfully and without complaint undertake work of the most trying and often revolting nature, who devote the best years of their lives and who not infrequently lose life itself in the interests of the suffering poor, our nurses serve you conscientiously in all points and never spare themselves in their kindly efforts to restore health to the sick, or to ease the pain of the dying.

She recalled that during her years of tenure seven nurses contracted typhoid and two died.

Alice Martelli had given more than three years' faithful service, during which she had not 'grudged her time, health and intellect, in the service of the Hospital…' and that the work had been the greatest interest in her life. Not all members of the Committee had been negative, with some still retaining confidence in her. She was asked not to resign but, upon asking for a reference, was given a lukewarm letter of few words.

She went on to be quite successful and ran a private practice with the former matron of the Alfred Hospital. An eloquent witness at the Royal Commission into Charitable Institutions in 1890–91, Martelli's evidence contained damaging information about the Children's Hospital, exposing the sixteen-hour days, 6 am to 10 pm, with half an hour for meals. She said: 'No young woman should have to work those hours. Nine hours was enough.' In April 1890, the nurses' hours were changed to nine-and-a-half-hour shifts; 'the night nurses to come on duty at 10 pm and leave off as soon as possible and not later than 7.30 am'.[27]

The first certificated nurses

The Nursing School was inaugurated on 16 April 1890. After the prescribed course of two years' lectures, a certificate was issued showing attendance at the prescribed courses: twelve months' lectures of anatomy and physiology, and general nursing at the Melbourne Hospital for Sick Children. The first successful candidates were Grace Jennings Carmichael, Eleanor Goddard, Margaret Price and Alma Packham.

Interestingly, in 1891 the next batch of thirteen nurses listed Sarah Bishop, who was by then fifty-five. Another was Nurse Esther Dorothea Harcourt Vernon, who migrated to Australia alone at the age of seventeen, from Blackburn near England's Lake District, with 'five pounds sewn into her stays'. She had seen an advertisement for nurses in an English newspaper. She lived exclusively at the Children's during her training; some years after graduation she became a private nurse and then the guardian to William Snowball's children after their mother's death.[28]

The Nursing School had been slow to develop for many reasons. The building of a Convalescent Cottage at Holyrood Street in Brighton in December 1884, and in 1886 the second storey extension in Carlton, caused a shortage of money, chaos and disruption. Lack of a Nurses' Home severely hampered the Hospital's ability to recruit and train a suitable number of nurses. But by 1890 the rules were re-organised, the training time was extended and the Hospital was staffed by a group of competent certificated nurses. In 1891, Grace Jennings Carmichael wrote: 'The struggle is by no means over yet…nursing has been placed on a much higher level within the last few years, and recognised as a profession demanding refined and intelligent students'.[29]

The nurses' badge carried the motto 'By Labour Must the Prize be Won'.

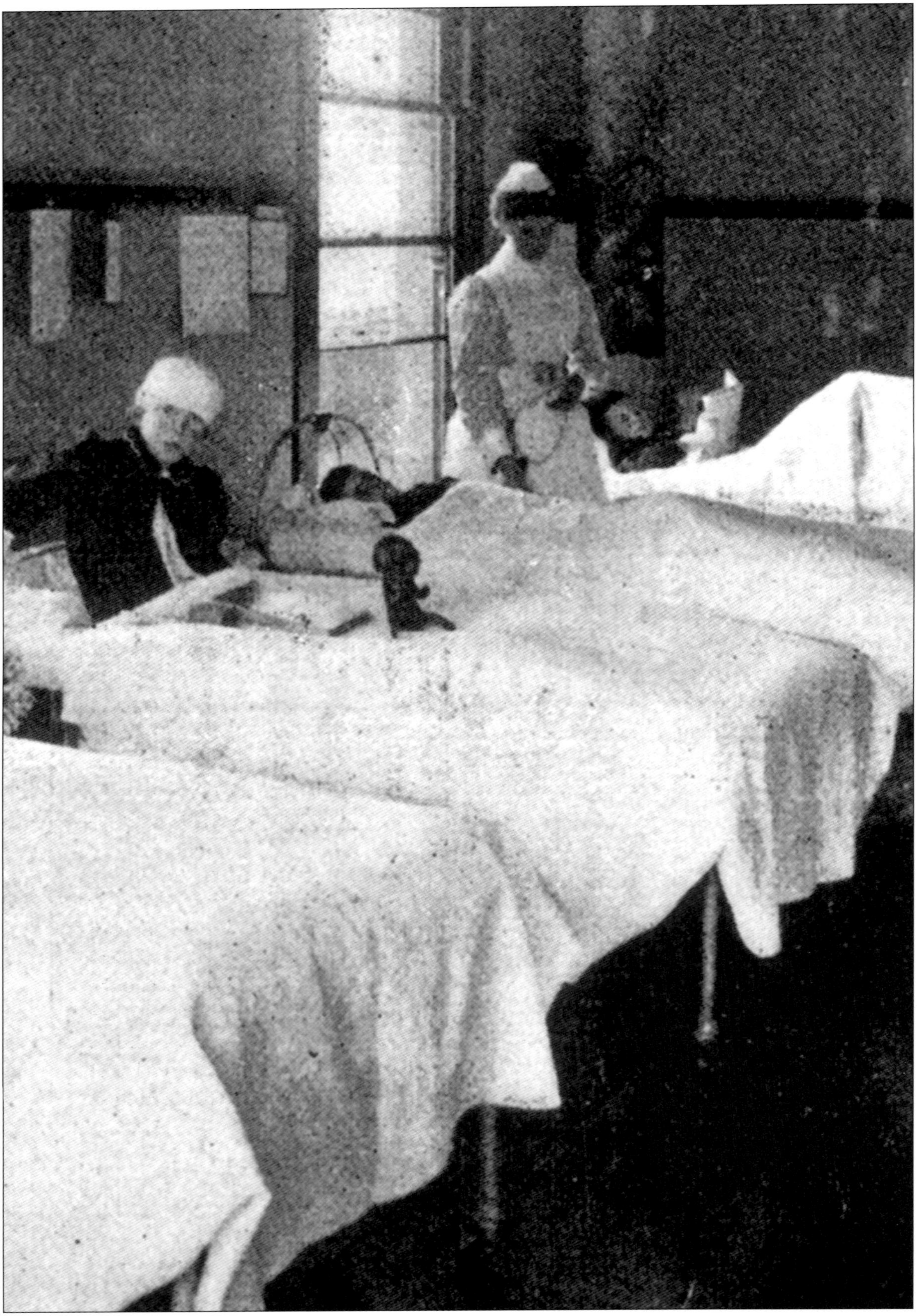

CHAPTER 3

A Growing Workforce

the 1890s

When Sybil, Lady Brassey, the fifth Patroness of the Children's Hospital, arrived in Melbourne in August 1895, the Australian colonies were emerging from the worst economic crisis in their short-lived history. Victoria, and Melbourne in particular, had experienced grim times as financial institutions crashed following the land boom; people lost fortunes, jobs, property, businesses and savings. The poor continued to struggle with unemployment and poverty; charity hospitals remained in a financial mess, and the Children's Hospital was experiencing the worst epidemics of infectious diseases since its foundation.

Unlike her predecessors, Lady Brassey was not merely an appendage to her husband. In her thirties with a young child, she was the second wife of the Governor of Victoria, Lord Brassey, and twenty-three years his junior. A model of English womanhood with the traditional upper-class virtues of warmth, enthusiasm and energy, she also had a quirky sense of humour. Although politically discreet as the Governor's wife, her behaviour showed signs of a 'New Woman' in tune with the 'woman questions' of the 1890s: the right to vote, to enter the professions, to earn a living, to gain independence and to attend university. She rode a bicycle, a symbol of women's emancipation. More than once she even wrote and delivered her own short speeches.

Elizabeth Ward, Carlton, 1902.

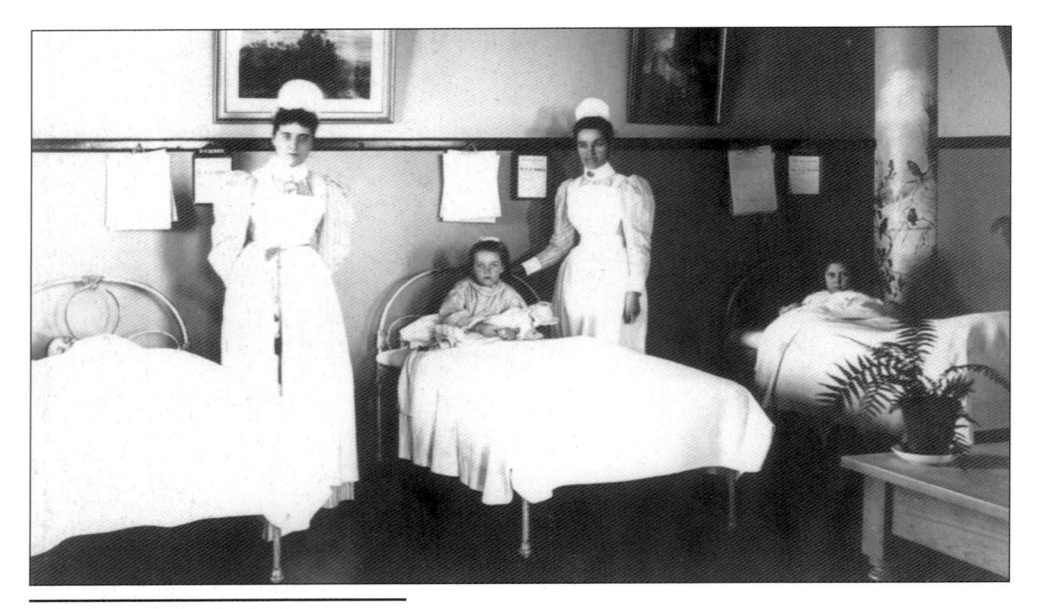

Sumner Medical Ward, 1895.
Bailleau Library, Views of Melbourne, AMA Collection.

Her support for good causes made Lady Brassey a popular figure, and her abiding love of children played out among activities in women's health and child welfare. She attended functions and meetings and listened to women's conversation.[1]

On her first visit to the Children's Hospital, Lady Brassey promised to attend meetings and become a regular visitor.[2] She encountered young nurses of good education from south and east of the Yarra and took a keen interest in their well-being. As she did with university women undergraduates, she invited Children's Hospital nurses 'to afternoon tea at Government House and other entertainments'.[3] Her term of office at the Children's Hospital could not have been more auspicious. Her suffragette image reinforced a new generation of assertive, well-educated and dedicated young women. Nursing had been recognised 'as a profession demanding refined and intelligent students'.[4] For those daughters of the well-off who might ordinarily have engaged in social charity work and other good causes, the depression had made the prospect of earning a living an economic necessity. Nursing was one avenue open for a professional future.

The emergence of nursing as a profession

With the introduction of the first Nursing School, the image changed. As medicine and surgery advanced, the Hospital world became more complex and, in keeping with the times, examinations for nurses became more technical. Qualifications were

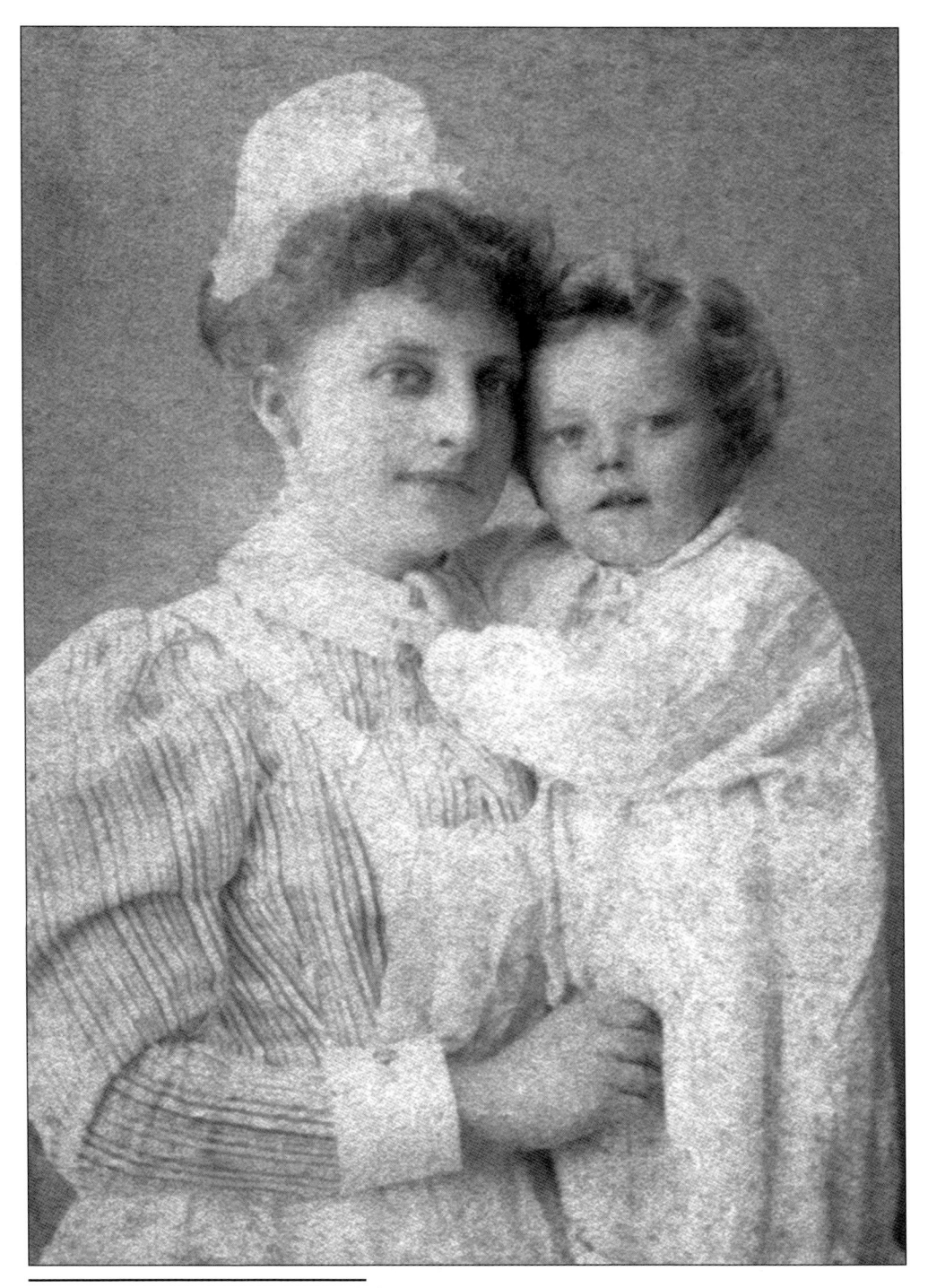

Nurse Florence Bullivant and child, 1897.
RCHA/Bullivant Collection.

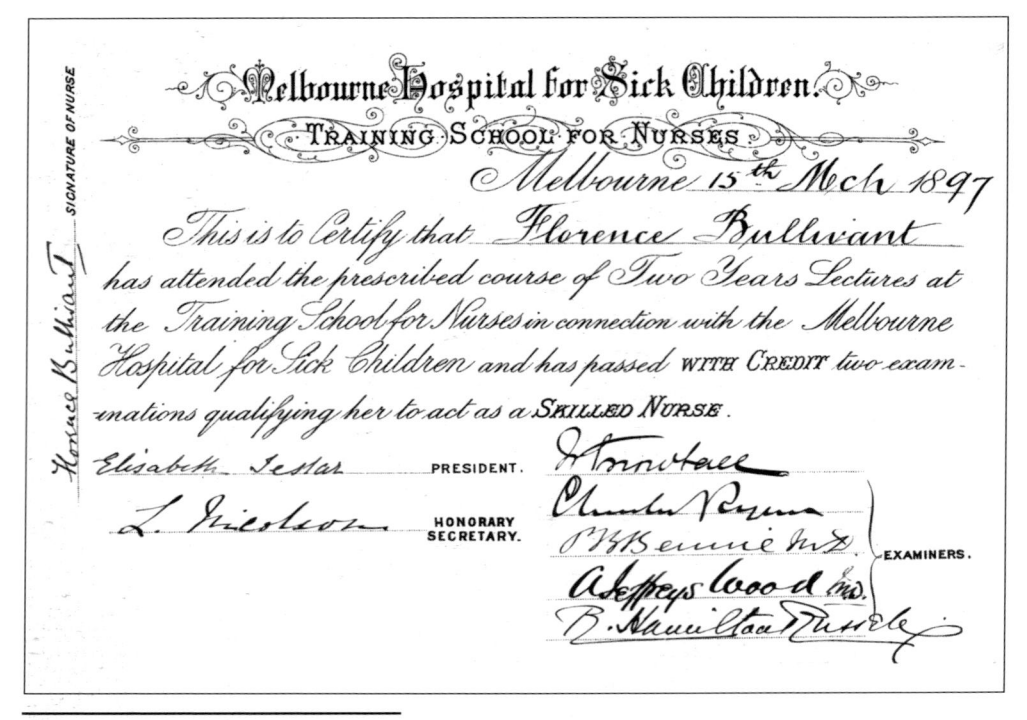

Certificate, Florence Bullivant, 1897.
RCHA/Bullivant Collection.

greatly sought after. The Hospital Annual Reports published the names of those who completed their training and received certificates. This gave nursing the status of a discipline to be studied like other professions.

Rules were re-written: no probationer could enter before the age of twenty-one years or beyond thirty and she was required to undertake a three-month unpaid trial, presumably to weed out those who were not suitable. In June 1891, the 22nd Annual Report announced that the Committee recognised the importance of efficiently trained nurses and 'had extended the term of training to two years'. It was also noted 'that better arrangements for obtaining thorough practical and technical knowledge have been made'.

The Report also noted that 'an urgent necessity for improved buildings for patients and nursing staff will engage the attention of the Committee during the coming year'.

We can see from the meagre registers that survived from the 1890s that the applicants were not merely restricted to the working-class areas of Melbourne. The families needed the means to support their daughters during this time and almost without exception they were from Protestant, well-off families from the suburbs and country regions: Toorak, St Kilda, Box Hill, Malvern, Elsternwick, Kew and Glenroy,

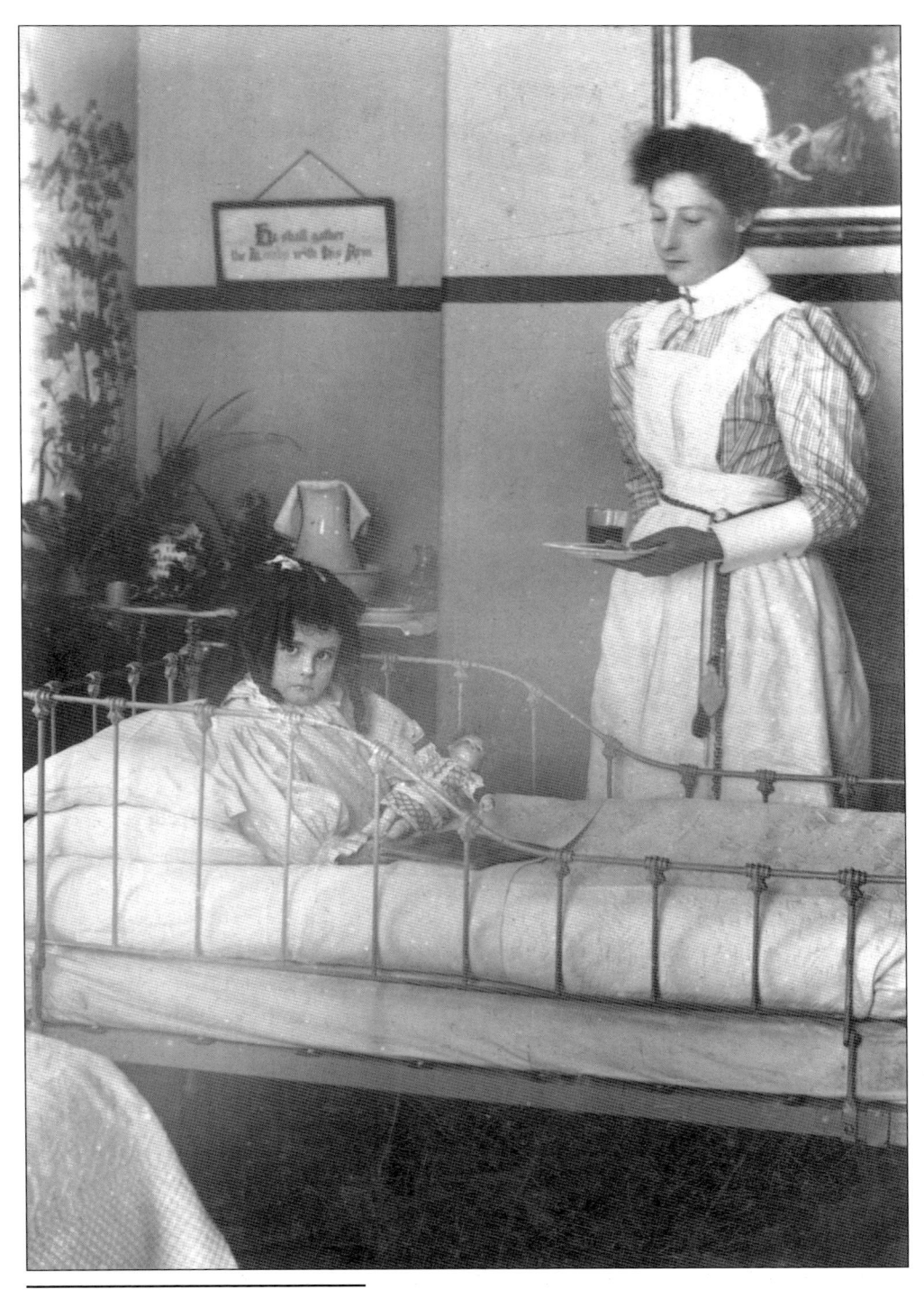

Time for medicine: A cot in the North-West Ward, December 1895.
RCHA/Bevan Collection.

as well as Beaufort, Casterton, Beechworth, Ballarat and Warrnambool. Some even came from New South Wales and Tasmania.[5] Later in the decade, enquiries were received from the Pacific, from Suva, and two sisters applied from Tokyo. The Children's Hospital became quite famous, attracting the best and the brightest medical people and educated women, and it was emulated by the establishment of children's hospitals in other states.[6] In 1897 a writer to the *Age* newspaper noted that many nurses were related to members of the Committee and the medical staff.[7]

Women in leadership

New Zealand-born Evelyn Augusta Conyers began her training in 1892 at the Children's Hospital at the age of twenty-two.

When she entered the Hospital, working conditions were restrictive and pay was a token; first-year nurses received an amount equal to that of a domestic servant, at £20 per annum, and there was nothing for probationers. Despite the long working days and nights and a high rate of infection amongst the nurses, nursing was popular and several hundred applied each week. The waiting list was suspended several times. This pattern continued for many years and, in March 1896, with fifty on the list, the books were closed.[8] Registrations did not reopen until June 1897, when fifty applications were immediately received. Whether it was the intimacy of a smaller establishment or the desire to work with children, we shall never know. Perhaps it was a sign of the lack of opportunity for women to engage in satisfying pursuits.

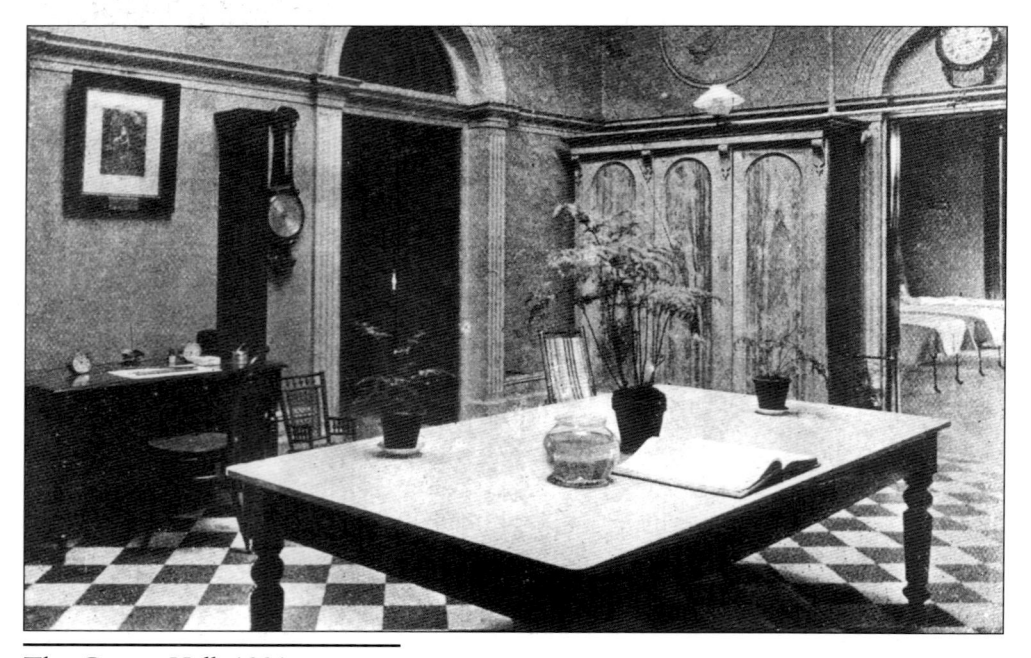

The Centre Hall, 1901.

Evelyn Conyers was born in 1870, the daughter of William Conyers, an engineer, formerly of Leeds in England, and his wife Fanny Mainprize. Her education was taken in New Zealand at Invercargill Private Girls' School and Dunedin Girls' High School and she moved to Australia with her family in the early 1890s.[9] Evelyn's nurse training days were completed without incident and she left no memoirs, so we have to look elsewhere to understand what she encountered in the Hospital.

EVELYN AUGUSTA CONYERS OBE, RRC 1st class with Bar, Florence Nightingale Medal, Diploma and Medal (International Red Cross Committee at Geneva). First Matron-in-Chief, AANS Member of Council of the Victorian Trained Nurses' Association 1903–42.

Evelyn Conyers became an Army Nursing Reserve in 1904 and was an original volunteer with the Australian Army Nursing Service. She travelled in the troopship *Shropshire* at the outbreak of World War One to Egypt. Appointed to Australian military headquarters in 1916, she became responsible for all Australian Army Nursing Service Imperial Forces in London and one of the most highly decorated nurses of the Great War.[10]

When Evelyn began nursing, the physical structure of the old Hospital remained visually beautiful but nurses were crowded three and four to a room. More than forty children were accommodated in the big, sunny, upstairs ward with the balcony adjacent to the operating theatre that faced Pelham Street. Through the windows, the children could see their pals in the playground of St George's School and hear the noises from the Rathdowne Street State School. Medical cases, about thirty a day on average, were in the spacious downstairs rooms off a central hall from the main entrance.

Lady Hopetoun and a few celebrities visited on 11 May 1892 and were highly pleased.[11] But Mrs Austin, the Deputy President, was not so impressed. Visiting during that week she found the children dining on cold mutton. There was a little unpleasantness when Dr McKay and the Matron came before the Committee where they stated that 'cold mutton was seldom given…that green vegetables were not suitable for many of the children'. The reality was children were very ill and ate little.

Two cases of scarlatina were presently in the 'house' and a child was dying of tubercular meningitis. Dr McKay reported that 'he was obliged to admit an infant a few weeks old on Saturday brought in by the Police in a starving condition'.[12]

About ten cases of typhoid were admitted each week while more than eight hundred were seen as out-patients in a conglomeration of buildings at the rear facing Pelham Street with a separate side entrance. Two extra Honorary Doctors, Stawell and McKay, were appointed to the Out-patients Room because of the large numbers of children.

Evelyn Conyers completed her training and then gained adult experience at the Melbourne Hospital. Despite her varied working life, she never lost sight of her mission for the causes of children and for the Children's Hospital and the welfare of Returned Nurses. She became the first Matron of the Queen's Infectious Diseases Hospital at Fairfield in 1904, and, after returning from war service, the proprietor of a private hospital. In 1921, she founded the Royal Children's Hospital League of Former Trainees. She devoted her whole life to nursing. On her death in September 1944, the *Australasian Nurses' Journal* commented: '[H]er special qualities were her knowledge and interest in the profession, her outstanding gifts as an organiser, her balanced mind, her strong sense of justice...made her an outstanding figure in the nursing world.'[13]

In 1893, the depression caused the Committee to reduce wages and the nurses received £5 less, that is, £15 a year. By 1893, probationers were only being registered if they agreed to work two years without pay but by 1894 many were leaving to be governesses, to take work in other hospitals and for private nursing positions. Despite the lack of monetary reward a large number of applicants continued to grow.[14]

The Boer War volunteers

Frances (Fanny) Hines and Janie Lempriere trained at the Children's Hospital (in 1893 and 1896 respectively) and were volunteers with Queen Alexandra's Imperial Nursing Service at a time when the Nightingale legend was very strong. They travelled at their own cost to Africa for duty in the Boer War. Women had to be well-off to go as volunteers as there was no Australian Nursing Service.

The impetus for sending Australian nurses to the Boer War came from the nursing profession itself, supported by a 'jingoistic public'.[15] For whatever reason, they were willing travellers with an abiding sense of adventure. All of these women expected to nurse wounded not sick patients and much to their surprise, their expectations were wrong. Epidemics of typhoid or enteric fever, spread by contaminated water caused two-thirds of the twenty thousand deaths that occurred on the British side.

JANIE MCROBIE LEMPRIERE was born in 1872, the daughter of a wealthy mercantile family. She grew up in St Kilda and received her education at a small private girls' school, Fairlight. After training at the Children's 1894–96, and further experience at the Alfred Hospital, she went to the Cape, South Africa, in 1899, paying her own fare in steerage to offer her services to Sir Alfred Milner, the British High Commissioner. She served with distinction at No. 2 BGH Wynberg, and in several other military hospitals.

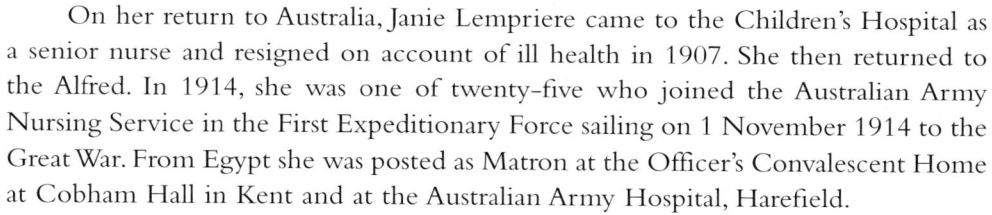

On her return to Australia, Janie Lempriere came to the Children's Hospital as a senior nurse and resigned on account of ill health in 1907. She then returned to the Alfred. In 1914, she was one of twenty-five who joined the Australian Army Nursing Service in the First Expeditionary Force sailing on 1 November 1914 to the Great War. From Egypt she was posted as Matron at the Officer's Convalescent Home at Cobham Hall in Kent and at the Australian Army Hospital, Harefield.

Janie Lempriere never married but adopted two boys when she was in her forties. She died in Melbourne in 1950.[16]

FRANCES (FANNY) EMMA HINES
On the east side of the corridor in the old Nurses' Home in Carlton, a brass plaque honoured Frances (Fanny) Emma Hines, who died at Bulawayo on 7 August in 1900, aged thirty-six. Her friend, Julia Anderson, wrote: 'she died of pneumonia contracted in devotion to duty. She was quite alone with twenty-six patients at any one time; no possibility of assistance or relief, and without sufficient nourishment'.[17]

We know very little about Frances Emma Hines, who was born in 1864. She entered the Children's Hospital Nursing School in 1893, devoting several years to children's nursing. Sailing from Australia with nine other nurses in March 1900 as a volunteer for South Africa, Sister Hines apparently worked alone before rejoining her group in Bulawayo where she contracted pneumonia and died. She was buried with full military honours, the only Australian nurse to have died in this war.[18]

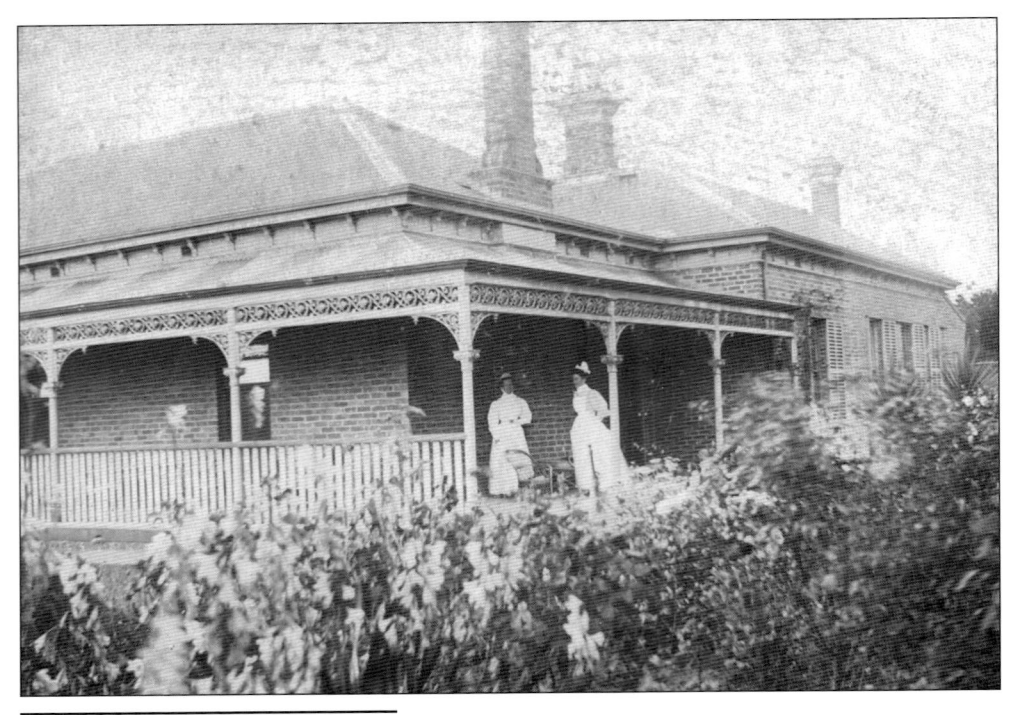

Nurse Ida Bevan on the veranda at the Brighton Convalescent Cottage, 1908.
RCHA/Bevan Collection.

Brighton Convalescent Cottage

The 1890s produced remarkable women, some of whom worked largely unsupervised at the Brighton Convalescent Cottage. A most difficult problem for the Committee was the maintenance of the small establishment where some twenty-two frail children, many from deprived slum areas of the inner city, were cared for by a series of housekeepers and one nurse. The staff changed with great regularity. The nurse was expected to assist with cooking and washing all the children's clothes as well as caring for quite ill children, entertaining them and attending to all their needs. But the hardest to bear was being 'on call' day and night. The Committee took a narrow view on time for relaxation: instructions were 'that the Housekeeper and Nurses are not to entertain friends at the Cottage except to the extent of afternoon tea occasionally or for light refreshments'. It is no surprise that Ada Hardy, a trainee, resigned 'not being strong enough for the work'.

A Sub-committee of ladies attended each week at Brighton. Despite all good intentions, the Cottage was a running saga of mismanagement with violations of the most basic rules of good housekeeping. In March 1890, the Sub-committee reported on a special inspection. They found 'the pantry in a neglected and dirty state, a jar of mouldy treacle full of flies on the shelf with the fresh milk and food in daily use, weevils in the oatmeal, barley and flour, ants in the sugar...the bread cupboard infested with mice and a quantity of infestations of mice. And on the top shelf a collection of rubbish...'

The Committee resisted sending a trained nurse to Brighton for many years despite the call of the medical staff to allow chronic cases to be placed for 'a change of air, good food and rest at the seaside...and a trained nurse to apply bandages, splints and so on'. The lonely location on the wind-swept coast of Brighton was out in the sticks. A definite improvement occurred when Nurse Alice Mowbray Flack was posted there but she suffered from nervousness on account of being in so lonely a position at night and 'on account of the fright she received at the Hospital some time since when a burglar was found in her room'.[19]

There were many nuisances: the gatekeeper at the train station allowed his goats and cow to trample the vegetable garden at night. Somewhat unkindly, it was recorded in August 1897 that 'Mrs Downes of the Committee regrets that Sister Mowbray will be compelled to resign as she is afraid of being in so lonely a position at night'. But Alice Mowbray Flack was too valuable to let go and she returned to Carlton where she was appointed to a senior position, the first nurse to be called 'Sister'. She became assistant to Miss Hilda Player in 1907. Following the incident with Miss Flack, the Committee did finally connect the telephone for security purposes.[20]

The charge position at Brighton fluctuated between Hilda Burn, Mona Kerr, Cathleen Massie and Mona Kerr, until finally Matilda Danaher was appointed as the Nurse-in-Charge. A very experienced nurse from the Training School of 1891, she resigned in sympathy over the Barlow case previously mentioned. But, as the Committee was so short of staff, she was recalled and became one of the Hospital's most valuable assets. Her career continued at the Carlton hospital and finally at the Brighton Convalescent Cottage. She stayed for twenty-two years.

Education of nurses

The Nursing School closely followed the Nightingale model, but never adopted the two-tier system taken up by some other hospitals: the 'lady probationer' who paid an entrance fee, and the assistant who did not. At the onset of the economic depression in 1893, a wholesale reduction of wages occurred with retrenchments. First-year nurses were not paid at all, and in 1899 an entrance fee of half a guinea was imposed for all probationers. Despite the depression, the nurses' training was improved and in 1894 fifty-one lectures were given by the honorary and resident medical staff as well as numerous bedside clinics.[21]

A common public perception of nurses was one of self-sacrificing 'guardian angels'. However, in reality some were not afraid to speak their mind. As previously mentioned, the assertive character of Alice Martelli, the Head Nurse who resigned in protest at the 'heavy-handedness' of the Committee, gave the members a great deal to think about. Throughout the 1890s, grumbles gathered momentum about the food and conditions. Matron Bishop was able to keep most of the complaints under control with attention to the nurses' dining table, stating that the night nurses were supplied with a hot, fresh cooked dinner with vegetables and that the second relay of day nurses were also supplied as far as possible.

Several Committee ladies mentioned that reports were circulated outside that meals and allowances were not sufficient.[22] Several nurses were called in so that their views could be heard. Matilda Danaher had no complaints, while Nurse Flack stated 'everything was very nice, much better than when she came to the Hospital five years ago'. Nurse Lempriere disagreed: 'When on night duty there was not always enough supper at 12 o'clock; on duty 9 pm to 6 am—dinner at eight, supper at 12.30, bread and butter and tea at 6.30 am'.

Technical education of nurses was completely under the control of the honorary physicians and surgeons, while the teaching of bedside care, simple procedures, and some domestic services such as feeding of children and dietetics were left to seniors and trainee nurses on the job. With a mind to future employment prospects for children's nurses, Dr Snowball continued to urge the Committee that probationers should be instructed 'in household duties and invalid cooking'. They could then easily be employed in the homes of socially prominent families. He stressed tuition in 'their duties and bearing towards employers when engaged in

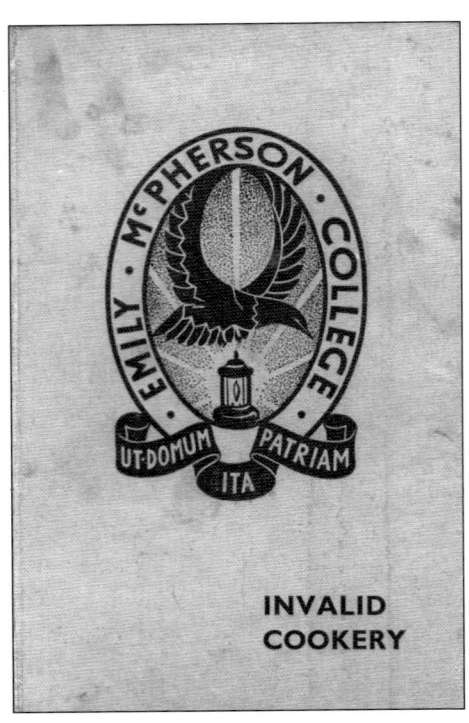

INVALID COOKERY

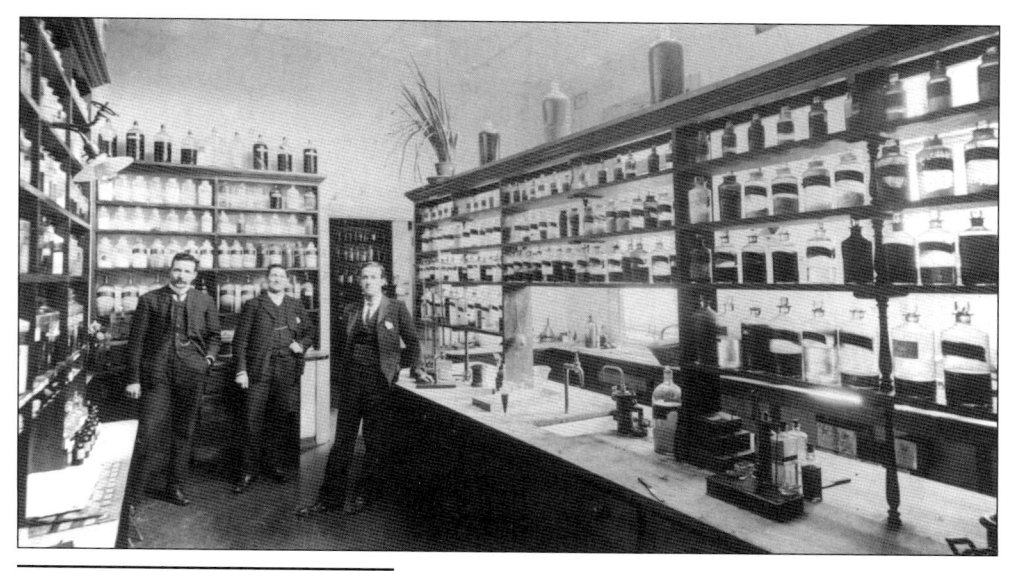

Pharmacy. Alfred Heath (right). Mid-1890s.
RCH/Caccetta Collection.

private nursing'. He explained that many nurses 'upset household arrangements when private nursing, from want of knowledge and other causes'.[23] What those 'other causes' were, we have to imagine.

Some in the medical profession wished to control training schools and knowledge. In 1880, the *Australian Medical Journal* warned about 'modern ideas...ending towards a great change in the personnel and tone of hospital nurses...ladies have in some places taken the field and performed the duties with more or less success. Experience had shown that lady nurses thought too highly of their own skill and exhibited tendencies towards diagnosing and prescribing of a very free description.'[24]

We know that at least one of the textbooks used by a Nurse Topp at the Children's Hospital perpetuated this idea. The foreword stated that 'the more highly trained the nurse the less likelihood there is of her attempting to usurp the role of the medical man.'[25] The supposition appears to be that the more knowledge the nurse had, the more her need for competition with medicos would be satisfied. But there was little evidence of tension between nurses and doctors at the Children's Hospital despite the curriculum being tightly controlled by the Honorary Medical Staff. Matron or her deputy and Head Nurses supervised general nursing procedures. The Honorary Medical Officers met on a regular basis within their own circle and actually devoted a substantial amount of time to planning and delivering lectures. In 1898, Dr Officer suggested that nurses should have oral and written as well as practical exams.[26]

Nurses' accommodation

The cramped conditions of nurses' rooms and their proximity to the wards led to a high incidence of illness among nurses. While the bedrooms for day nurses were comfortable and not very crowded, with ample fresh, clean linen, the night nurses' bedrooms did not favour rest and sleep. A laundry with a lift adjoined with a day nurses' room and a servants' room on the other side. Underneath was the doctors' and Matron's dining room, with smells rising three times a day and the echo of voices.[27]

In 1892, the Board of Health advised 'that the nurses' quarters' should be away from the Hospital. But it was a scathing report of the Inspector of Charities, tabled at a special meeting in February 1892, that caught the Committee's attention. Nevertheless, a new Nurses' Home appeared to be a low priority.

The issue did not come to public notice again until the Annual Report of 1898. The Children's Hospital came under the jurisdiction of the Melbourne City Council and was frequently visited by the Health Officer. The Mayor of Melbourne reported that 'the nurses' accommodation was unsatisfactory'. The Committee responded that 'a building was underway for the new out-patients block with provision on the upper floor to house some of the nursing staff'.

In 1899, a few nurses moved into the new building—a tall, red, brick Tudor Gothic building with small dormer windows particularly unsuitable in the scorching summer heat. We can speculate about the noise and discomfort: the building faced directly on to Drummond Street where more than one thousand children, accompanied by their parents and siblings, came through the front door to the Out-patients Hall each week.[28] By night, this was a 'red light district'.

The purpose-built Nurses' Home in Rathdowne Street was completed in 1908, sixteen years after the original report of the Inspector of Charities. For the intervening years, the Committee rented several houses adjoining the Hospital in Rathdowne Street, which were later demolished to make way for the Nurses' Home. In 1902, they bought 'Elmira', a terrace which, like so many of the old Carlton houses, was run-down and rat infested. Eventually restored to its former glory, 'Elmira' became the senior nurses' accommodation and remained so until the 1950s.[29]

Three years' training

In 1895, the Victorian Government added a clause to the *Factory and Shops Act* stating that no nurse in a charitable institution was to work more than one hundred and sixty-eight hours in any twenty-one days. The Children's Hospital was well prepared. Unlike some other Melbourne hospitals expecting crippling financial consequences, the Children's Hospital Committee did not resist. The 27th Annual Report of 1896 stated that 'arrangements are being made to reduce the working hours of nurses which are at present 10 and a half hours per day' but, 'with due regard to the welfare

> **Melbourne Hospital for Sick Children.**
>
> OUT-PATIENT FORM.
>
> Ladies,
>
> I beg to recommend
>
> residing at
>
> who is unable to pay for medical attendance, for child, as Out-Patient of the above Institution.
>
> To the Committee,
>
> MELBOURNE HOSPITAL FOR SICK CHILDREN.
>
> Signature and Address of Contributor.
>
> day of 188
>
> Mr. a'BECKETT attends on Mondays and Thursdays at 2.30. | Dr. WIGG attends on Tuesdays and Fridays at 2.30.
> Mr. GARRARD attends on Wednesdays and Saturdays, at 1.
>
> Contributors, before signature, are requested to ascertain, from personal enquiry, that the case is one needing charitable relief, and that the Declaration on back hereof is duly signed by applicant.
>
> OVER.
>
> *(Stamped across form: PATIENTS MUST PROVIDE THEIR OWN BOTTLES. NO MEDICINES DISPENSED IN DARK OR SODA WATER BOTTLES.)*

of the patients, the alterations will extend the time of training from two to three years'.

There had already been moves to reduce the working hours following unwelcome publicity at the Royal Commission into Charitable Institutions in 1890.[30] Three commissions were held during the nineteenth century recommending changes to the 'so-called' voluntary system and reform of charities. Alice Martelli, the Head Nurse who resigned in protest over the Barlow case, was called as a witness to explain her experiences of long working hours. She revealed that '…at the Children's Hospital… nurses used to work from 6 [am]–10 [pm] with a half-hour for meals; lately that has been altered—they are allowed alternate days off at 6 pm…young nurses from the fact of their youth should not have to work so long'. Her opinion was that three months' menial work was quite enough. A certificate should be drawn up with qualifications, character and temperament: 'Get those who lecture them to sign the certificate and the standard would be better. Stop the gossip about one hospital being better than the other.'[31]

The Committee, sensitive as ever to public criticism, changed the night nurses' duty hours to start at 10 pm and to leave off as soon as possible, not later than 7 am.

The end of an era

Sarah Bishop was born at the time of the foundation of the colony of Victoria. She witnessed the development of the Children's through the most difficult of times. At her retirement in 1899, Robert Murray Smith described her as:

[T]hat excellent lady who for twenty-four years filled her responsibility and frequently hard-worked office with unfailing tact, and courtesy, watching the establishment grow. She assisted in its progress with every means within her power. It was a small place when she took charge in 1875; when she resigned in 1899, 'it had become foremost among kindred institutions in Australia and might worthily rival those of the mother country.'[32]

The gentle demeanour, kindness and empathy of the Children's nurses became legendary. With the publicity surrounding the fundraising for the rebuilding of the new Hospital, a torrent of articles appeared about Hospital children and their nurses in school papers and journals. In 1900, for example, following a decade of intolerable child mortality from infectious diseases, and despite a deteriorating complex of old buildings, the Committee managed to project appealing images of youthful, healthy young women in crisp uniforms and badges tending to angelic children in little beds.

In 1900, a 'visitor' wrote a glowing report as he followed his guide into the large building to the staircase:' The room was lofty, light and perfectly ventilated; the walls had a warm and cheerful colouring; there were plants, flowers, toys, a bowl of gold fish here and there, and the children were looking at picture books and Christmas cards…there seemed to be a good many children, but they were wonderfully quiet.' Small convalescents sat around the high stove fender or at low tables in happy and intimate silence. 'As the bright-faced Sister and nurses in their blue and white uniforms passed a group or a cot, some pale little face would light up for a moment at a caressing touch or a playful word.'[33]

The reality was, infant mortality continued to be undesirably high. In Dr Arthur Jeffreys Wood's view, 'advances in the world in the care of sick children were deplorably slow' and 'Melbourne shared in this lamentable state of affairs'.[34] There was little difference in the distribution of incidence of infectious illnesses; every family, rich or poor had at least one child who died in the early childhood years.

Nurses were susceptible to serious illness. A dedicated nurse, Blanche Fowler died at the Children's Hospital in August 1897, her long illness ending with an intestinal haemorrhage resulting from typhoid. As a mark of respect and sorrow, the Committee paid her funeral expenses.[35] She served four years as a nurse at the Hospital.

Special appeals for donations for the Hospital came flooding in and very soon the Hospital was in a strong position 'to go it alone…as the great sympathy of the public and especially the young people would be lost otherwise'. The Children's Hospital was a special institution appealing to all persons in the colony, altogether different from other hospitals, and had already received many offers of entertainments and other supports which would undoubtedly have been lost by joining others with a general appeal.[36]

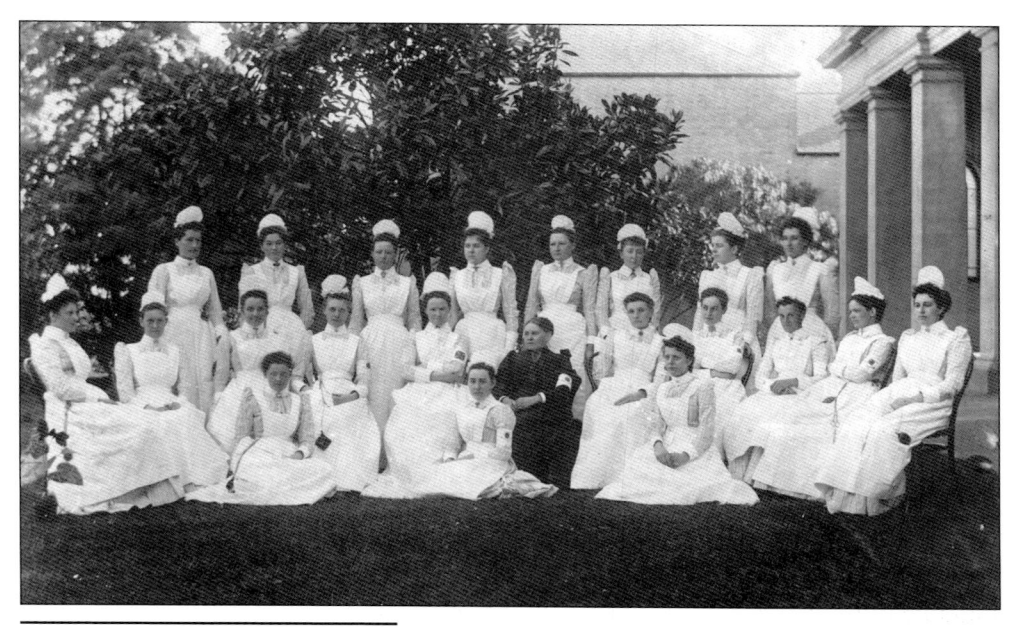

Matron Bishop and her nurses in the walled garden, 1893. Grace Jennings Carmichael, standing (right).

A reference from Dr A. Jeffreys Wood was insurance that Children's Hospital nurses would be welcome wherever they travelled in the world. A Children's nurse with the appropriate training could easily progress to private nursing and was in demand in the homes of the families who could afford to keep a nurse.

A treasured, rare document left to the Children's Hospital nursing archives is such a testament. Constance Mary Murray entered the Children's Hospital Nurses' Training School on 29 October 1900. On her departure for England, Dr A. Jeffreys Wood wrote: 'Constance Mary Murray is thoroughly trustworthy, careful, sympathetic and bright, and she is an ideal nurse…'[37]

By the twentieth century, eighty-two nurses had been trained at the Children's Hospital.

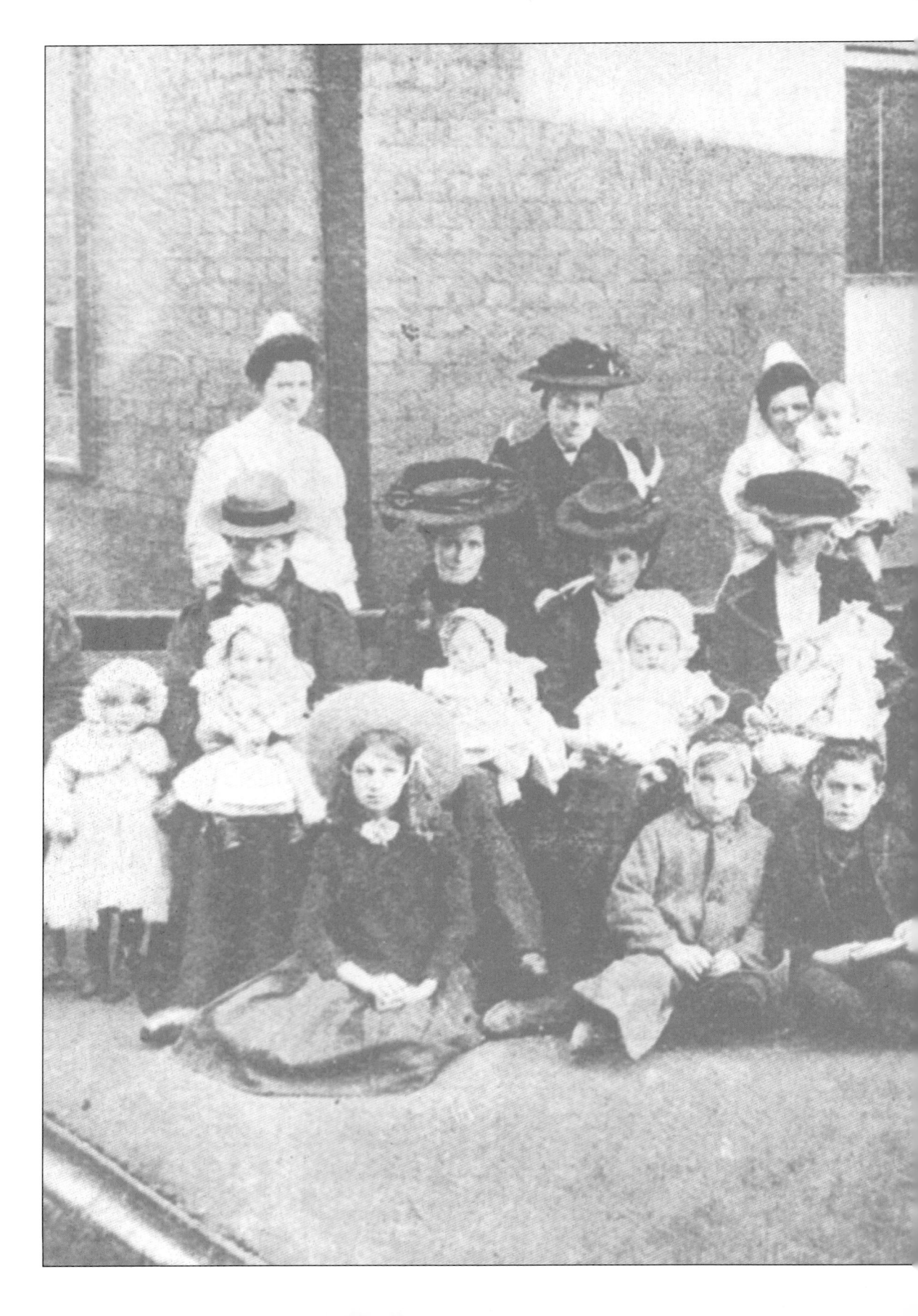

Part 2

1900–1924

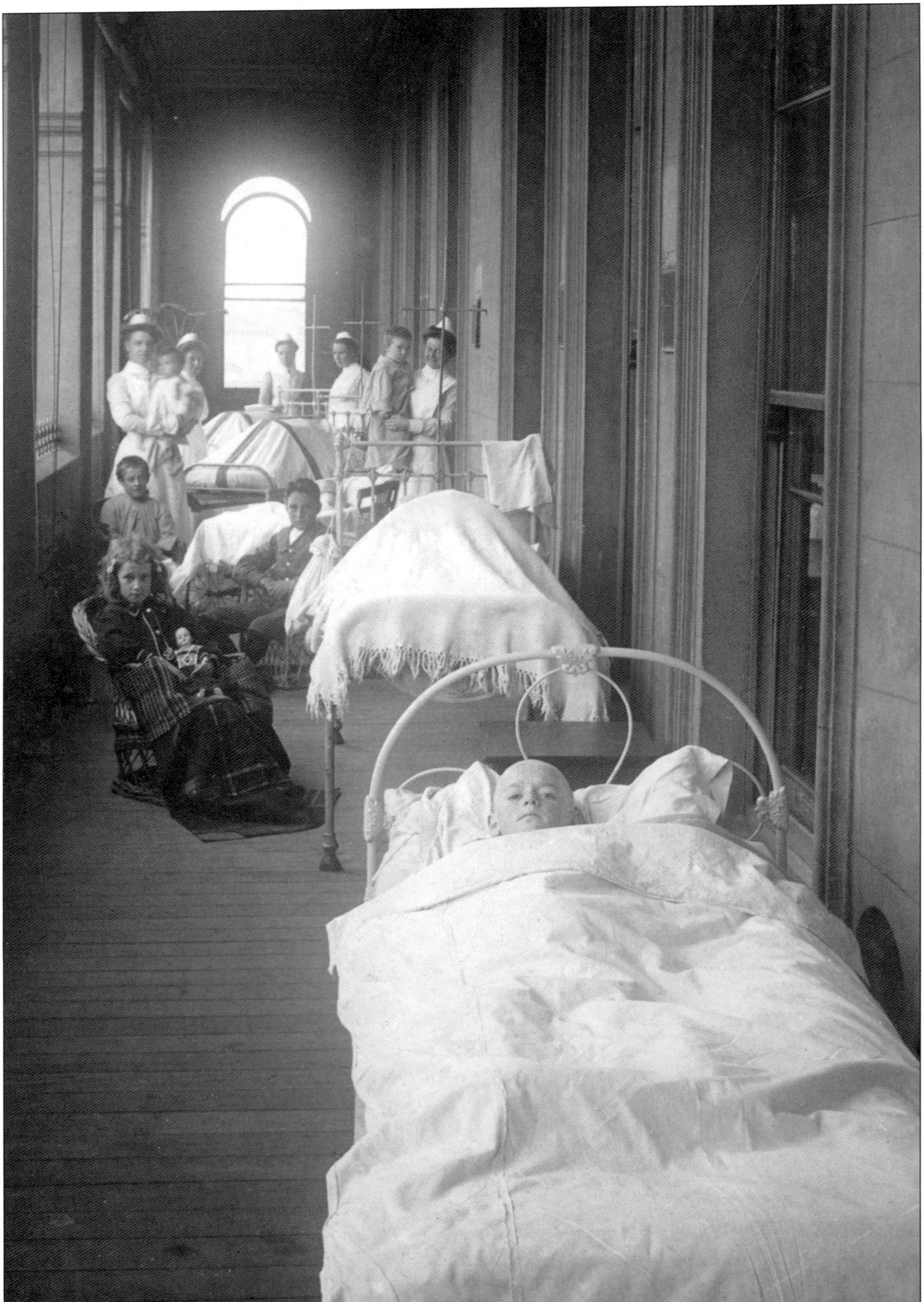

CHAPTER 4

The Years of Miss Player
1900–1922

It shall be the duty of every nurse to watch and attend the children with care and kindness, inability to amuse or render contented the patients may be regarded as sufficient grounds for dismissal.

Nurses' Rule Book, Children's Hospital, 1902

The new century brought challenges for Australian women. They won the right to vote, to own property, to travel and run their own business. Some entered the professions and went to war; for the first time, middle-class women had a chance to choose between marriage and the freedom of a career. In 1921, the first woman entered Parliament.[1]

Melbourne had come far; the excitement, the viceregal presence and the pomp and glamour of Federation promised a more civilised and gentler society. However, for the poor working class of the crowded inner suburbs, conditions were little different from the depression of the 1890s. The tragedy of infant mortality and maternal disadvantage was unaltered in grossly unhygienic slums.[2] The chance of having a decent start in life was negligible in housing with no bathrooms or kitchens, backyard pan lavatories, poor drainage and damp floors.

This was a time of greater awareness of children's needs. In 1904, a Mrs Edwards, the Lady Superintendent of the Victorian Infant Asylum and Foundling Hospital, gave a talk to the Royal Victorian Trained Nurses' Association entitled 'The Feeding and Management of Children'. She referred to the 'age of the expert' in the care of babies, often relegated to some inexperienced and untried young women

---

Balcony of the Surgical Ward, 1905.
RCHA/Collins Collection.

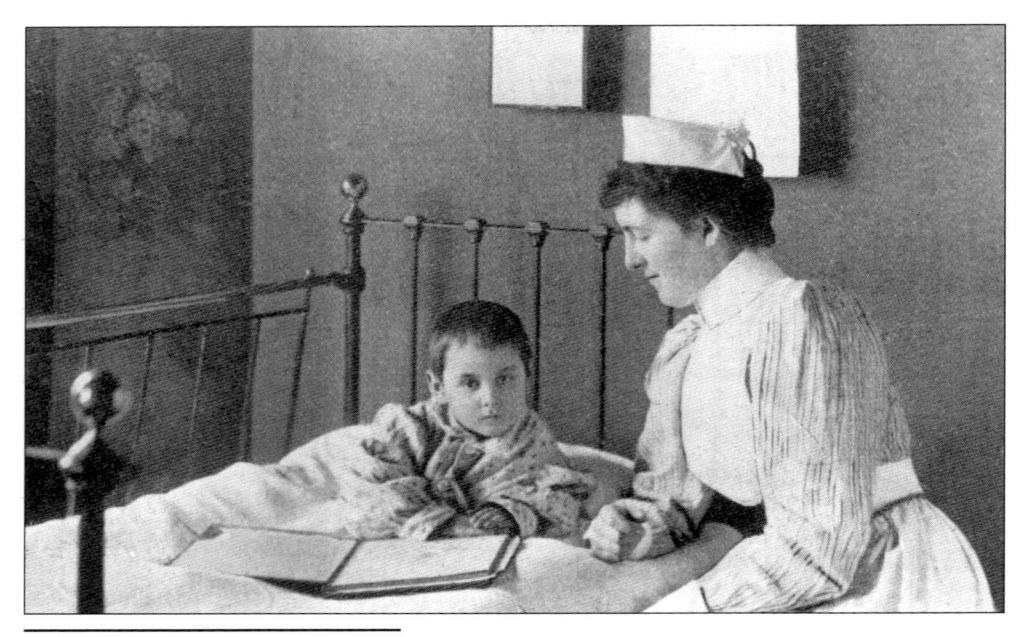

A cot in the Centre Ward, 1902.

who 'act' as nurses. She argued for children's nurses to be qualified comparably to adults' nurses, hoping that 'there will be in every State an organization for the training of baby nurses'. The necessary qualities for those receiving the training would be a 'love of children, unlimited patience, great firmness, and with an understanding that a mother's first duty to society is to nurture her own child'.[3]

The medical staff had long recognised the role of advocacy by the Children's Hospital in issues of public health, better housing, clean milk and, by example and education, the prevention of malnutrition and accidents. Early in the twentieth century, provision was at last being made for babies, long excluded except for surgical emergencies. The risk of cross-infection, lack of suitable artificial feeding and lack of accommodation for breast-feeding mothers had concerned the medical staff for thirty years. When planning the new Princess May Pavilion in 1901, Dr Arthur Jeffreys Wood's request for eight baby cots and an extra five nurses was denied for some unexplained reason, probably a lack of finance. However in 1903, two babies were admitted to each of the two wards in the new medical building. This was the beginning of the long tradition in the research and care of babies, particularly those with the killer disease, summer diarrhoea.

The increasing admission of babies over the following twenty years presented many problems, not least being the intensive staff requirements and the need to develop satisfactory infant feeding. The person to lead the Hospital in these complex challenges was Hilda Player.

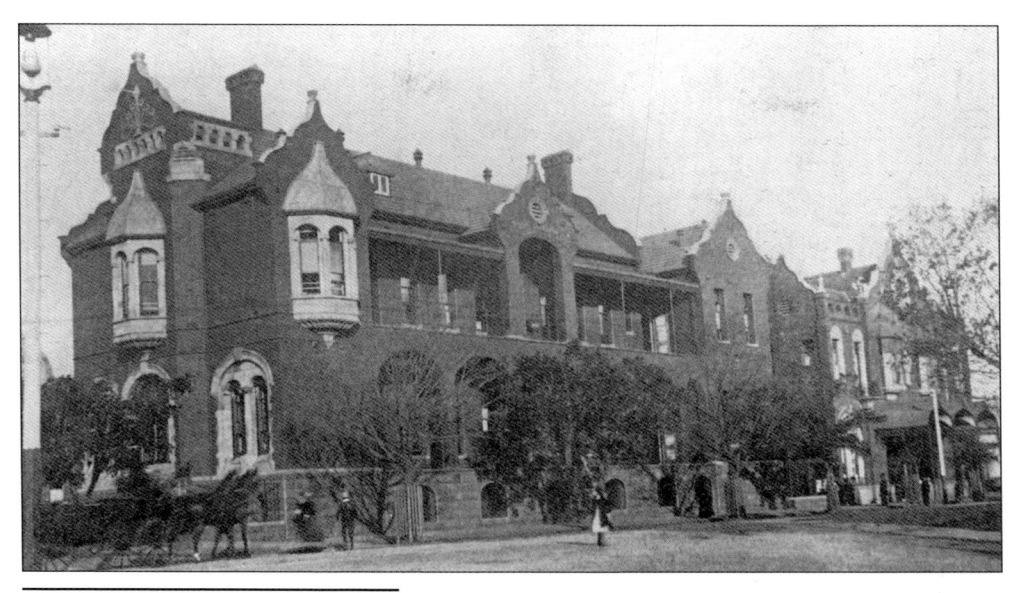

Princess May Pavilion 1907, Wards 7 and 8.

Hilda Clara Player succeeded Mrs Bishop in 1899 to become the third Matron of the Children's Hospital. An Englishwoman by birth, she came to Australia at a young age, and in the 1890s trained at Sydney's Royal Alexandra Hospital for Children. Her remarkable ability was recognised in 1894 when she became their first trainee to take the position of Deputy, then Matron at that hospital. An ambitious woman, she gained two years' adult experience at the Melbourne Hospital and also private nursing.[4]

We know of Miss Player's personal characteristics, that she was immaculate in appearance, rather slight in build, fussy and strict. The surviving photographs show her dressed in clinical white from her cap to her shoes, a contrast to Mrs Bishop in widow's black. She proved to be an outstanding administrator, teacher and advocate for the advancement of nurses, regularly contributing articles and 'social' news to the emerging Victorian Trained Nurses' Association Journal, *UNA*.[5]

Well-qualified and experienced, Miss Player could be a firm negotiator, never afraid to speak out. For the first time in the history of the Hospital, the position was given the English honorary title 'Lady Superintendent' rather than Matron. The inference was that nursing reform could only be effective if a well-educated woman of a superior class was in sole charge of the nursing and domestic establishment. By implication, the Lady Superintendent had independence from hospital physicians and direct access to Committees and Boards of Management.[6] In fact, Miss Player took on huge responsibilities. There was no hospital manager or medical superintendent, in the early days.

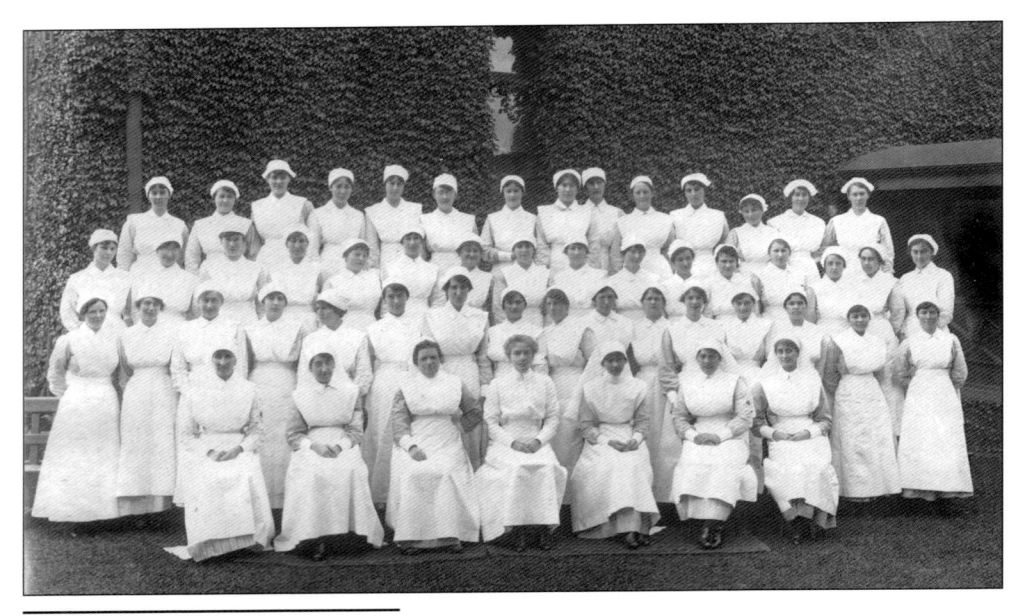

Matron Hilda Clara Player (centre) and her nurses. Maria Thomas, Assistant Matron and Out-patient Sister (left) of Matron, c. 1910.

Before the end of Miss Player's three months' trial, she made recommendations for the re-organisation of the nursing staff. By 1902 she left no doubt about her role and status. The Rule Book for that year stated: 'The Lady Superintendent was Mistress of the Household.' Those nurses who broke the rules were treated harshly; for example, an inability to amuse and make the patients contented was likely to be regarded as grounds for instant dismissal. Nurses' behaviour was expected to be exemplary. They were to practise 'quietness and decorum and to wear noiseless slippers when in the wards'. Orders went up the line: resignations and complaints were to be directed in writing to the Lady Superintendent herself who then reported to the Committee.

The Lady Superintendent's responsibilities were very wide. Known as a reformist, Miss Player took new initiatives, including relieving nurses of dirty, menial work and introducing new titles such as 'Sister' and 'Staff Nurse' to indicate the level of proficiency and responsibility the individual had acquired. The former position of Head Nurse, denoting seniority without certification, no longer existed. Staff Nurses were required to take the load off the Sisters for teaching and supervision of probationers. The use of the title 'Sister' signalled the final resistance of the charity hospitals to the similarity and symbolism with the Catholic orders.[7] These women quickly became administrators, delegated to be responsible for the orderliness and cleanliness for their own areas, Medical and Surgical, while the overall responsibility for the nurses and their training was delegated to a Deputy Matron.

After 1904, Miss Alice Mowbray Flack, a Children's Hospital nurse trained in 1891, took charge of some of the household tasks: catering and domestic arrangements, laundry, linen and the sewing room as well as the welfare of the nurses. Hers was therefore the forerunner of the position of Home Sister.

For the probationers, the dreaded split shifts, already in place for decades, stayed. Nurses worked 7 am to 10 am with a break until 1 pm. With a half-hour break for tea, the same nurses then gave the children their supper and put them to bed. In later years the hours were reduced to 9 pm. In the 1960s these shifts were still in place, the only concession, a straight 7 am to 5.30 pm shift before their one day off.

It was not all plain sailing. Initially the longer-serving nursing staff did revolt against change they considered was grossly unfair. When their precious one day off a week was changed to one day a month, seventeen nurses out of twenty-nine wrote to the *Argus* voicing their extreme anger.[8] Despite a promise to review the matter in three months, there is no record that the rules were changed. Instead the nurses were severely reprimanded by the Committee for their 'lack of *esprit de corps*'.

Miss Player was sometimes called upon when there was social need. In May 1901, a child from Deniliquin had stayed six months at the Children's Hospital and had nowhere to go. The police were contacted and her father called for her. Miss Player also reported 'that the child Kelly's mother was in the Women's Hospital and very poor'. Miss Player was directed to write to the mother 'if she wishes the Committee to find a home for the child?' The mother wrote back, stating that 'she would be glad if she could be placed in a home until the winter is over. She only earned 3/- a week and was in delicate health.'

Miss Player does seem to have made the Hospital her life. As one of the new disciplinarians, a phenomenon that developed in the profession following the formation of the Australian Army Nursing Service in the Boer War years, she was in stark contrast to her homely, motherly predecessor. Nevertheless, her kindness and concern for the well-being of the children and the nurses was remembered. Mary Wilson, a twenty-year-old country girl, began her probation in April 1915 and Miss Player encouraged her and her fellow nurses to take two hours off during the afternoon to go on the cable tram to St Kilda 'for some air'.[9] She remembers nurses too sick to work being treated sympathetically. There is some evidence that in the early days of her appointment, Miss Player met with the nurses socially and invited several to her house at Frankston.[10]

Raising the profile of the Hospital was certainly one of Miss Player's goals, for she was also extremely class conscious. The introduction of the entry fee for probationers, initially half a guinea, increased to £10 in 1904, and ten guineas (£10/10/-) in 1907, eliminated poorer girls with no social status. Entry was refused to a probationer in 1909 because, the Committee said, 'she was not the class of nurse the Matron liked'.

An elderly doctor, a Resident at the Hospital before World War One, commented that 'the nurses here, unlike those at the Melbourne and the Women's Hospitals were girls one would meet socially'.[11] One problem with this was that the nurses, once trained, had no need to stay at the Hospital for employment and often returned home or married. The trainee staff at that time numbered fifty-three and five Sisters.[12]

Generational change

When Miss Player was appointed in 1899 the Hospital had expanded to seventy-two beds. There had been little change in the Committee members and Honorary Doctors since the foundation of the Hospital nearly thirty years before. She entered a world with a particular culture, an intimate, cosy establishment of gentle old-fashioned women and ageing doctors. Her path was eased by the changes in the Committee of Management and the widening circle of new young medical appointees.

Catherine Austin, a wise and experienced socially prominent woman from the Western District and Toorak, the mother of eight children, succeeded as President of the Hospital in 1899.

Dr William Snowball was succeeded by Dr A. Jeffreys Wood, another popular children's doctor and a public health advocate. He showed willingness to assist with the training of nurses.

Of the notable physicians and surgeons who left the Children's after 1900 to take up adult surgery at the Alfred and the Melbourne Hospitals, Charles Ryan was one of the most interesting, regaling the student audience with his tales of adventure and flamboyant manner.

CHARLES RYAN, Honorary Surgeon 1878–1914, 'was a picturesque character, known for his blustering bonhomie and breeziness'. A consultant surgeon to the Children's Hospital 1890–1914 and popular Collins Street surgeon, he was connected to Lady Janet Clarke and father of Maie Ryan (Lady Casey). Educated at Melbourne Grammar School and Melbourne Medical School, he finished his degree in Edinburgh, graduating in 1875. After studying in Bonn and Vienna he joined the Turkish Army at the commencement of the Russo-Turkish War, returning to Melbourne 'in a blaze of publicity'.[13]

The most admired surgeon was the gentle and aesthetic Hamilton Russell, distinguished and handsome, who arrived in Melbourne in 1890. He directed his work to the children of Carlton until 1901; afterwards at the Alfred Hospital and some private practice. Returning to the Children's Hospital intermittently until World War One, Russell's willingness to train theatre nurses and his good nature were said to disperse around him such an atmosphere 'that surgeon, sister, resident, dresser and probationer alike were bonded in the great task of healing'.[14]

Russell took up a further appointment at the Children's towards the end of his professional life in 1920. The nurses knew him affectionately as 'Hammy', and deeply admired his wonderful and courageous surgical skills.

HAMILTON RUSSELL, Honorary Surgeon to the Children's Hospital 1892–1901, 1905, 1920–25. Born in England in 1860. He studied medicine at Kings College Hospital, London, and was the first dresser and House Surgeon to Lord Lister.

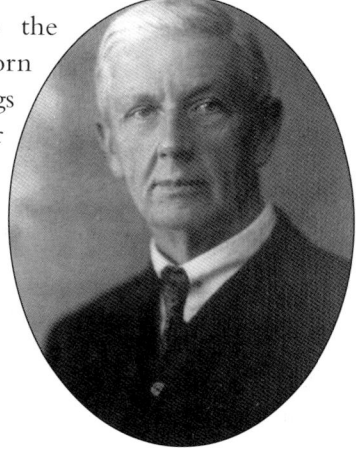

Theatre work

Nurses loved the excitement, atmosphere and drama of the operating theatre. By the very nature of children's vulnerability and the standards of the day in the use of primitive anaesthetics, the surgeons acted swiftly.

Interior images of the operating theatre of the late nineteenth century show that gloves and masks were not introduced until 1908. Russell was known to swab carbolic into the open wound and therefore had a low rate of post-operative infection. In the sunny upstairs operating-room, the windows opened to Pelham Street catching the northern light. In the event of a night time emergency, surgery was carried out by gas-light. Electricity was connected in 1913 to the new surgical wards and the operating theatre.

Despite their love of the work, theatre nurses were not short on complaints: tired feet from standing for hours on the hard terrazzo floors, serious damage to their hands from the constant use of carbolic, the pervasive and nauseating smell of the antiseptic sprayed on walls and tables affected their health.

A nurse's life

Some of the most archaic rules governing nurses evolved during this period; for example, the ritual of attendance and supervision by senior nursing staff at mealtimes to 'overcome difficulties'. These appeared to centre on the nurses' food, or lack of it. Throughout 1907, food supplies were particularly short, the monotony was terrible and nurses were simply hungry. Constant complaints were finally heard when nurses fell ill with ptomaine poisoning. The President, Mrs Gavan Duffy, interviewed eight nurses, six senior and three second-years. The results were found to be: no butter for breakfast and none for latecomers at tea, the meat was gristly, the porridge lumpy. The nurses were tired of milk puddings.

Following an enquiry by Dr A. Jeffreys Wood, the matter was cleared up and Matron arranged for the Night Sister to stay on to supervise the breakfast table. Dr Wood had second thoughts about the ripples he caused and wrote 'he had only enquired about the butter for the patients initially, but also noted how pleased he was that dripping had disappeared from the nurse's dining room'.

Working in the Out-patients Hall was quite an experience. If anything epitomised the busyness and colour of the Children's Hospital in the landscape of Carlton in the early 1900s, it was this new department. The red-brick building, a local landmark in Drummond Street, received hundreds of visits of patients a week and thousands per year. In 1908, the year of the first recorded polio epidemic, there were 18,000 visits.

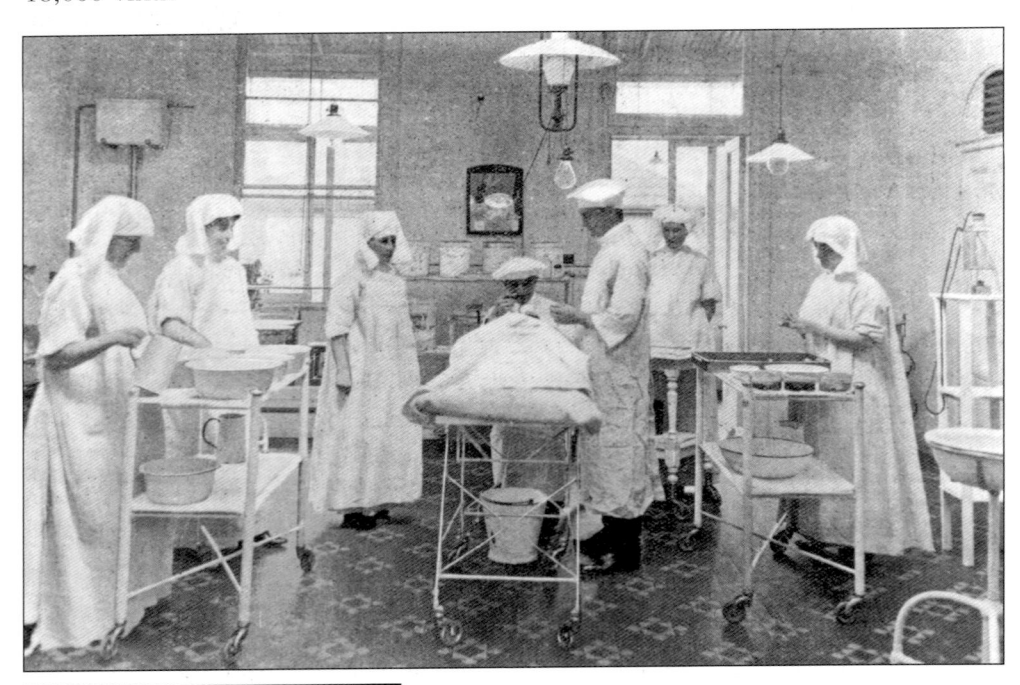

Operating theatre, 1909.

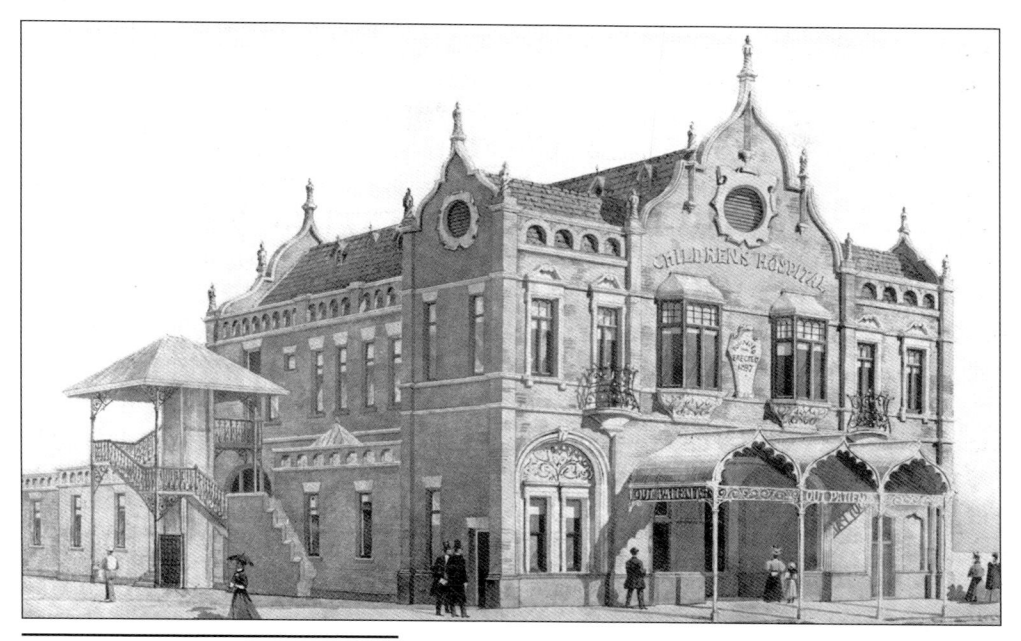

Out-patients Department, 1899. Drummond Street with nurses' entrance, left.

The building had no facilities for visiting parents: few toilets, no changing rooms, no canteen and nowhere for sick children to lie down. The hard wooden benches were rarely empty of seated people. If a child or mother wanted to go to the toilet, the mother had to have someone to keep the seat warm or lose her place, sometimes for several hours. Unusual incidents were a never-ending source of amusement to the staff; the same families returned many times, as in a general practice.

In 1921, fifty years after the foundation of the Hospital, the Auxiliaries under direction of Miss Mary Guthrie, introduced a simple canteen in the basement of the Princess May building on Drummond Street. A penny could purchase a bun and a cup of tea; to warm babies' bottle, a half-penny.

Mary Grant Bruce, author of the Billabong Books, wrote an article on the Hospital in the magazine *The Woman*.[15] She described the atmosphere in the Out-patients Department where 'children of all ages—wee babies to big boys and girls are objects of keen interest to the other urchins of Carlton's teeming streets'. A little girl of seven had Billy, two years younger, in tow. Two terrified little faces peeped over the counter. 'Billy's swallered 'is sixpence', said the small girl. 'Mum sent us out shopping an' 'e put it in 'is mouth an' its gone down! Mum says if y' don't get it up she'll skin, 'im.'

The resources of medical science were instantly at Billy's disposal but the X-ray failed to divulge any hidden coin, and science stood baffled. At this point, Billy, in wholesome fear of more drastic exploration, collapsed, and confessed he had not swallowed his capital at all. It had disappeared in the more ordinary way, but the 'wrath of Mum' was imminent, and the Hospital's proximity suggested a way out. One of the staff gave Billy sixpence, and he went forth a restored solvent.

The Victorian Trained Nurses' Association (VTNA)

Nineteenth-century nursing reform centred on the establishment of standard training and registration. In July 1896, a meeting occurred between the Melbourne, Alfred and Children's Hospitals to discuss the establishment of rules for nurses and the desirability of a Central Board of Examiners, but came to nothing. For several years the idea lapsed. It was not until 1901 that the newly formed Victorian Trained Nurses' Association (VTNA) called a meeting between representatives of Melbourne's leading hospitals. Then it was resolved that 'there shall be one final examination for all nurses, five examiners be appointed, one from each of the three hospitals: the Melbourne, the Alfred, the Sick Children's and two examiners from the VTNA'. In July 1902, Dr Peter Bennie, a leading physician and surgeon at the Children's was appointed as the Hospital's representative. Other notable representatives from the Children's were Dr W. Atkinson Wood, brother of Dr A. Jeffreys Wood, and Miss Evelyn Conyers, a former Children's Hospital nurse and private hospital proprietor, a foundation member of the VTNA, Matron of Fairfield Hospital and Army Reservist. Evelyn Conyers remained a loyal advocate and important figure in the progress of nurse registration in Victoria and a friend to the Children's Hospital nurses all her life.

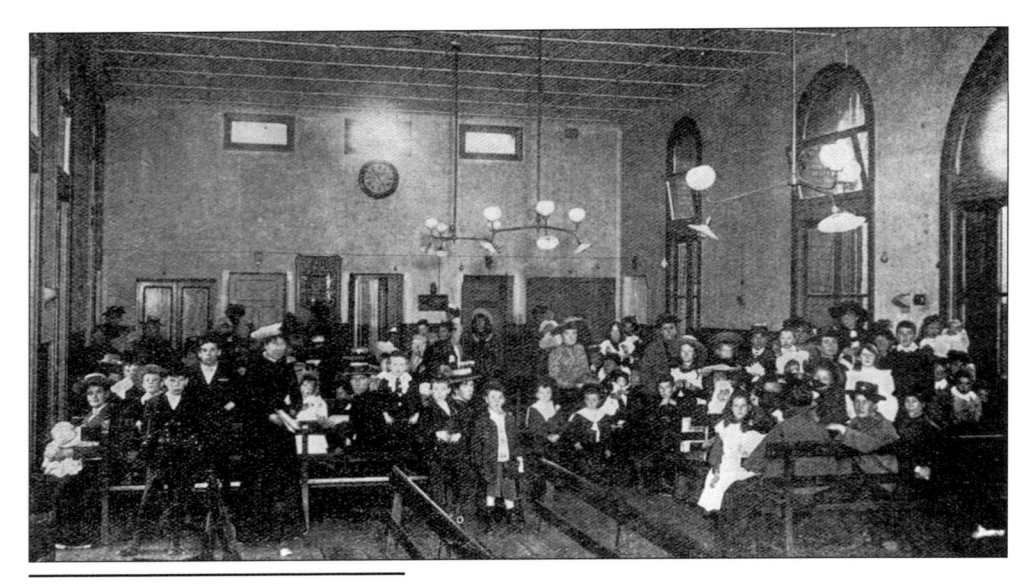

Out-patients Hall, 1906.

The VTNA nursing syllabus was based on three years' general training in a public hospital and did not recognise a special class of patient or their diseases. For example, the Women's Hospital, the Eye and Ear, and the Queen's Memorial Infectious Diseases Hospital (Fairfield) did not qualify. For some inexplicable reason, the Children's Hospital was classified as a general hospital.[16] One possible explanation was that the medical discipline of paediatrics had not yet come into its own and, for purposes of classification, children were treated as small adults. More likely were the powerful influences on the VTNA Board.

But a particular problem for Children's Hospital nurses became evident: the ability to move from one hospital to another for further training and advancement; if Children's nurses did move, they were required by that hospital board to train all over again. This caused many nurses to become discouraged; some stayed at the Children's for years without venturing into the wider community. The Committee suggested that those Children's Hospital nurses holding the Hospital certificate should be able to obtain a certificate in another hospital by serving only one additional year instead of two. Nothing came of this. Many nurses moved on to the Alfred and the Melbourne, became settled and never returned.

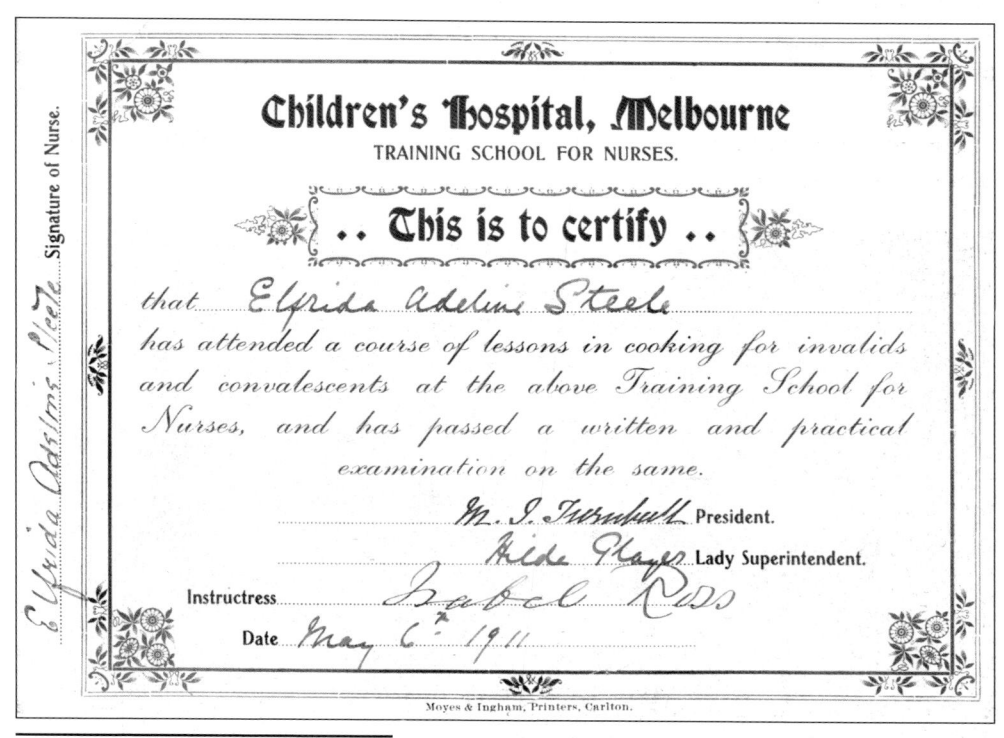

Children's Hospital Certificate, 1911.
RCHA/Steele Collection.

Registration of Children's nurses was controversial. Although the certificate of competency complied with the principles of general nursing, the ambivalence on the part of the Committee of Management that the Nursing School be kept in line with mainstream general training and also remain 'special', came to a head with the introduction of the Nurses' Registration Bill in 1923. It was not until the *Nurses' Registration Act 1924* that the status of the Children's Hospital Nursing School was examined in detail. Following an amendment to the Act in 1929, Children's Hospital nurses were required to complete three years of adult nursing at the Homeopathic (Prince Henry's after 1934) or at the Women's Hospital. This caused further debate and was found wanting because there was no male nursing, the very reason that many parents approved their girls taking up children's nursing in the first place. It was not until 1939 that further enquiry resulted in a reciprocal arrangement to rotate nurses from the Melbourne Hospital, the only hospital without children, for three months at the Children's, and Children's Hospital nurses for six months at the Melbourne Hospital.[17]

The decline of Miss Player

Hilda Player epitomised the professional image of a twentieth-century Hospital Matron, a dedicated, outstanding nurse, administrator and teacher. Within fourteen years, the total number of nurses increased from twenty-nine to more than seventy, the Hospital was rebuilt, and many reforms took place.

Unfortunately, the brave new vision was overshadowed by the sadness of World War One and the impact on the Hospital community, and the death of two nurses, one from unknown causes, the other from typhoid fever. Several war deaths were connected to the Hospital: the brothers of several nurses, two sons of Committee member Mrs Gavan Duffy, the only son of Justice and Mrs Higgins, two of Dr Snowball's sons and two former Resident Medical Officers, were killed in action.

As the years went by, Miss Player's sense of humour deserted her and she became intolerant of anyone having fun. The inbred nature of the small Hospital community encouraged gossip and a lack of privacy; Matron's quarters were adjacent to the doctors' in the lovely building in Pelham Street. She made a few sacrifices during the war when asked to share a bathroom with the lady doctors but her tolerance was stretched to the limit by the male doctors. Returning from the theatre one Friday night at 11 pm, she heard 'considerable noise'. On investigation, three Residents were entertaining lady visitors at supper, and the noise continued after 11.30 pm! Although the matter was reported to the President, all would have gone into history but for a new twist. Six months later, Matron found Dr Spargo visiting two final-year nurses in the nurses' sitting room at the Isolation Ward. Both nurses were suspended, and the doctor resigned.[18]

The question of nurses' salaries was never quite resolved; often at the whim of the Committee, a long-serving nurse might be lucky. In 1918, for example, Sister Danaher's pay rose from £84 to £100, the first increase for many years. She had been at the Hospital since 1889, a period of twenty-nine years, in charge of the isolated Convalescent Cottage at Brighton for twenty years.[19] Miss Player's salary was raised for her contribution to the war effort and in 1920 raised to £250 'for her skilful management in the Spanish Influenza epidemic'. Sister Belstead was appointed to the position of Home Sister and assistant to Miss Player at £80 per annum in 1917.[20] From 1901 all the Sisters were on an equal footing, the only claim to seniority being length of service.

The Children's Hospital continued to function as the local general practice well after the war, a place to go for charity when life was tough. Such was the reputation of the Children's that many mothers, themselves undernourished and unable to breast-feed their babies, presented their child with summer diarrhoea, grateful to hand over to the nurses with their kind eyes and gentle touch. A clean bed, tender loving care, adequate feeding, clean milk and water, warmth and shelter, made up for the ineffectiveness of medical treatment.

At the close of World War One, the nursing staff was sadly depleted. The Hospital buildings and the Nurses' Home were run-down and shabby. Miss Player suffered ill-health, and her long-serving Sisters Thomas, Danaher and Mowbray Flack were at retirement age. The lack of suitable lecturers for the nurses had occurred when all the male doctors departed to the war and the difficulties of maintaining services lowered morale. Despite six months' leave on full pay, Miss Player's health deteriorated. She had little time to go, and in July 1920, she officially retired, unable to give her best leadership. The chronic and debilitating skin disease that caused her great suffering despite the best medical care was seemingly incurable.

Upon her resignation, the Committee praised Miss Player as a 'most highly efficient, loyal and faithful servant of the Hospital'. Her great friend Maria Thomas, the Out-patients Sister for twenty-two years, was appointed Acting Matron but she stayed only until 1922, and then became carer and companion to Hilda Player who died in 1925.

The Committee was aware of the need to adjust to the post-war years and almost immediately, from a wide field of applicants, Miss Grace Wilson, CBE, RRC, was approved to take up the position of Matron and Superintendent. Miss Wilson was one of Australia's most distinguished World War One army nurses, a woman of great strength and charisma.

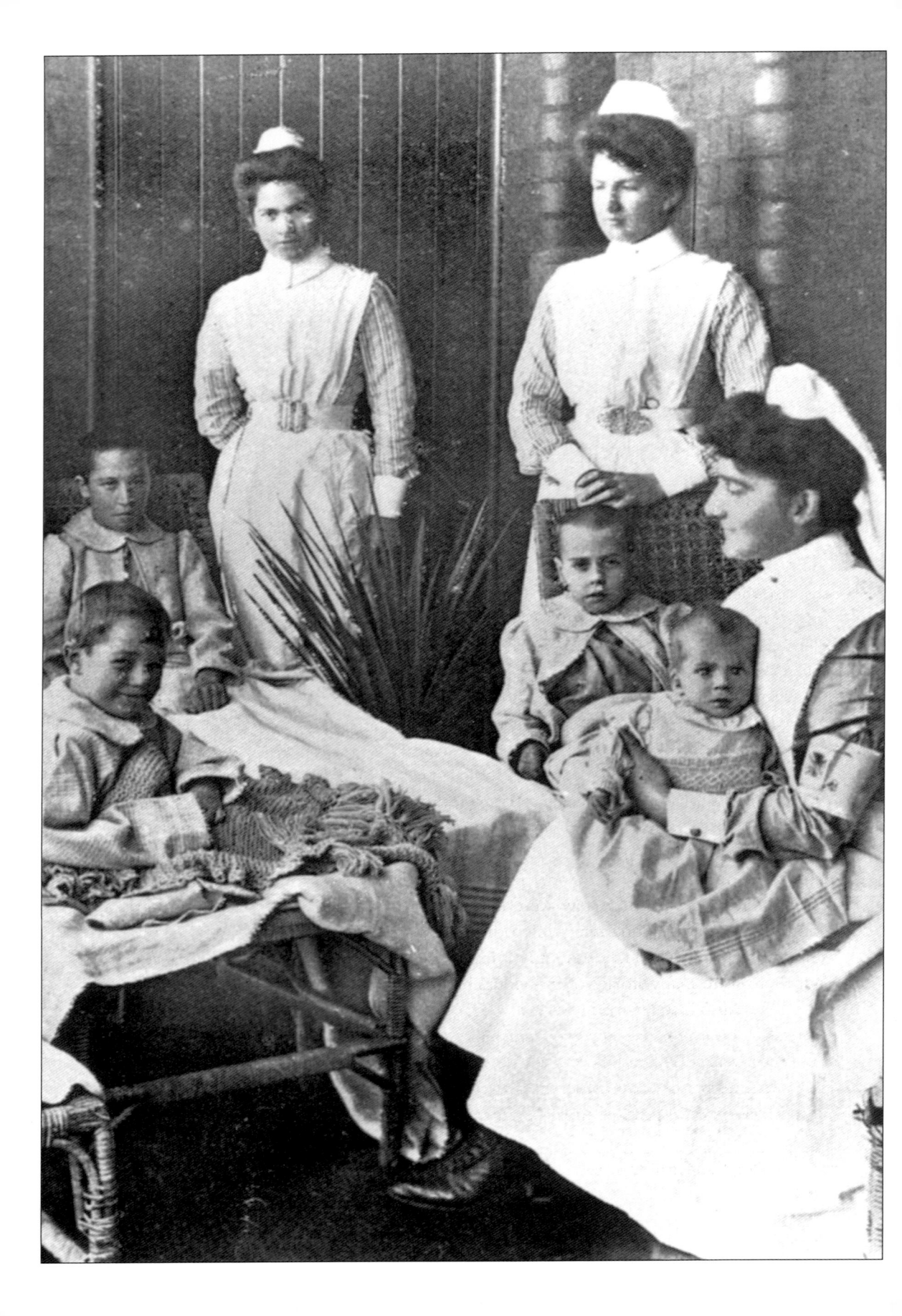

CHAPTER 5

The War Years

1914–1918

*O*n 15 August 1914, in support of the 'mother country' Great Britain, Australia declared war on Germany. The involvement of Australia in World War One had profound consequences for the country and an unsettling effect on the nursing profession. The Australasian Trained Nurses' Association and state counterparts volunteered the services of their members, but the full effect of the conflagration on the other side of the world was not immediately apparent until the horrors of the Gallipoli campaign unfolded in 1915.

In total, about 2,139 Australian nurses served overseas in the Australian Army Imperial Force, through Burma, India, the Persian Gulf, Palestine, Egypt, Salonika, Italy, France, Lemnos Island and England; about 130 were seconded to the British Nursing Service while 423 remained in Australia.[1] In reality, the majority of the Australian Army Nursing Service Reserve (AANSR), as part of the Australian Army Medical Corps, served on the periphery of the war zones, in field hospitals and casualty clearing stations. A few were in the midst of the action; some remained in administration at headquarters while others staffed evacuation hospitals, the hospital ships and troop ships. They saw only a fraction of the wounded, sick and suffering. But there were many stories of individual bravery and stoicism.[2]

The Australian Nursing Service began in 1899. After the Federation of the Australian colonies, the newly established Australian Army Medical Corps of the Commonwealth Military Forces set up the Army Nursing Reserve. During World War One, nurses of the Australian Army Nursing Service (AANS) volunteered as a part of the medical units of the Australian Imperial Force (AIF).

Nursing staff and patients, 1907.

Nurses at war

Children's Hospital nurses, no less than the medical staff, were swept up by the patriotic fervour of the times. Only graduate general nurses were eligible and, for the first time, the suitability of Children's Hospital nurses seriously came into question. Within four months after the declaration of war, the President of the Hospital Committee, Mrs Hilda Turnbull, interviewed Dr Fetherston (Lieutenant General, Director of Medical Services, World War One)[3] and protested against Children's Hospital nurses being regarded as less completely trained than those from any other general hospital. The position was apparently resolved when the Committee decided that the Hospital would fall in with any offer made by other Hospitals to instruct women for military purposes. Between 1915 and 1918, eighty-nine Children's nurses served in the Great War.[4]

Janie Lempriere joined the AIF, sailing in the first convoy on 8 October 1914 for Egypt. She already knew the hardships, the camp conditions, the dirt, the lack of supplies and feelings of helplessness while nursing young men in the Boer War. Typhoid, a disease very familiar to Children's Hospital nurses, was responsible for more than two-thirds of the 22,000 deaths among British and colonial forces. Initially, only those Children's Hospital nurses with years of experience in adult hospitals were accepted for enlistment. In 1915, Miss Lempriere achieved a senior post as Matron at the English mansion 'Harefield', converted to a Convalescent and Rehabilitation Home for Australian Officers in the English countryside. Later in the war, she accompanied many wounded and sick men on hospital ships returning to Australia.[5]

Evelyn Conyers, one of the very first to join the ranks of the Australian Army Nursing Service Reserve in 1903, joined the AIF on 11 October 1914 as the Senior Sister. She sailed on the *Shropshire,* one of a convoy of seven ships among which twenty-five Australian nurses were distributed. Her nursing staff of three was kept busy inoculating troops against typhoid, carrying out other vaccinations, assisting at surgery and nursing twenty cases of measles.[6] On arrival in Egypt she was despatched to Cairo for urgent duty in the Egyptian Army Hospital, Abyssia, to nurse New Zealand troops. She rejoined the 1st Australian General Hospital (AGH) at Heliopolis on 10 July 1915, to take over the most daunting of tasks, the position of Night Superintendent.

Following the Gallipoli disaster, Dr Fetherston re-organised the administration of the Australian Army Medical and Nursing Services and created new positions. One of these positions, Acting Principal Matron, AIF, went to Evelyn Conyers who was appointed to Surgeon General Neville Howse's staff in Cairo. By then, a mature and very experienced woman of forty-five, Miss Conyers' superb organisational abilities were duly recognised and on 12 January 1916, she was promoted to Matron-in-Chief, AIF.

The next move in May of that year, to AIF headquarters in Horseferry Road,

London, widened her responsibilities for posting, promotion, pay, discipline, leave and other concerns for all Australian Army Nurses in Egypt, England and Europe. Her negotiating skills became legendary; not only did she reconcile differences between nurses and medical officers, but she also encouraged good relationships between British and Australian nursing services personnel.[7] Unfortunately, Evelyn Conyers left no personal records of her extensive Army experience in the Middle East and is believed to have destroyed records of nurses under her command.[8]

Ina Annie Laidlaw came from the Western District in Victoria and began training at the Children's in 1913. She joined the AANS in June 1917 and when posted to India, served in military hospitals in Bombay and Poona. One of the very few to return to Melbourne at the end of the war, she resumed her civilian career eventually becoming Assistant to the Lady Superintendent at the Children's Hospital and Lady Superintendent of the Frankston Orthopaedic Hospital until 1942.

The only death among Children's Hospital nurses in the Great War was Beatrice Middleton Watson. The service memorials have long since disappeared but for those who can remember the entrance to the old Nurses' Home in Carlton, an Honour Roll listed the eighty-nine nurses who served with the Imperial Forces 1914–18.[9] Sister Watson's memorial, a brass plaque in the north–south corridor, on the centre of the eastern wall of the Home, was unveiled on 2 June 1923 and read:

> To the dear and honoured memory of Beatrice M. Watson, who died on Active Service at No.1 Stationary Hospital, Ismailia, Egypt, and June 3rd, 1916. Sister Watson, deeply grieved by her fellow workers, was a woman of bright personality struck by a sudden and short illness and untimely death.[10]

Her military funeral was held 'in a beautiful oasis in a lonely desert country'.

In August 1916, the Children's Hospital Committee presented to the Hospital a handsomely carved board with the names of forty nurses on active service 'so that the good record of the Children's Hospital Training School should be perpetuated'.[11]

Life at the Hospital in war time

War began when the Children's Hospital was set for expansion: the Annual Report shows that in 1914–15 there were 2,156 in-patient and 80,000 out-patient attendances. By 1915, recruiting for the Army Nursing Service was in full swing, with no definition of what the destination would be. From their recruitment at Garden Island, some Staff Nurses and Sisters returned to show off their uniforms, but Hospital nurses thought them 'very dull and strange'.[12]

At the close of 1916, the Hospital was seriously depleted of staff, and women doctors, many of whom the Hospital had previously denied appointments, made up the entire medical staff. Dr Vera Scantlebury was appointed Senior Resident Medical Officer in December and Isabella Younger, Ellice Davies, Annie Bennett, Janet Grieg, Helen Sexton, Helen Kelsey and other sessional women kept the Hospital going. The nurses became devoted to these medical women; when Vera Scantlebury became very ill with diphtheria, she was lovingly nursed for many weeks in the Isolation Pavilion (Ward 16). As the war dragged on, fifth-year medical students were seconded into sessional out-patient clinics. But the cosy domesticity of the institution was severely disrupted when staff left for war service.

The pride and joy was the new Edward Wilson Surgical Pavilion of sixty beds. Known as Wards 9 and 10, they provided an additional sixty beds. Not since the opening of the Princess May building on Drummond Street, some years previously, was there such an important event. According to the press of the day 'the doors were 'thrown open' on the 6 August 1913 by no less than the Governor General Lord Denman'.[13] Seventy medical beds were constantly occupied in Wards 7 and 8, and the basement served as a Massage and X-ray Department. Such was the demand that the nurses' sitting rooms in these wards were converted to bathrooms for infants and emergencies. The Committee believed the nurses did not need sitting rooms in the wards and had the nurses' consent for the change.

By mid-1915, very few Resident Medical Officers, Senior Sisters and Staff Nurses remained at the Children's. Management was encouraging staff to enlist but at the same time their attitude was ambivalent. When senior Sister Belstead was released to join the Army on a month's leave with full pay, her position was kept available, possibly in the expectation of her early return. Her departure was a severe blow to Miss Player, as she was losing one of her senior assistants. Although there were more probationer applications than ever, very few senior nurses returned to their old jobs; a few of the trained nurses of the 1890s, were nearly ready for retirement but stayed on.

An outbreak of eighteen cases of diphtheria in 1912 lingered on into the war years. It was a disease with a long recovery period that required careful nursing, and the transfer of children to the Convalescent Cottage at Brighton was not always successful.[14] The journey was quite a challenge for the nurse accompanying the child: a Cottage Committee member, Mrs Higgins reported that a child had coughed out its tracheotomy tube while being transferred. The rules for transfer were reviewed but we are not told how such an event could be avoided. In 1914, thirty-three children had been resident at the Cottage for more than three months because their homes were unsuitable. There was nowhere for them to go.

Miss Player had been Lady Superintendent for almost fifteen years when war was declared and during this time the rule was reinforced that 'the Resident Medical Officer has no control over the duties of the Nursing Staff. Any complaint about the nursing was to be referred to the Matron.'[15] The Committee of Management had knowledge of all facets of Hospital life: the Sub-committees dealt with areas of special

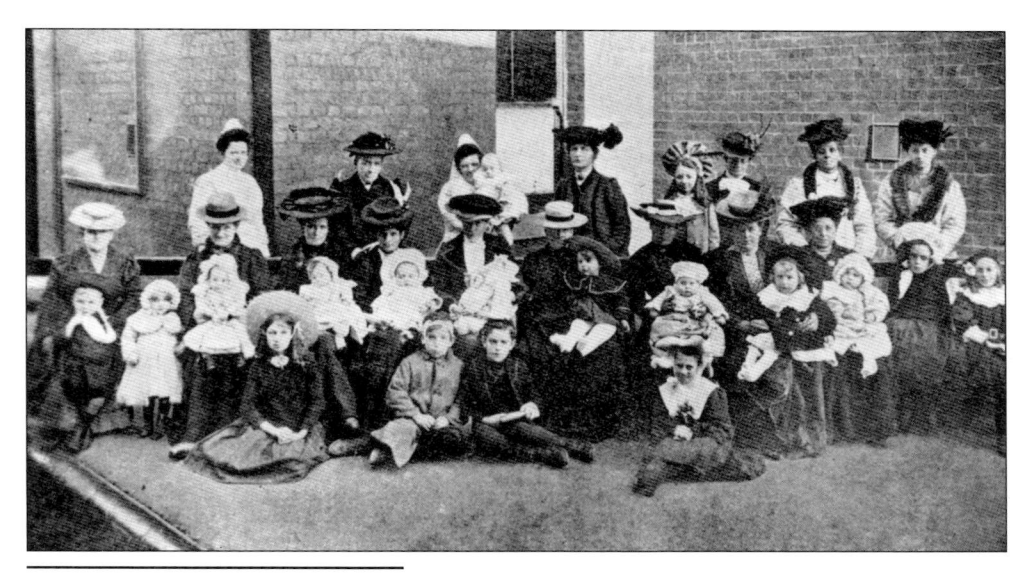

Plaster cases. Out-patients, 1907.

interest and Matron controlled the nurses in matters of discipline. Where an event was likely to go public or protocol was undermined, a nurse was in trouble. One seriously over-stepped the line: in order to facilitate enquiries by telephone about the condition of children in the wards, a telephone list commonly sent to the clerk was left on the table in the enquiry office. The nurse unfortunately placed the word 'pegged' on the list after the name of a child who had died. She received three months' suspension.[16]

The Nursing School, prestigious and fully subscribed with well-educated girls from middle-class backgrounds, expanded to seventy including four Staff Nurses and seven Sisters. Perhaps to keep up morale during the war years, the nurses' uniforms were reviewed to keep up with fashion and comfort, and the result was a change of colour and dress material, lowered collars and elbow-length sleeves. The teaching syllabus had not altered; Honorary Medical Officers delivered the technical, scientific and medical content on a rotation in their own time. Ward Sisters and Staff Nurses carried out general nursing instruction under the watchful eye of Matron Player. To show appreciation of her good service and economical management during the war, Miss Player's salary was eventually increased to £175 per annum.[17]

But working conditions were not always kept up to standard. Many of the male staff helping around the Hospital disappeared as the war progressed. The Committee had in 1913 implemented the removal of bodies to the mortuary by a mortuary attendant rather than a nurse, but unfortunately, this rule was waived. In the case of a death through the night, the night sister had to take the body to the morgue, 'a long dim trek to that out of the way ghostly place'.[18]

Parts of the building structure also presented danger. In the linen room of the Princess May Pavilion, a nurse had fallen off the top of the stairs and narrowly escaped being thrown through the window into the well of the food lift. Iron bars fixed across the bottom window prevented any possibility of such a thing re-occurring but no further modifications to the stairs were carried out.

The war years created confusion and some anxiety; most Hospital rules were unchanging but others became controversial depending on the preference of an influential Committee member and reflecting the tension of the times. During the war, the Hospital, historically non-sectarian, had the controversial, long-running saga of the presence of a Catholic priest in the wards. Before the war, a Committee lady of some influence, Mrs Gavan Duffy, asked 'that in cases where Roman Catholic children in the Hospital are in a very critical condition, could her son, a priest at St George's Church be informed in order that he may visit'. The Committee gave permission but in 1915 she reported a further difficulty 'when Roman Catholic children are in *extremis*'. The Reverend J. H. O'Connell had complained that due attention was not given to priests at this Hospital and on two occasions nurses had been very rude. Mrs Gavan Duffy was very ruffled. Dr Bullen had acted as peacemaker and explained that the condition of a child in question had caused the night nurses great anxiety; they had no time to call a priest. The Committee made it quite clear that each case of cerebrospinal meningitis occurring in a child of Roman Catholic religion was 'to be reported at once to Father O'Connell'.[19] This issue re-emerged in the later decades of World War Two when the Parish Priest from St George's often visited at night, sitting for hours by the beds of very ill children and acted as friend and advisor to the young night nurses.

Nurses' work and conditions

Their numbers badly depleted, nursing staff were literally run off their feet. Sometimes unfairly, they were charged with inattention. In January 1916, a three-year-old child fell off the balcony, but luckily was not seriously hurt. The Committee investigated applying safety netting for the balconies but ultimately blamed the nurses for lack of supervision.

The strict economies practised by the Committee often devolved on nurses' living conditions. Concerned at the cost of hot water, the Committee decided to install showers in nurses' bathrooms, presumably to save the amount used in the baths. When the telephone bill for the Nurses' Home came to £11/5/- (about 5,000 calls) and only £3 had been put in the coin box, it was resolved that unless each user placed one penny in the box, the telephone service would be discontinued. As the telephone was the only outside link, this seemed particularly harsh. Many nurses had brothers at the war and two were notified of their deaths while on duty.

Reports of nurses' work and conditions trickled in; outsiders complained of the

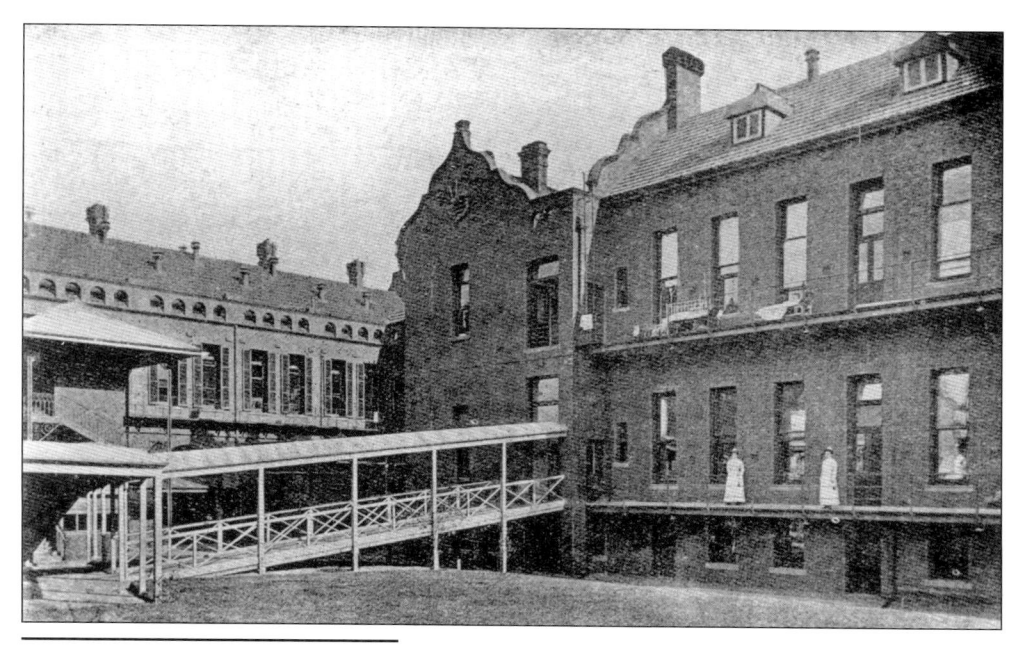

Pavilion Wards 7 and 8, dispensary and Isolation Ward, 1905.

heavy work nurses were called upon to perform. The President, speaking for the Nursing Committee, showed that 'the duties here entailed less menial work than obtained in other hospitals, and that…their training should be instructed as the nurse would have to do in a private house'. But Mary Wilson (née Alderson) found the work very heavy when she began at the Children's in August 1915 at the age of twenty-one. Of very short stature, small and delicate, Mary found that the physical demands took a great toll on her body. She complained after one week to her stepmother, 'I wanted to be a nurse but really, I am just a housemaid'. One of her vivid memories was 'pushing a great padded red gum slab of wood on a handle each morning through the ward to polish the floors like a mirror'.[20]

The nurses' official starting time was seven in the morning but most juniors came on duty at six to ensure everything was in order: the children's breakfasts, the cleaning, the bedpans, all ready and quiet for the Doctor's rounds. In the long Snowball Ward 7, Mary said the children 'would all be calling out at once for bedpans. The tiny bathrooms were a long way down the ward and the work was terribly hard.' Vague about some of the children's illnesses, she did remember there was plenty of diphtheria. But her most vivid memories were of the terrible accidents, especially burns and scalds, 'with the skin hanging off, the bones showing through on the child's back, the screaming at dressing time'. There were many childhood accidents at the wharves along the river where children from the slums played. She said, 'it nearly made me cry'.[21]

Mary Alderson's stay at the Children's was short-lived; the records show she was almost continuously ill with tonsillitis and needed extended leave to recover. Her idol was the strong, vibrant, lady-like third-year nurse, Ina Annie Laidlaw, who took a liking to Mary—they were both adventurous country girls—and supported her strong desire to go to the war. Mary's brother, Arthur, had already enlisted, shipping his horse to Fremantle. She said, 'I wanted to get over to England, get to Germany, see the world'. Matron Player was uneasy; she absolutely ruled it out. Mary was 'not to go' because she was not trained, but, defiantly in the end, she just ran away. Reporting to the recruitment officer at Port Melbourne barracks, Mary was immediately rejected because of her size: the officer said she looked like a child herself. Mary returned to the Children's for a short time but left the Hospital as 'unsuitable' and eventually trained as a midwife at the Women's Hospital.[22]

Many people had sympathy for the nurses. Mrs William Smith gave £100 towards providing extra comforts. Another £10 was to be spent on lounges for the sitting room in the Nurses' Home. For years, certain members of the Committee considered the breakfasts set out in the Nurses' Diet Book quite unsatisfactory; German sausage for breakfast was insufficient. Matron attended a meeting about the matter and stated that 'nurses had expressed their liking for some of the items referred to and in the event of their not liking tomatoes, eggs and so on, they could easily have cold meat. Nearly all took porridge, considered to be quite satisfactory.' After much procrastination, the Committee resolved to concentrate on improving nurses' food, especially by including butter and, periodically, fresh fruit.[23]

As well as supervision of the nursing staff, Miss Player oversaw the long-serving and loyal domestic and laundry staff. Julia Ryan and May Shine worked and lived in at the Hospital for twenty-one and sixteen years respectively; their last pay rise was to £36 in 1911.[24] By 1914, the domestic staff had expanded to such a degree that the conditions for maids were poor: four rooms with four beds to a room. Other tiny rooms had three beds. The furniture was good but very shabby. Miss Mary Guthrie, a notable volunteer and friend of the Hospital, proposed partitioning to provide single rooms to improve the accommodation for the twenty-five maids.

The war created a surge in applicants for nursing but almost all nurses enlisted as soon as they received their certificates. The numbers of Hospital patients escalated but nursing staff numbers remained the same and the Committee was forced to review the situation. In July 1916, the training period was extended from three to four years, the justification being the improvement in the quality of nurses. In reality, this was a way of keeping senior nurses on to maintain a pool of trained staff.

For nurses, doctors and particularly the Lady Superintendent, restrictions on Hospital supplies during the war were severe. In December 1914, Miss Player was instructed to refrain from purchasing surgical supplies from Plisch, Kliger or any other German firm, while Miss Danaher, the Charge Sister at the Convalescent Cottage, was directed to refrain as far as possible from ordering any imported articles.

MARY GUTHRIE was a very important figure in the life and development of the Children's Hospital for three decades of the twentieth century. As the founder of the Auxiliaries she kept a keen eye on the administration, the welfare of the staff, nursing, medical and domestic, and the comfort of mothers and babies. She campaigned for the establishment of the baby wards following World War One. As the grand-daughter of Mary Reiby, the Tasmanian convict and emancipist who later became one of New South Wales' most successful businesswomen, Mary Guthrie inherited the family drive to achieve. She was born in East Melbourne in 1860 into a family of wealth; her father was a grazier. In 1894, she joined the Children's Hospital Committee and remained a member until her death in 1931.

The cerebrospinal meningitis epidemic

The most sinister war-time disease struck Melbourne in 1915–16. Common in crowded areas such as army camps and jails, cerebrospinal meningitis, sometimes known in children as 'spotted fever' or the meningococcal strain, was particularly swift and deadly. Meningitis, more than any other disease except poliomyelitis, created panic due to its severity, suddenness and fatal outcome, particularly in children.

A disease characteristically associated with overcrowding and conditions of stress and fatigue, meningitis was particularly prevalent in the Boer War and World War One; in Melbourne it was connected to the Broadmeadows Army Camp.[25] In 1915–16, a total of eighty-six cases were treated at the Children's Hospital. The death rate was 46 per cent.[26]

During the epidemic, attention centred on a building at the Children's Hospital called the Medical Flat. This was a free-standing isolation room partitioned into three wards sited in the centre of the Hospital grounds (in later years converted to a tennis court and car park).

The nurses were alone on night duty but during the day three nurses staffed each room. The Flat was to become the subject of intense medical and public speculation. From the public point of view, the controversies came from fear and ignorance and the inability to cure the disease.

Because the Hospital was severely understaffed at this time, junior nurses were forced into senior positions, therefore putting a great strain on the Hospital system of teaching; these young girls were sometimes forced into situations for which they were not prepared. Hilda Lindsay began nursing at the Children's early in 1915, and takes up her story:

[O]ne day about 5 pm I was told to go to my room, pack all my belongings, have a good sleep, then move to the Medical Flat, for duty at 10 pm. I had never been in the building. I found to my horror when I arrived that I was to be the only nurse on duty. I was there for twenty-one weeks…eight-hour shifts with no days off…the first days in the wards the work was hard…some times heart breaking. When at the end of my time I requested days off I was told 'but you only worked eight hours a day'. I pleaded the restrictions of isolation and was granted two days off, and able to mix with my fellow human beings again. [27]

Nursing meningitis was a challenge; Children's nurses became very familiar with the signs: high temperature, irritability, arched back or opisthotonos with retracted head, legs drawn up, eyes rolling and, in young babies, convulsions. Nurses became very skilled at observing Kernig's sign that allowed the doctor to make a diagnosis.[28] An inability of the patient to take fluids caused great dehydration and suffering and the hygiene of the mouth with glycerine and borax was of the greatest importance. High temperatures in children were a challenge for nurses; care was taken with regular sponging, giving aspirin and sips of fluid. Intravenous infusions were not common, the most routine medical procedure in the days before antibiotics being the lumbar puncture to release cerebral pressure, often with perilous results. Nurses learned to set up the lumbar puncture tray under the most sterile conditions, a test of the great efficiency.

Meningitis was of particular interest to pathologists and a great deal of activity and interest centred on the Medical Flat. Hospital doctors and the pathologist were in constant attendance, handymen delivered firewood to heat the rooms, maids delivered meals and cleaned and—most controversially to the public—parents were permitted to visit.

The Children's Hospital became the subject of a vitriolic campaign in the *Age* newspaper, that too many resources were concentrated on the few, to the neglect of other aspects, particularly the nurses and their working conditions. An article headlined 'How Meningitis Spreads' mirrored public fear. It described how two breast-feeding women walked from Lygon Street to nurse their babies in the Hospital, and walked back to board the tram, therefore carrying 'germs'.[29] Dr Jeffreys Wood, very keen to promote breast-feeding, emphasised that nursing mothers were encouraged to come and go as they pleased. He pointed out that the three-roomed, medical, self-contained flat at the Children's had three wards, with sixty-five admissions at that time, accommodation for three [night] nurses and that none of the nine nurses had died or even contracted the disease.[30] All the nurses had received vaccination against meningitis.

In July 1916, the press condemned the Children's Hospital for allowing a child to write to its parents, the implication being that germs may have been transmitted

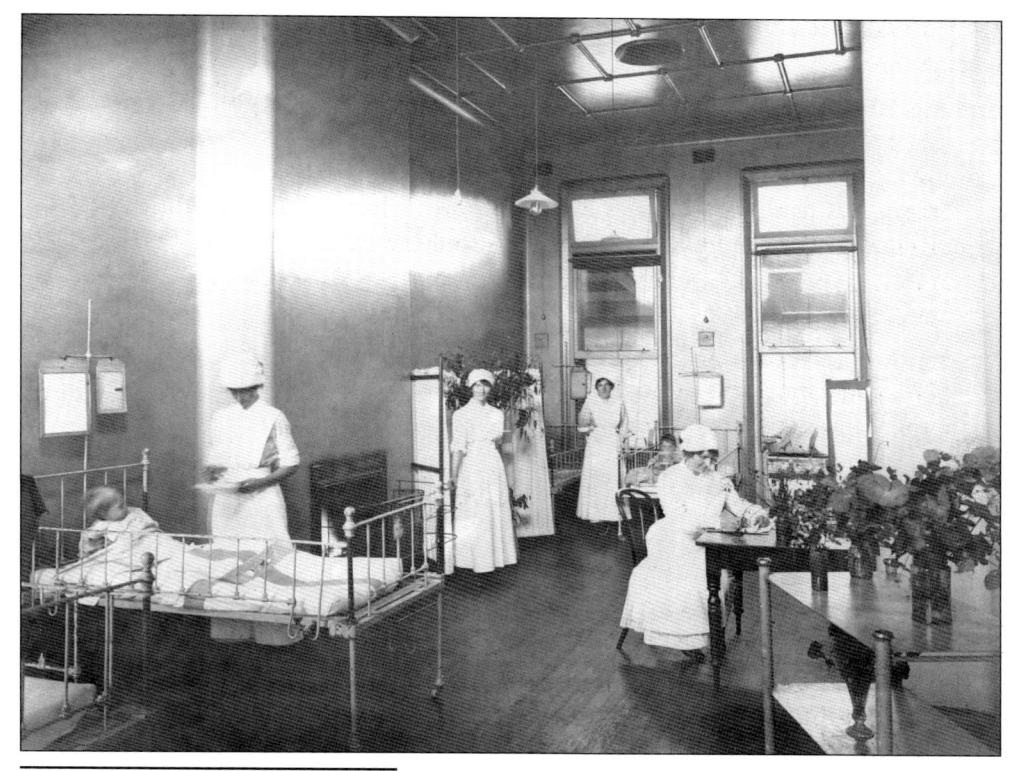

Medical Flat, 1910.

through the writing paper. In response to the critics, Dr Reginald Webster, the Hospital Pathologist, stressed that 'there was no danger, but in deference to public opinion, the practice [of letter writing] had been stopped'.[31]

By 1917, the situation had eased and Fairfield Hospital opened a ward to cerebrospinal meningitis cases. Children's Hospital nurses were sent to assist at Fairfield and stayed three months.

Being a country girl, Nurse Hilda Lindsay had not met many hazards in the way of infection or built up antibodies. She took some time to complete her training: her first year stretched into one year and seven months. On resumption of duty, Matron Player greeted her kindly, but with regret: 'I was regarded as not strong enough to finish my training.'[32] Pleading for another chance, Hilda proved them wrong. Not only did she finish her training during some of the most difficult years ever experienced by nurses and Hospital administration, she followed this with a staffing year.

The end of the war

The Hospital was in a difficult financial position and stringent measures had come into force; the boiler was turned off at night to save coal, a gas steriliser was installed in the operating theatre for emergency night-time operations, a maid had been sacked and the position of House Sister abolished.

In addition to their normal work, nurses found time to collect funds to buy material for bandages for the Red Cross, and the Committee donated a piece of calico. One of the most trying problems for the nurses was the shortage of children's clothes. Constant appeals through the *Argus* yielded 485 flannel jackets. However, not all gifts were useful for needs in the wards: Lady Mackinnon gave a bean slicer, the Railways donated half a ton of mild steel of varying sizes for splint making. But a distinct highlight occurred with a donation of poultry for the nurses' and doctors' Christmas dinner.

Hospital buildings deteriorated and the Nurses' Home became neglected; the furnishings were shabby. Food was short and subject to inflation. Supplies of blankets, sheets and uniform materials were scarce and subject to continuous price rises.

Miss Player's health deteriorated. In her memoirs, Hilda Lindsay acknowledged that the Hospital and the trainees owed a great deal to Matron Player and Sister Thomas, the Sub-matron, who had given many years of service. A time of acute shortages of staff and equipment, Matron's frequent saying was 'a good nurse can always improvise'. The reply was, 'what with?'

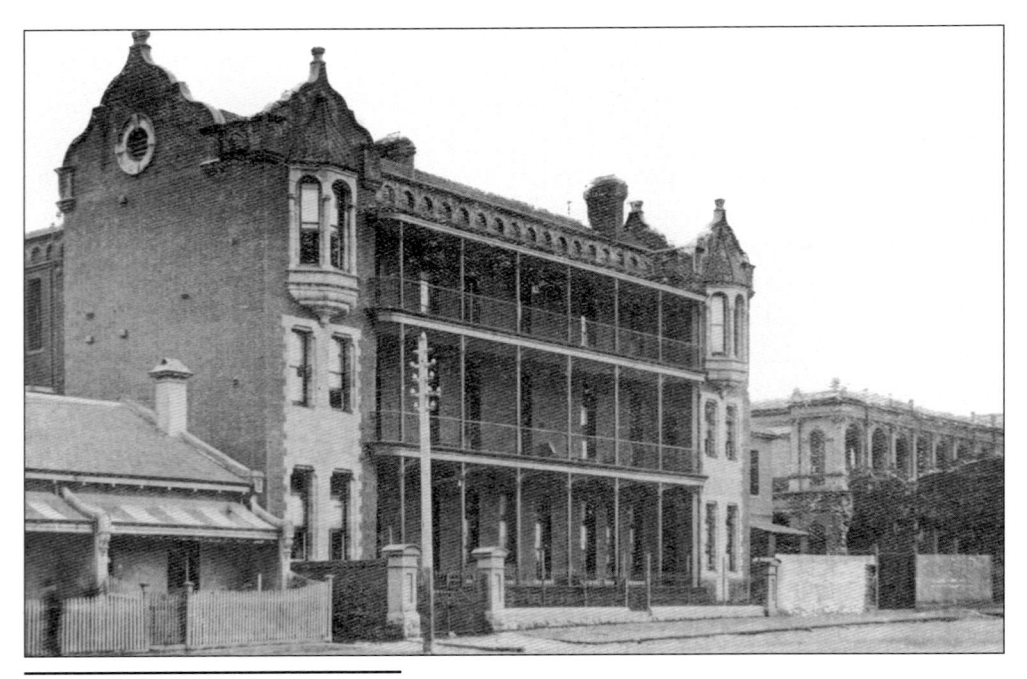

John Robertson Nurses' Home, 1908.

Many nurses left never to return, but the Committee was undaunted. While practising the 'strictest economy', the Hospital was involved in 'Baby Week', already planning baby wards and a new kitchen while the Medical Flats were being made ready to use for treatment of infantile paralysis.

An additional telephone line was installed when the main line, central 927, had been 'engaged' eleven times in one day. Most of the female doctors left as male doctors returned. Dr Annie Bennett resigned as Senior Resident Medical Officer after residency for nearly two years and was replaced by Dr Kingsley Norris.

But new medical challenges were on the horizon for nurses. On 14 November 1918, as a direct result of the war, an unwelcome development occurred: escalating cases of venereal diseases. In keeping with the *Venereal Diseases Act 1916*, notifiable cases in babies and children, previously distributed between the Royal Melbourne, Women's and Alfred Hospitals were, for lack of facilities, to be treated at the Children's Hospital.

There was also little understanding of the pandemic sweeping the world. In August 1918 word reached Melbourne that, 'quarantine regulations should be made ready for the expected outbreak of Spanish Influenza'.[33]

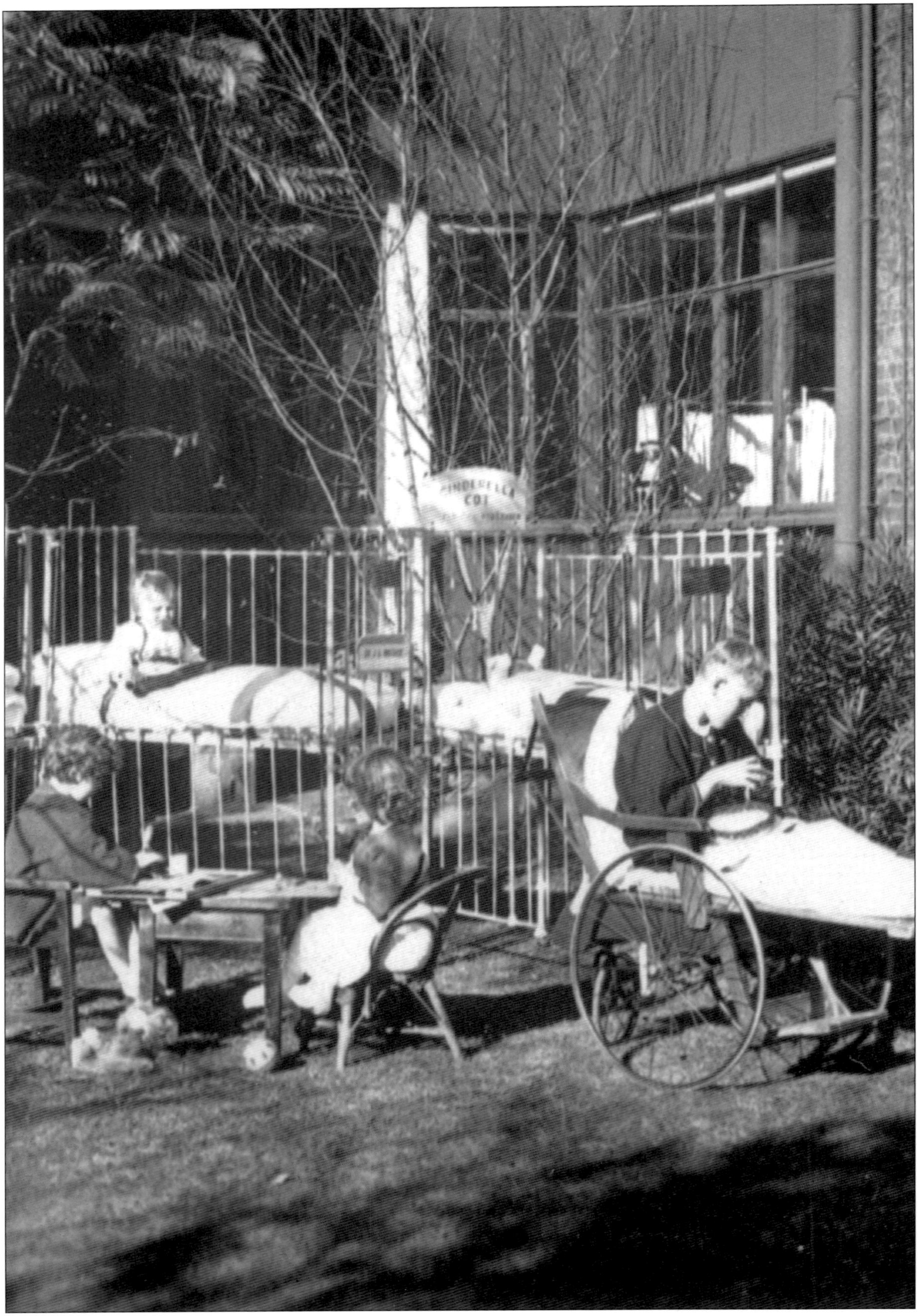

CHAPTER 6

War Nurses Return

1918–1924

For many nurses returning to civilian life, the Great War was a turning point in their desire to create a better future for children. Medical science benefited from the war years but for those who resumed their working lives at the Children's Hospital, many challenges awaited them.

Three main issues confronted staff and management at the Children's Hospital: facilities for management of children with venereal diseases, the influenza epidemic and the ability to care for babies and very young children.

In May 1918, the *Argus* ran a campaign:

Venereal Disease: children catch it by contact with sponges, towels and other articles handled by infected adults.

Dr Robertson from the Board of Public Health reported that all cases recorded from July 1917 to April 1918 numbered 6,346 in the state, 5,217 males and 1,129 females with 230 in the country. It was not clear how many children were infected.[1] One of the most difficult diseases to treat, syphilis appears to have been largely ignored in the nineteenth century with only an occasional reference in the Hospital records. The worst form in children was congenital syphilis contracted in utero, but not easily diagnosed at birth. The disease became evident in infancy when children commonly died. From 1906, the Wasserman test became almost universal in children

---

Children enjoying the sunshine outside Ward 10.
RCHA/Aicheson Collection.

presenting to Out-patients; mercury treatment was given orally or by injection to those returning a positive test and achieved some success. Dr Jeffreys Wood treated the mothers but 'working class fathers remained elusive'.[2] More often than not, the infection was reproduced in each succeeding pregnancy. The arsenical drug, Salvarsan, most commonly administered as a subcutaneous injection, was moderately successful. Following years of continuous treatment the disease, thought to be cured, commonly reappeared in old age.

Children with these diseases were kept out of sight until the *Venereal Diseases Act 1915* came into full effect. The Children's Hospital could not refuse admission but three years lapsed before the Victorian Health Department agreed to finance a treatment ward.[3] The free-standing building at the rear of the Hospital was an isolated, stark, cold and dreary little place with wide-open doors regardless of the weather. Soon, about thirty little patients filled the beds, many of them girls with gonorrhoea. Dr Robert Southby was the honorary physician associated with the care of these children for many years.

The details of the nurses' working day in the ward are not clear at this distance in time but Jean Hardham remembers as a junior in the 1920s that:

> Ward 13, the Syphilis Ward, was next to Ward 16 [Infectious Diseases], behind the tennis court. You did a certain time down there under supervision of course. The syphilitic babes, oh, they did not last very long. However, these little tots with gonorrhoea were put up in lithotomy and we gave them warm douches every day. We always wore gloves and gowns. When you think of it now there was really no treatment, little could be done. So it was a tough life but it [nursing] was something I always wanted to do and I loved the children. It didn't matter what they had you were there, you had to watch them, you had to observe them, but they very quickly deteriorated. It was interesting, part of the training.[4]

As punishment for misdemeanours, Matron Walsh was known to threaten junior nurses with a tour of duty in the gonorrhoea ward, known to the nurses as 'Siberia'. Away from the mainstream activities of Hospital, life was lonely. A nurse was left for five months, forgotten.[5] In November 1919, a severe shortage of nurses prompted the Honorary Medical Staff to put a list of recommendations with a view to stringent modification of the staffing of the venereal diseases ward and the operating theatre:

> Only acute infectious cases for which the wards were established were to be admitted.
>
> That only those nurses who had completed at least two years training and had in addition, theatre and out-patients experience be allowed to work there.

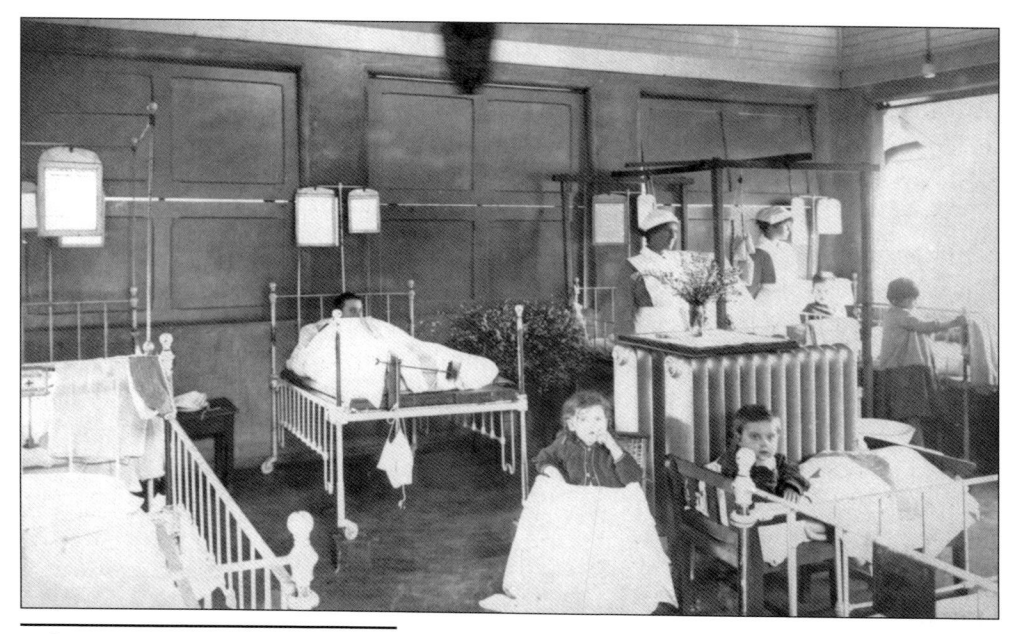

Infectious Diseases Ward, 1905.

> That the full strength of Sisters be restored, an operating theatre sister be appointed responsible for all theatre instruments and the training of nurses, in the management and preparation [of the Theatre].

So unpopular was the ward where nurses could be called as 'extras' for other duties, that many nurses were on sick leave on 1 July 1920 when the VD (Venereal Diseases) Ward was officially opened. But Matron was asked to ensure there was always enough staff to meet demand.

The influenza pandemic

Plans for expansion of the baby wards were thwarted when the most serious post-war emergency occurred. Hospital authorities were instructed to prepare for the influenza pandemic sweeping the world. The first cases expected with the arrival of the troop ships crossing the Indian Ocean were delayed for a few months by Commonwealth quarantine regulations, but in January 1919 were admitted and isolated at the Melbourne Hospital.

In the meantime, the State Government requisitioned the Children's Hospital Secretary Mr Robert J. (Jim) Love,[6] 'in regard to equipping all Melbourne Hospitals to cope with influenza'.[7] This new viral strain, the Spanish flu, unknown to medicine, had sudden onset, with symptoms of debilitating pain, fever, blinding headache, a dry cough, nasal bleeding and pneumonia. Lethal to all age groups but particularly young adults, the pneumonic form of the disease killed fifty victims in Melbourne by the end of January 1919. Officially, the Children's did not take infectious cases but such was the reputation of the nurses that the Lady Mayoress asked them to give a demonstration of nursing influenza. The Committee reluctantly consented 'in view of Miss Player's eagerness'.[8] The treatment, little different from most treatments of the day, consisted of strict bed rest, keeping the chest warm, fresh air, light nourishment and free evacuation of the bowels.[9]

Dr Webster's Pathology Department inoculated the nurses and, although some became ill, none died. Nurse Hilda Lindsay recalled that her training continued free of illness until 1918, her staffing year, when she became so ill with influenza that she decided to leave.[10] The Children's could not take many extra admissions due to the lack of nurses, as almost half of the 133 probationers who entered during the war had left.

The Medical Flats and several wards were prepared. The Children's Hospital did not play a major role in the drama, but overall treated more than 600 patients. Life went on; the day-to-day difficulties did not lessen: ongoing outbreaks of diphtheria and scarlet fever caused great anxiety.

Public buildings became emergency hospitals. Schools, halls and places of entertainment closed. The majority of influenza victims were admitted to the Melbourne, Alfred, Homeopathic and Fairfield Hospitals. Near the Children's Hospital, the Exhibition Building was duly prepared for the transfer of convalescents. Such was the escalation of cases that the Exhibition was quickly filled with acutely ill patients, and became a *de facto* hospital. More than 4,000 soon packed the vast hall. Horse-drawn ambulances with masked drivers and attendants arrived at the Nicholson Street entrance in the February heat with stretcher cases, many of them mothers with at least one child.[11] The dreariest sight was the removal of the dead at the rear gate. The death rate varied in all hospitals but averaged about 9 per cent.[12]

Save the Babies campaign

In October 1918, the *Herald* newspaper revitalised the 'Save the Babies Appeal' from the first decade of the twentieth century: 'Infant Wards to have 85 cots'.

> Babies are to be saved by the Children's Hospital. The infant death rate in Victoria at 69 is higher than all other states. The chief categories of death are diarrhoeal diseases, failure to thrive or wasting, pneumonia and prematurity. The baby wards will have baths and changing rooms arranged on model lines, with an electric lift, a flat [sun] roof, wide balconies and extra accommodation.[13]

Donations to the appeal escalated from to £3,000 to £30,000 and on 14 December 1921, the *Herald* reported the sequel to the Babies' Campaign launched by the Children's Hospital three years before:

> Lady Forster opened the new babies' wards to handle 1,400 sick babies under two years, victims of gastric and diarrhoea problems in the summer which bring about such heavy infant mortality and in winter, broncho-pneumonia.

Of all the problems confronting hospital authorities, these diseases widened the role of paediatric nurses in a public health education campaign. Support of mothers through Baby Health Centres and the emphasis on the benefits of preparing clean milk were seen as necessary steps to improve children's health.

In September 1923, the new Baby Wards were not being fully utilised because there were no laundry facilities for them: nurses carried heavy buckets to the sluice to rinse and scrub lethal stools that cultured *salmonella* and *shigella*. Under huge, boiling hot water taps their hands became raw. Filthy nappies were thrown into the large bins ready for the wardsman to transport to the main hospital laundry. This was not the last time the nurses carried out this task, introduced in times of stringency.

A fresh approach and new ideas

The Committee wasted no time replacing Miss Player, who retired in 1920. Grace Wilson, a tall, beautiful and physically strong woman, was forty-one when she commenced at the Children's Hospital on 1 December 1920. Quick to appraise the situation, she delivered a report within a few weeks:

> We are seriously short of nurses, those on duty are, I consider, being overworked. And probably there will be better health among the nurses when they are relieved of extra work. They are going on duty earlier than they should and coming off later. I cannot stop this as the necessary work must be done. The general care of the wards is being neglected simply because the nurses have no time for this work, all the time must be spent on the children.[14]

Probationers were applying at the rate of three a week but that was not enough. The most far-reaching and important reform implemented in Miss Wilson's time was the abolition of the £10/10/- premium entry fee for probationers, which resulted in a wider range of applicants. She introduced new rates of pay: for first-year £20, second-year £25 and for third-year, £30. A nurse was not to receive any payment for the first three months, but if she signed on, the payment would be forthcoming. A two-week holiday for every six months was a welcome introduction. Miss Wilson went to pains to acquaint herself with the nurses, inviting them for tea, arranging outings and generally getting to know them.

GRACE MARGARET WILSON (1879–1957), CBE, RRC, FNM
Matron and Lady Superintendent of the Children's Hospital Melbourne. November 1920–October 1922. Life member of the Australian Trained Nurses' Association (ATNA), Council Member of the Royal Victorian Trained Nurses' Association (RVTNA), sometime President, Royal Victorian College of Nursing (RVCN), trustee of the Edith Cavell Fund, Life Member of the Returned Soldiers, Sailors and Airmen's Imperial League (RSL). Miss Wilson was also active in the Girl Guides and the Red Cross Society.[15]

Grace Wilson was described by colleagues as a magnificent-looking person, a tenacious fighter for nurses' rights with a strong personality. Particularly active on many nursing organisations such as the RVTNA, she was always present at Anzac Day commemoration services. In her short time at the Children's, she promoted the League of Former Trainees, advertising the inaugural meeting at the Hospital through *UNA*, the journal of the Victorian Trained Nurses' Association. Although she was at the Children's for less than two years, she made a significant contribution, and paid special attention to nurses' recreational needs. She was openly critical of the Committee of Management's style.

Grace Wilson was educated at Brisbane Girls Grammar School and entered the Brisbane Hospital as a probationer in 1908. She gained her midwifery certificate at Queen Charlotte's Lying-in Hospital in London and joined the National Hospital for the Paralysed and Epileptic (Albany Memorial). Returning to Australia, she became Matron of the Brisbane Hospital in 1914.

When war was declared, she joined the Australian Army Nursing Service, being appointed Principal Matron of the 1st Military District. In April 1915, she transferred to the Australian Imperial Force as Principal Matron of the AIF 3rd Australian General

Hospital, first at Lemnos, the clearing station for Gallipoli casualties, then Abassia in Egypt in 1916, and Abbeville in France where the AGH unit expanded to 2,000 beds. Miss Wilson was discharged from the AIF in April 1920. She became Matron-in-Chief of the Army Nursing Reserve in 1925.

Her resignation from the Children's Hospital was a great loss, although she would not have fitted into this particular type of management. In the 1930s, she took up the post of Matron at the Alfred Hospital to build up their nursing school. An orientation course, a training school committee and tutor sisters were just a few of her innovations. Miss Wilson served in the Middle East with the AIF in World War Two and in 1954, at the age of seventy-five, married Robert Wallace Bruce Campbell in London. She died three years later at Heidelberg Repatriation Hospital and was cremated with full military honours after a service at Christ Church, South Yarra.

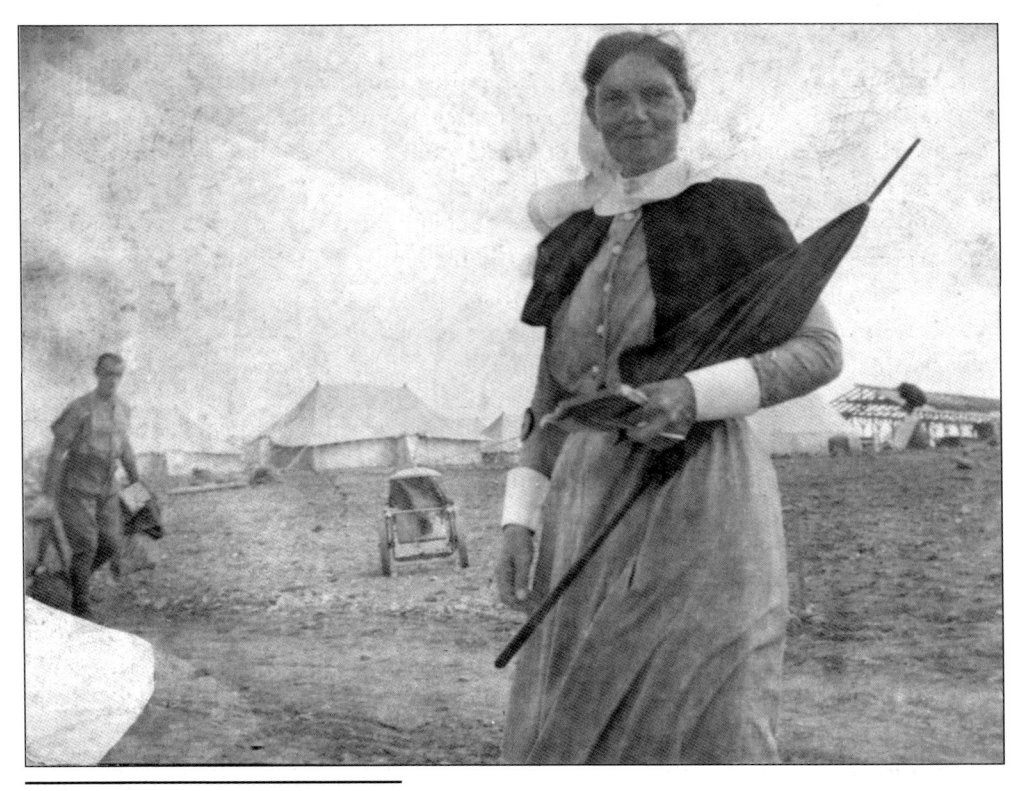

Grace Wilson.
Australian War Memorial, Canberra A05332.

Miss Wilson's path at the Children's Hospital was not easy. Her recommendations were resisted; for example, the Committee would not accept her suggestion that children be given their dinner at 4 pm to fit in with reduced hours for domestic workers. Honorary staff thought 4.45 pm best and the Committee endorsed this. She suggested that trained nurses be engaged from the Alfred and the Melbourne Hospitals to boost the complement of Staff Nurses. This matter was deferred. Permission was given to advertise, as so much of Sisters' time was now taken up with doctors' rounds, and proper supervision could not be exercised over junior nurses and would be aggravated when the new curriculum was in force. On night duty, when an emergency operation had to be done, the Night Sister had to go to the theatre.[16] Miss Wilson also cleaned out the 'deadwood', explaining to the Committee that a probationer of six weeks' standing had, on Saturday night, brought wine into the Nurse's Home and become intoxicated. The probationer was asked to leave. Matron also asked the Committee to take some action in regard to Miss Thomas, the long-serving—for more than twenty years—Out-patients Sister, explaining that:

> [T]he work of the OP Department was not being well done. The doctors are complaining and Sister Thomas disregards instructions.[17]

The Committee hoped things would improve, but Sister Thomas resigned after serving thirty-two years and six months at the Children's. In her favour, she was given six months' leave on full pay. Miss Wilson also asked to be relieved of the responsibility 'of teaching Nurse Iris Smith who was untidy and incompetent'. After one month's warning to improve, Nurse Smith finally left. When a nurse was found to have taken cocaine, her father was advised immediately to take her away.

There were more niggles but the climax came when the Committee was upset that Matron went to Ballarat for a nursing examination. Her instructions were that she was 'not to leave the Hospital for more than a day without permission of the Committee or the President'. She also allowed the final-year nurses to hold a dance in St Kilda without seeking permission. Matron duly apologised.

Fears were prompted not only by the shortage of nurses but also by controversies. In February 1921, the RVTNA wanted the Children's trained nurses to do an extra year of general training before receiving their certificate. But the formation of the Trained Nurses' Guild, an organisation formed in January 1921 and granted registration in the Arbitration Court, opposed much of what the RVTNA stood for. The members of the Guild were demobilised nurses, of whom there were 1,000 in Victoria. Upon their return they found industrial conditions depressingly the same as when they had left several years before. The RVTNA had never regarded material reward as inimical to the true spirit of nursing, but believed that public acclamation was enough. The members of the Guild found the Association out of date, old-fashioned and unprogressive. This was also reflected in press reports of the day. The

Royal Victorian Trained Nurses' Association.

MAY 1924.

**Abbreviations must not be used:
All questions of equal value.**

SURGICAL NURSING.

1. How would you prepare the following for use at an operation? (*a*) Plain Catgut, (*b*) Rubber Gloves, (*c*) Hypodermic Syringe, (*d*) Scissors.

2. How would you prepare for operation and nurse after operation—a patient with Hæmorrhoids (Piles)?

3. What are the chief points to observe in nursing a patient suffering from a Fractured Spine in Lower Dorsal region?

4. Describe how you would prepare and administer Saline solution by the rectum giving strength and temperature.

5. What could a nurse do for a patient in a case of severe vomiting after a major abdominal operation?

RVTNA surgical nursing exam paper, 1924.
RCHA/Ivy Flower Collection.

Age, on 27 March 1922, carried a banner: 'Pity the poor nurses sweated working conditions.'

One hundred nurses from the Alfred, Children's and the Melbourne Hospitals banded together to form the 'Guild'; to lobby for an eight-hour day, with the intention of taking nurses into the industrial arena, the Wages Board and the Arbitration Court. Intrinsic to this was the notion of revitalisation and adaptation to new conditions and advancement of nurse education. Consequently, the nursing world was in a state of great ferment. This was reflected in the concerns of the Committee that

> [S]hould a log be presented by the Nurses' Guild and made law, pay of trainees will be much higher, and the hours of work shorter than at present, the latter making it imperative that the nursing staff be considerably increased.[18]

The Trained Nurses' Guild fizzled out as government legislation, introduced progressively in 1923, culminated in the *Nurses' Registration Act 1924*. The RVTNA subsequently lost power and influence for some years but re-emerged as the College of Nursing in 1934.

For returned nurses who had travelled the world, the small community, the enclosed and narrow life with the rigid hierarchy and parsimonious attitudes of the Committee, was cloying and stifling. Conditions were stagnant. World War One had accelerated progress in science and medical specialties: the introduction of blood transfusions, improved anaesthetics and a wider knowledge of pathology attracted young doctors to the Children's where medical practice was vibrant and exciting. This air of optimism pervading the medical world did not extend to nursing, which was depressingly the same. While the medical profession benefited immeasurably from modern developments, this was not reflected in nurse education and practice.

There was little hope of advancement and the wider world beckoned. Many nurses believed they could do more good in private nursing, in community work among mothers and babies and in remote nursing.

Miss Wilson's appointment to the Children's Hospital was short-lived. Her reforming management style led to so much friction with the Ladies' Committee, about whom she was openly critical, that in 1922 she resigned to run a private hospital. Her resignation left the way open for the Committee to revert to their old ways of control. Nevertheless, such was the good reputation of the Hospital that there was no shortage of applicants for the job of Matron.

Nurses make their mark in community work

In March 1922, the *Age* ran a series of letters, regarding 'sweating conditions', at the Children's Hospital where probationers were working twelve hours a day for 'a few shillings a week'.[19] At this time the exodus of nurses to marriage and community work was noticeable. Children's nurses were particularly suitable in the natural progression to preventative health education in the Baby Health Centre movement, to Bush Nursing and to work in private homes. For a small subscription, families could transfer to a safe haven of a Cottage Bush Nursing Hospital where babies were born, and children were admitted for tonsillectomies, emergency procedures and minor accidents. Bush nurses required enormous energy and courage. Those Children's Hospital nurses who retired from the job, married and lived in a country area, often continued to be called out in emergencies. Their work took them to remote parts of Victoria with primitive transport. Reliance on assistance 'in kind', such as fresh eggs and firewood, supplemented their primitive living and working conditions.

Ann Milburn trained at the Children's Hospital from 1921 to 1924 and worked for many years in the remote and rough logging areas of the Otway Ranges. Her presence was reassuring at bush camps and farms where she attended accidents, illness and home births, as well as providing comfort to isolated families. She is also remembered in later years as the Sister-in-Charge of the Children's Hospital's Sherbrooke Convalescent Annexe in the Dandenong Ranges. From 1936 to 1952, she provided a home for generations of city children with chronic chest diseases.

Ella Grace McNeill (née Robinson) recalled her years at the Children's as a trainee from 1921 to 1925, as a Staff Nurse and Home Sister. At the conclusion of her training, she became the second nurse to be awarded the Jeffreys Wood Gold Medal and, in January 1930, resigned to study for the Infant Welfare Certificate. In 1931, she joined the Bush Nursing Association of Victoria where her long years of training were really put to the test. Ella had never heard of her first post, the small country town of Cressy, far from city life. The only means of transport, a horse and jinker, was an adventure when the horse had a mind of its own. Ella travelled long, dusty, treeless roads against cold, prevailing winds, visiting mothers and babies on isolated farms when times were tough (1931–33).[20]

The maternal and child health movement gained momentum after the Great War but its genesis was at the Children's Hospital with the work of Drs A. Jeffreys Wood, R. Atkinson Wood, Hobill Cole and others. The infant welfare movement began in the inner suburb of Richmond amid deep concern for the high infant mortality, family deprivation, poverty and isolation. Muriel Anna Peck completed her training in 1907 and devoted her life to the welfare of mothers and babies. The Baby Health Centre Movement began in Victoria in June 1917. Dr Isabella (Isabel) Younger Ross, a former Resident Medical Officer at the Children's Hospital, initiated the first Baby Clinic in Richmond, assisted by Muriel Peck.

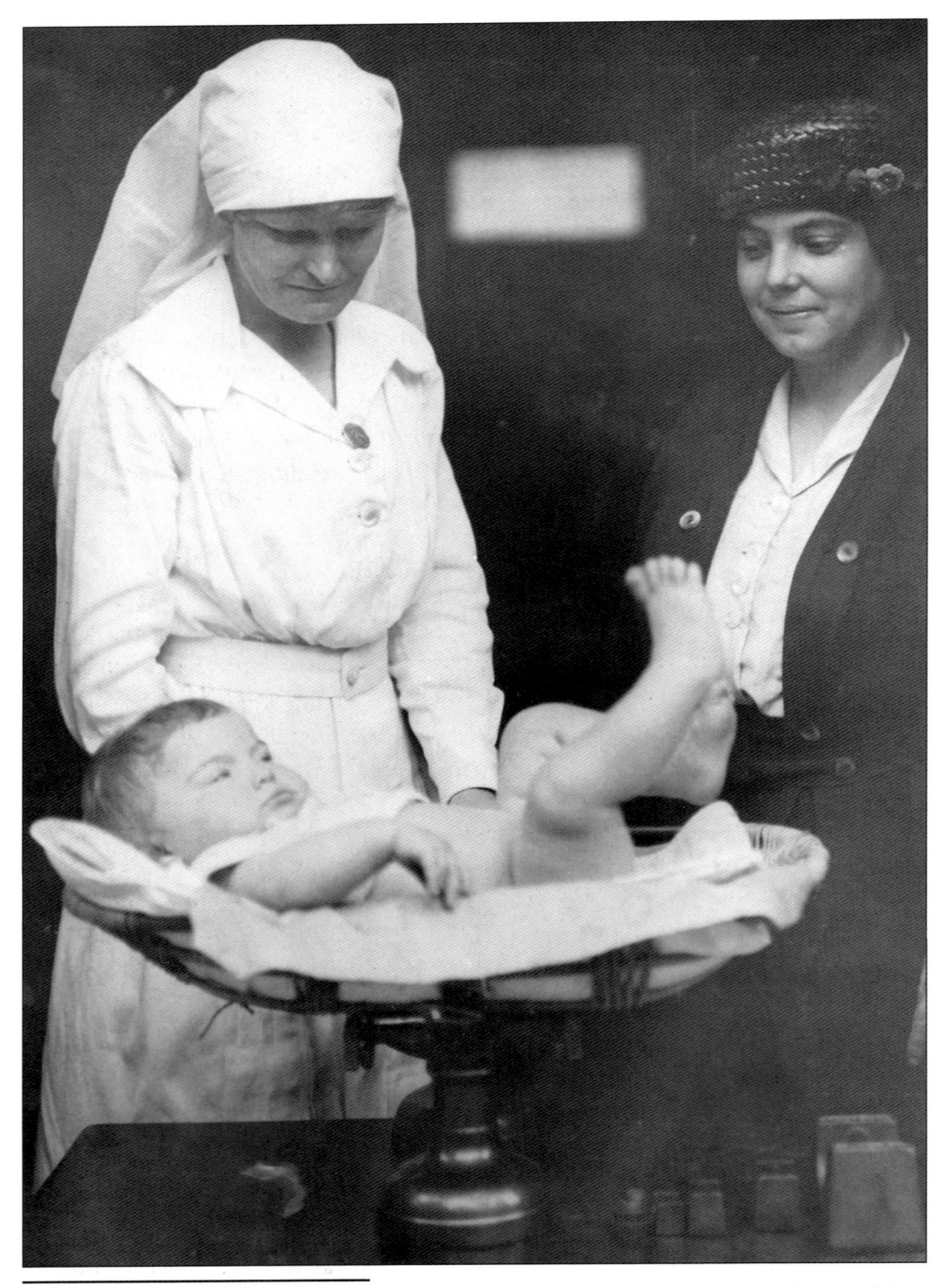

Muriel Anna Peck (RCH 1904–07), founding Sister of the Victorian Baby Health Centres Association (1918), with mother and baby.
La Trobe Australian Manuscripts Collection, State Library of Victoria.

MURIEL ANNA PECK (1884–1947), a trainee of the Children's Hospital and a pioneer of infant welfare prior to the introduction of Baby Clinics in 1917, was the first Baby Health Centre Nurse (modern day Maternal and Child Health). A role model for nurses, Muriel Peck had a serene manner and calming influence. Her rare gift for teaching baby care and feeding assumed central importance to generations of mothers.

Sister Peck made twenty-three trips on the Better Farming Train for the VBHCA and continued for ten years with the Infant Welfare Department. She became assistant to Dr Vera Scantlebury Brown, acting as an Inspector, giving advice on buildings and equipment and as an intermediary between municipalities and the State Government. She became a State Examiner of Infant Welfare and Mothercraft Nurses and, in the 1930s, a Baby Health Centre was named in her honour: 'The Muriel Peck Cottage' at Monbulk. She died after a long illness in 1947.

Miss Peck had extensive experience as a visitor for the Lady Talbot Milk Institute in Mulgrave. Milk was delivered from tuberculin-tested cows at the Model Farm at Caulfield to the Willsmere Dairy in Kew, pasteurised, bottled and distributed to poor women unable to breast-feed. In suburbs such as Richmond, where the council was able and willing to subsidise the scheme, the milk was delivered with a block of ice; the Talbot Society provided the ice chest. Sister Peck's job was to educate mothers with advice about hygiene and care of the milk and utensils.

Dr Arthur Jeffreys Wood retired from active involvement at the Children's Hospital in 1921 and remained a consultant until his death in 1937. A teacher of exceptional qualities, he was an active participant on the Victorian Baby Health Centres Advisory Committee. While the Committee of Management at the Children's was most concerned to build new and better facilities for sick babies, Dr Wood kept his vision firmly on the future of preventative services, through the growing Baby Health Centres network, and the important educative role of paediatric nurses. His memory remained in the Jeffreys Wood Gold Medal to the best Children's Hospital nurse, an annual award which continued until 1987.

The League of Former Trainees (LOFT)

The 1920s were a period of agitation for better wages and conditions for nurses everywhere in Australia. In August 1921, Grace Wilson placed a notice in the Nursing Journal, *UNA*, to advise of a meeting of past trainees of the Children's Hospital. In that year, a group of former Children's nurses, some of them returned from World War One, came together in the Fitzroy Gardens to form the League of Former

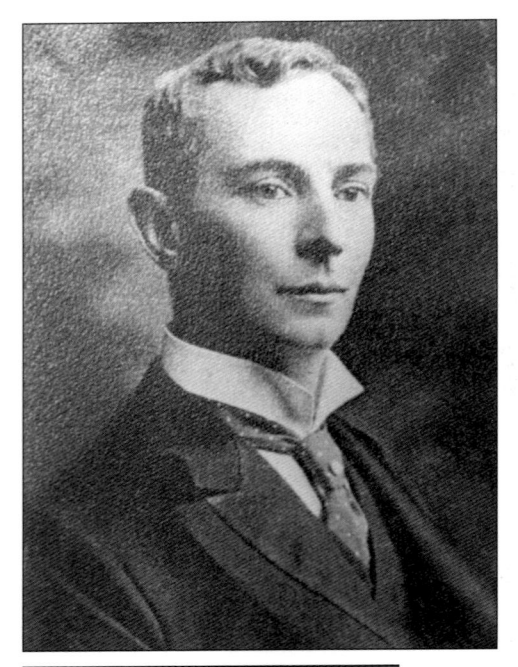

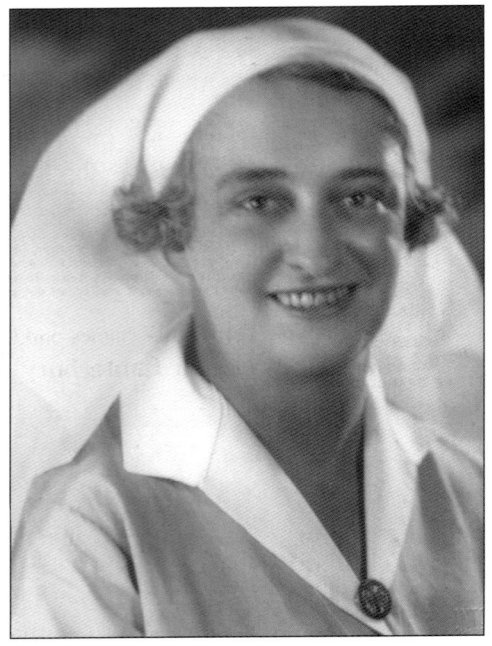

Left: Dr Arthur Jeffreys Wood.
Right: Muriel Lewis (RCH 1921–24), a pivotal figure at the Packenham Baby Health Centre and Packenham Bush Nursing Hospital, Gippsland, 1920s to 1945. *RCHA/Lewis Family Collection.*

Trainees (LOFT). The aims were to keep the past trainees together, to guard their interests and the welfare of nurses generally, to keep contact between the past trainees and the Hospital, and to support organisations that cared for the welfare of children.

Evelyn Conyers was a founding member of LOFT and, although she was by now running a private hospital in Kew and preoccupied as an office-holder of the RVTNA, her significant management skills helped to calm the waters between the opposing nurses' groups. She also upheld the profile of the Children's Hospital nurses towards general registration. When the *Nurses' Registration Act* was passed in July 1924, Miss Conyers became a founding member of the Nurses' Registration Board.

The League continued to meet twice yearly, in the summer months at the Botanical Gardens and in the winter, in the nurses' sitting room at the Hospital. At the July meeting of 1926, Miss Walsh was in the chair, and present were Miss Thomas (Vice-President), Miss Elsie Smith (Secretary–outdoors) and Miss Lucy Mackenzie (Secretary–indoors). Committee members included Miss Danaher, Miss Cook, Miss Laidlaw and Mrs Bernard Hall. The joining fee was set at one shilling for the first year and two shillings thereafter. A sum of £15/10/6 was contributed by members to the Hospital building appeal, and a memorial was proposed to Miss Player.

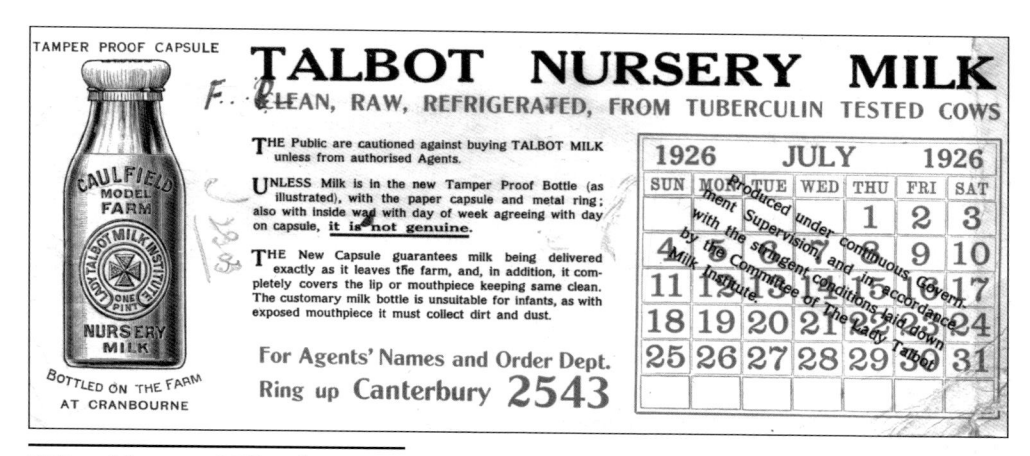

Talbot Nursery Milk advertisement.

Fifty members attended the meeting at the Botanical Gardens in February 1928, where catering was provided at one shilling and nine pence a head for tea and cakes at the Kiosk. The winter meeting held in the nurses' sitting room, brightly decorated with bowls of flowers, created a homely environment for the visitors beside a cosy fire. A short musical programme followed the main business. One of the new members to join that night was Muriel Peck.

The League had very generously raised funds to honour the long and devoted service of Miss Hilda Player. On 15 March 1928, the President Miss Walsh, on behalf of the members, handed over to the nurses' sitting room a handsome blackwood bookcase suitably inscribed as a memorial to the late Miss Player, Matron for twenty-two years.[21]

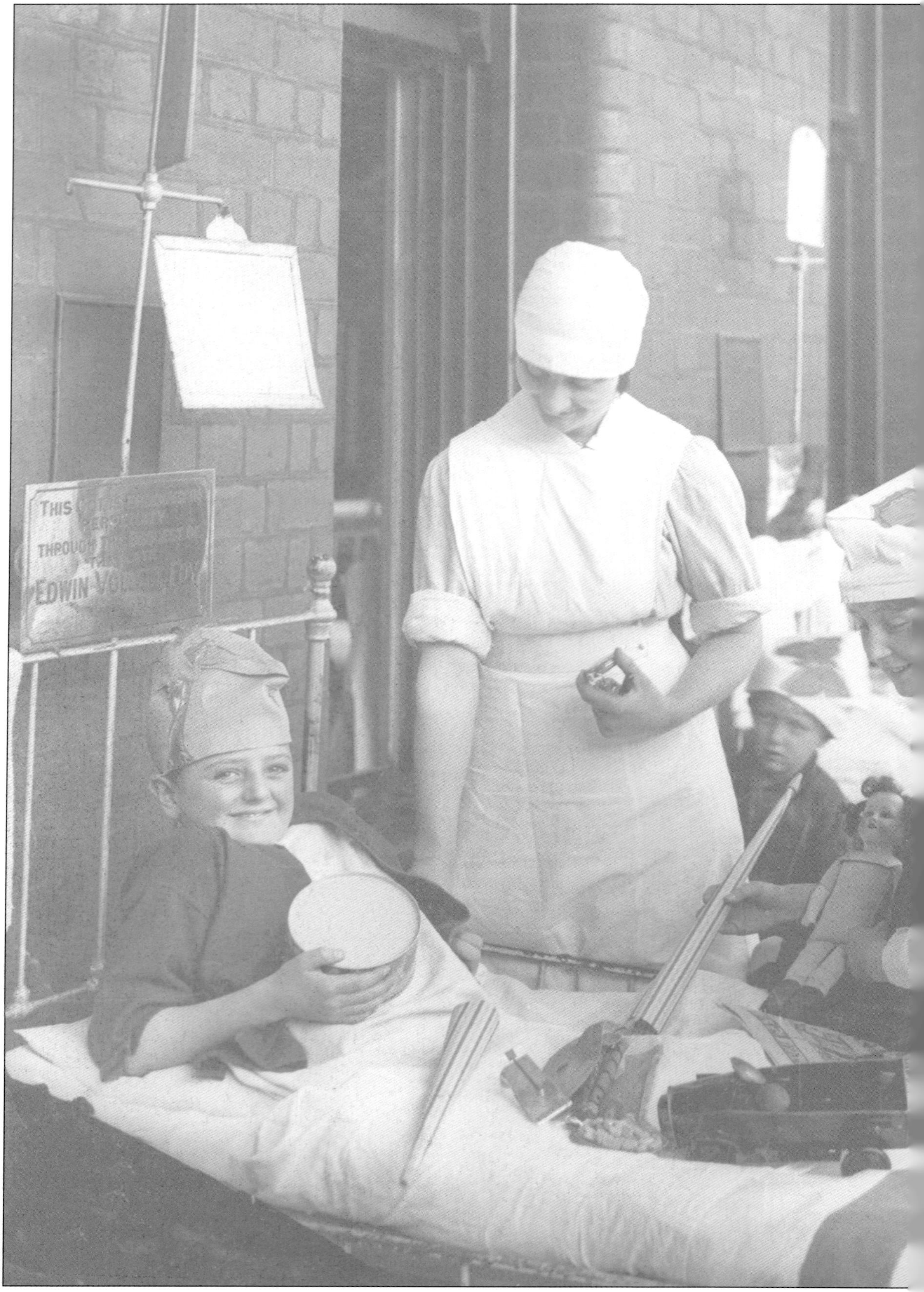
THIS
EDWIN

Part 3

1924–1947

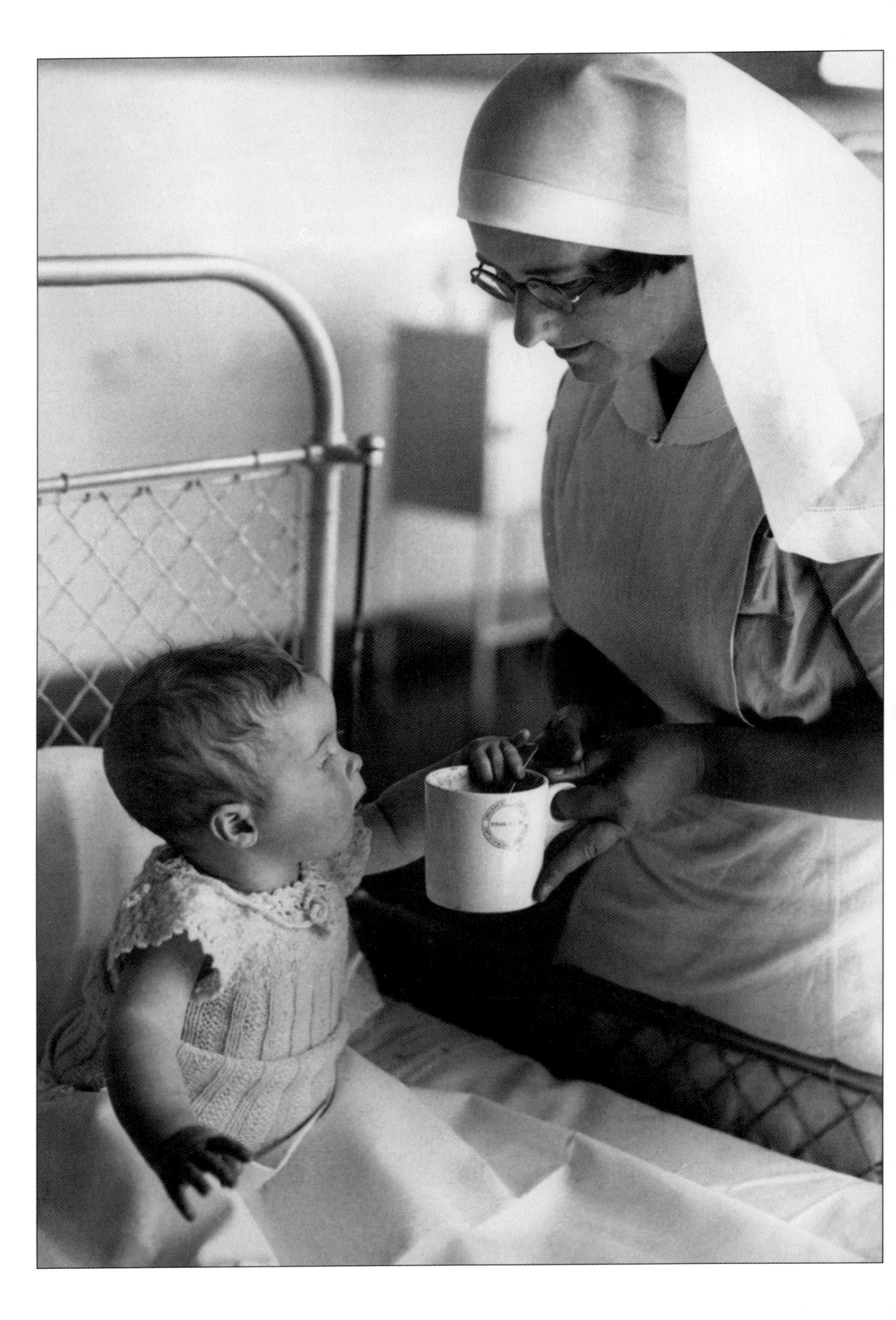

CHAPTER 7

Between the Wars

1924–1940s

This period in the story of nursing at the Children' Hospital must be seen against the extraordinary times of the Great Depression, the outbreak of World War Two, the public health movements and the beliefs of the times.

Sick children remained in the wards on average for about thirty to forty days, which gave the nurses every chance to get to know their patients. Until the 1940s, few medical treatments were available to assist recovery; procedures were less frequent and the pace of hospital life was slower. The wards were more peaceful, less hurried, with fewer people around. Upon admission, children were isolated from their families for about four weeks and thereafter parents could visit twice weekly—Wednesdays and Sundays—a time fraught with sobbing children distressed at their parents' departure. Careful bedside nursing, so necessary when children were admitted with severe and chronic illnesses, was the major factor in their recovery. During convalescence, nurses became the most constant factor in the child's world.

Despite the stringencies of the Great Depression, a modern orthopaedic hospital was established at Frankston in 1930 along the lines of the European open-air sanatoria. Children being rehabilitated from the aftermath of tuberculous diseases of the bones and joints and osteomyelitis became a public focus in the cause of the 'crippled child'. Trainee nurses worked in this institution and also, in the years of

---

Sister Estelle Davies feeding a child in bed. Nurses were not permitted to nurse the children out of bed. The rules changed after 1947.

World War Two, in the Convalescent Cottage at Sherbrooke Forest. Children were sent from the city slums to recover from debilitating chest diseases and other childhood illnesses.

The widespread poliomyelitis epidemics of the late 1930s created public pressure on the Children's Hospital to prove or disprove popular theories of treatment. 'Sister' Elizabeth Kenny was granted twenty-two beds at the Convalescent Cottage at Brighton, and two Children's Hospital nurses were trained in her special methods.

Within the context of the times, children's nursing, although distinguished by unchanging routine, became highly organised and efficient. Many women, disadvantaged by the Great Depression and lack of life chances, who would in ordinary circumstances have continued with their tertiary education, found in nursing an alternative for their considerable talents. These years—sometimes known for stagnation—were, in many respects, a time of progress in nursing at the Children's Hospital. They brought about the introduction of tutors, a Preliminary Training School, State Registration, rotation to the Royal Melbourne Hospital and a widening of experiences through rehabilitation medicine.

A nurse's life: 1920s–1940s

Isabel Pilkington recalls her life in the 1930s:

> It is difficult to compare the situation with the present. The world was a very different place. Basically, we saw it as our responsibility to get on with what we had to do. We did not expect many privileges, we rarely complained about our situation and by and large we earnestly applied what skills we had to the care of the sick.[1]

The qualification required to begin training was the Merit Certificate (Grade 8) issued at the completion of primary school, the equivalent today of Year 8. Few stayed at school beyond the age of fifteen or sixteen. This was a basic standard for the theoretical needs of the time. The rare candidate with secondary education did find the transition easier. Seldom did the idea to take up nursing come from newspaper advertisements. For most, it was word of mouth: the older sister of a school friend who had already begun nursing, or an aunt or mother. Many applied to adult hospitals, particularly the Melbourne, but were left with the impression that the Matron of that institution had particular preferences, such as family background and private schooling. In contrast, the most important requisite for entry to the Children's was a love of children. Applicants also provided a character and family reference from their minister of religion before an interview with Miss Walsh, and were required to have a medical examination by Dr Grieve, a senior consultant.

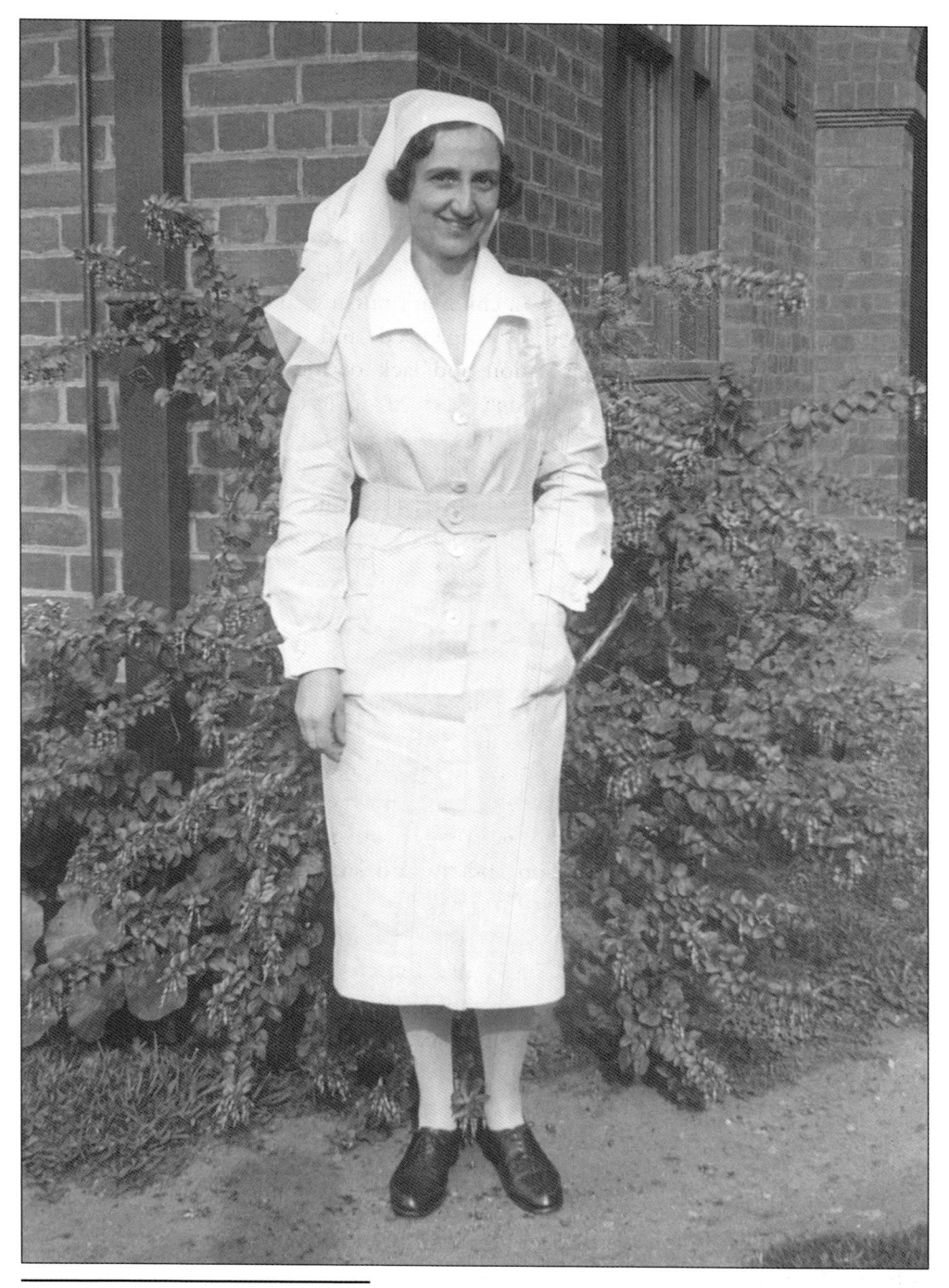

Isabel Pilkington, RCH 1932–35, Tutor (1938–43). Secretary to Mrs Lucy De Neeve 1951–60.

RCHA/Cunningham Family Collection.

Many girls longed to do children's nursing—there was no shortage of applicants. But for some country and interstate applicants the greatest stumbling block was their parents' fear of the seedy suburb of Carlton, then a slum with criminal elements. Three years was a long time and few parents expected their daughters to last the distance.

Patricia Thorburn's father objected to her career choice of nursing. She remembers his Victorian views on the matter. He was inclined to dictate his daughters' futures and it was usual for daughters to listen and take heed of fathers in those days. Nursing was no career, according to him. It was all hard work!

Patricia said:

By the time I finished my schooling I was sixteen and I just knew I wanted to be a nurse. Those various qualities that made me want to care for children were there within me from an early age. I thought about being a kindergarten teacher or a nurse, and being a nurse just seemed the natural choice. I knew I wanted to spend my life helping children.[2]

Because nurses lived in at the Hospital, Patricia could possibly be the first daughter to leave home. Yet none of the girls was supposed to leave until she was married. Her sister agreed: 'You know father likes us all around him. If he has his way he'll have the four of us fluttering around him all our lives.' Her mother was similarly upset with her choice. She delayed for two yers then, despite family opposition, began nursing in 1928 at the age of eighteen.

In the 1920s, the age to start nursing varied between eighteen and twenty-one. Her thoughts were: 'living in nurses' quarters was just like boarding school: lights out at nine o'clock; sign in, sign out; all sorts of rules and regulations'.

But being young, the probationers quickly figured out how to get around some of the rules and not spoil the fun. 'If we knew we were going to be late, we'd get someone to sign in for us—we didn't want to merry-dance with the Matron for being ten minutes late. Matrons really were dragons in those days!' There was little social life anyway, and, for the first six months, nurses were not paid. Patricia's father did not send any money because she was stubborn about nursing, '[b]ut Mum did; there is always someone to help you out. So a few of us would go down to Bourke Street and see a film for sixpence. We loved that, but we couldn't do it very often.'

Patricia was lucky; she could go home for a meal sometimes. Not so the country girls. The Nurses' Home became the centre of their lives, the weekly letter from home their only communication with the outside world. Visitors were strictly forbidden.

When pressured, nurses appeared for duty before the appointed time and stayed on duty until the work was done. Little consideration was given to personal lives; long-cherished plans and arrangements for a special day off could be rudely shattered by a move to another ward where it was not possible to be off duty on that day.

Jean Hardham was the second child in her family, and her parents thought nursing was too hard. They weren't keen. She made all the arrangements on her own. Her grandmother supported her, however, and was very proud to have a granddaughter training to be a nurse who was also able to give her injections for her angina. 'Mother and dad finally accepted it and I was given sixpence to get home from the Children's into town on the cable tram, then to East Malvern. They also offered an extra two shillings because we only got six a week.'

Jean voluntarily left the Anglican Girls' School, Korowa, at the age of fifteen before she did her Intermediate in 1926, to make way for the education of the younger children. The depression years loomed and her father lost his business. As there were six children to be educated after Jean, and although her mother wanted her to stay at Korowa another year, Jean insisted: 'No, I had three or four years and it is time I went to work.' Her family knew Sister Kathleen Shepherd at the Mission of St James and St John, and she was given a job as a nurses' assistant at the Arms of Jesus Babies' Home, where the Freemasons' is today.

During the economic depression and throughout the 1930s, employment conditions for Children's Hospital nurses stagnated. Salaries were paid monthly at six shillings and eight pence a week. By the end of each month, things were lean and nurses were not permitted to go to the dining room on days off. For country girls that meant starvation. Some received help from home, stamps or an occasional ten shilling note.[3] Jean Hardham remembers that she always brought a tin of biscuits from home after her days off and midnight feasts in the Nurses' Home were great fun. But unfortunately the crumbs attracted a rat in the night which bit her ear. She was severely injured. She remembers: 'It must have been serious because the consultant, Dr Grieve, was called to attend to my injury.'

The old Hospital buildings had not changed for many years and finding a way around the maze could be daunting for newcomers in the 1940s. Jeanette Pollock clearly recalled the night she started as a probationer at the age of seventeen: her mother, two sisters and the dog brought her into the Hospital where they were met by Miss Trixie Jarrett in her window box in the front reception area on Pelham Street. 'But', Jeanette recalled, 'the dog stayed in the car'. They all trooped over to the Nurses' Home and were shown into a three-bed room backing on to the boiler house. The beds were 2 feet 6 inches wide, with the thinnest horsehair mattresses:

> That was that! I said goodbye to my family. Kit Webster [the Home Sister] and the other girls came in and she showed us how to pull our caps on; we were just jibbering with nervousness. She went away and said we would be called at 6.00, have breakfast at 7.00 and Sister Morris who was the PTS [Preliminary Training School] Sister would collect us and take us to meet Miss Walsh.[4]

When Sister Webster left the room, one of the girls from the immediate PTS came in and said: 'Don't take any notice of what Sister Webster told you about your cap; this is what you do.'

Next morning the girls lined up outside Miss Walsh's door. Jeanette remembers thinking, 'I will never find my way back again. Everything is so spread out.'

Marjorie Allnatt said of her introduction to nursing in the early 1930s: 'There was no [preliminary] school then. You just entered. Someone finished the night before and you started the next day. Unusually two started together.' Both Marjorie and her room mate got off on the wrong foot from the start. The Night Sister's rounds included the early morning 'wake-up call' in the Nurses' Home; the banging on doors started at 6.15 am approaching down the passage. But the two were in Extension B; no one knew they were there and the call didn't come. They were not missed until breakfast. But it was all a new world and she said: 'That night we heard an ambulance. We were so excited we could hardly sleep.'

As a country girl from Swan Hill, Marjorie Allnatt had set her heart on a teaching career. With the expectations of a brighter student, she thought she would naturally move through Grade 8 to Leaving, to senior pupil teacher and, when old enough, to formal teacher training. During the depression, girls were disadvantaged

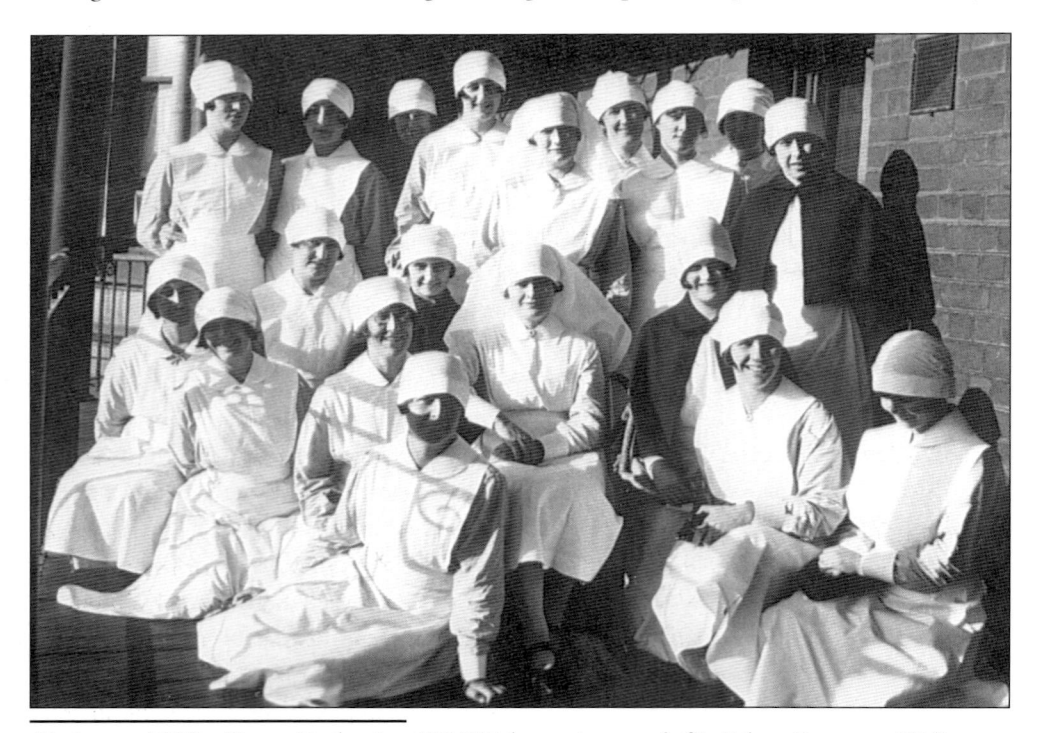

Trainees, 1930s. Sister Catherine 'Kit' Webster (centre left). Edna Curwen-Walker, seated (second right).
RCHA/Curwen-Walker Family Collection.

when recruitments ceased. Marjorie was extremely disappointed at her rejection. A series of articles on nursing in the *Age* inspired her to enquire at the Children's and the Melbourne Hospitals. At her interview at the Children's, Miss Walsh kept asking 'but why do you want to come to the Children's?' Her response, 'that she liked children', was apparently satisfactory. Her traineeship began in 1933.[5]

Nurses arrived on their first day with starched uniforms, white removable cuffs and collars, four pairs of navy blue bloomers, one eiderdown, one serviette ring, black stockings and shoes, and a small white cap to sit on the head at the correct angle. This sensible outfit was completed with the addition of one large red cape.

Dependent upon each other for company and fun, country girls could be very lonely on their day off when those they knew were on duty. With no relations to visit in Melbourne, days off were not as exciting as they were restful. Gradually, nurses were invited to each other's homes or on trips to the Myers cafeteria and the Athenaeum Theatre where the 'gods' cost 1/3d. The salary was 6/8d; an unbelievable bonus to them when it rose to 10/-. Marjorie Allnatt's parents always made sure she kept enough money to pay for the train fare home. Now and again, a pair of black stockings arrived in the mail or stockings for going out. Nurses borrowed from one another. Marjorie's evening bag was popular and did the rounds for anyone going to a dance. For going somewhere special, they always made sure they were dressed up, even if it was in other people's clothes.

There was a bit of pilfering that caused a lot of anger. 'You could lend it, but for someone to pinch it was the very worst thing anybody could do.'

For girls reared in big happy families on properties in country Victoria and Tasmania, where life was unchanged in harmonious and loving surroundings, the realities of a Children's Hospital and the convent-like life were overwhelming and depressing. Almost all were 'petrified of certain Ward Sisters', their harshness and sharp tongues. Una Wishart, a contemporary of Marjorie Allnatt, said, 'many cried themselves to sleep, had sleepless nights and stomach aches. One girl only lived at Kew and she cried all the time.'[6]

Fortunately with the way of youth most overcame these fears, 'to stick it out' so that their families could be proud, particularly those who experienced much parental opposition.

Unfortunately, nursing careers did not always end happily. The Committee became very disturbed by the high rate of illness, severe finger infections and death among nurses. A tragic example occurred in 1923. Nurse Holder of Fingal in Tasmania died after a short illness at the Children's Hospital.[7] Her parents, brothers and friends came to the Hospital to present a valuable gift of a cabinet Singer sewing machine to the Nurses' Home in memory of their daughter, sister and friend. The Reverend David Ross, on behalf of Nurse Holder's family, was present with Mrs Lauchlan Mackinnon, the Hospital President, and Mrs Butler Walsh, Vice-President. The Honorary Treasurer, Miss Guthrie, received the gift on behalf of the Committee, referring to the affection held for her by fellow nurses and her comments were supported by the Lady Superintendent, Miss Hilda Walsh.

Although there could be lots of fun in the Nurses' Home, life was sometimes bleak. Agnes Morris, a well-known and respected nurse, later a Tutor, thought the facilities were very poor. Shared bedrooms and communal bathrooms were only part of the story: 'It was very cold and they didn't feed us well.' Kate Menzies remembered 'We were always hungry…there was no heating in our rooms. We all had hot water bottles and rugs to wrap ourselves to study on morning or afternoon hours off.' Beryl White (née Letcher) recalled the rules and regulations were worse than boarding school or home. If your bed was not expertly made, it was sometimes ripped apart by the Home Sister and left in a heap, a nasty surprise when you returned from duty. One nurse returned to her room to find a note: 'You will not pass your exams if you make a bed like this.'

There were no facilities for tea-making. To discourage the use of the dining room, full uniform had to be worn at all times. In the 1930s, a disturbing incidence of tuberculosis among nurses caused great concern. Fewer cases continued until the 1950s. Dr Vernon Collins, a Resident Medical Officer in the 1930s and Medical Superintendent from 1937 to 1939, took a particular interest in the nurses' nutrition. In 1937, he recommended to the Committee that nurses be given cereals daily at breakfast instead of weekly, have a glass of milk a day, and cheese and fruit every tea time instead of twice a week. They were also to have potatoes every night.[8] The meals became more nutritious until the war years when Dr Collins was in England. During that time, many of his ideas lapsed.

For many young girls from the country and interstate with no means of emotional support, their contact from home was a weekly letter. If they were lucky, phone calls came through to the Nurses' Home, but this depended on whether the front office 'dragon', Trixie Jarrett, was in a good mood. Visitors were forbidden.

Despite the disadvantages, enormous camaraderie prevailed. An unloading of problems and hurts, anxieties and fears occurred on a regular basis. Today it is called debriefing or counselling, but then no one knew the burdens carried by these young women: the daily brush with death and parental grief, the harshness and discipline in the wards where they learned on the job.

Groups of friends in their immediate PTS supported each other. Mary McFarland said: 'We formed some long lasting friendships. Allowed one late pass a week, otherwise in by 10 pm and sign in the book—in hot weather we used to take the cable tram to the terminus and back just to get some fresh air.' Getting in late at night was not hard. There were plenty of ways: 'You would get someone in Ward 16 to leave the little gate open, or get over the mortuary gate.' The alternative was to walk boldly through the front office past the porter and the telephone operator. Then there was the fire escape in the Home and through the window on the first floor. 'The person sleeping under the window received a thump on the bed!'[9]

Marjorie Allnatt remembered her fear of coming home from the city:

> Running the gauntlet from the bus in Lygon Street, down that bit of Pelham Street—that was awful as there was nearly always someone there who would say 'Goodnight nurse' and you'd keep going. 'Goodnight nurse, aren't you going to stop and talk to us?' That was a hazard. I think we must have told someone about that because later on there were always policemen on bicycles there. Those few steps to the office—I have occasionally done those in one leap.[10]

The Home Sister, Ivy Flower, known to the nurses as 'Geranium', was a little person with a quiet and gentle manner. When she was appointed Deputy Matron in 1933, her successor to the Nurses' Home was Katherine Webster, fondly known to generations as 'Kit'. Everyone thought they were both terribly old. As they had trained at the Children's in the early 1920s, they were then in their mid-thirties to forty. With a dry sense of humour, while behaving at all times with the utmost decorum, Kit Webster warned the girls to 'draw down the blinds, under no circumstances dress or undress in front of the windows. There are peeping Toms lurking in the Exhibition Gardens.'

But Sister Webster also possessed a tremendous understanding of teenage girls. Many tried to trick her but she missed nothing. At each daily inspection the Home Sister and her Deputy wandered around the Nurses' Home and into the rooms; there were no locks and the courtesy of knocking was unheard of. Wardrobes were inspected and drawers opened. No one knew what they were looking for but strange things were there: besides the odd bottle of sherry poked behind the clothes, Kit once found a horses' bridle in the wardrobe belonging to a girl from the Western District who was known to have an Arab pony. Following inspection the door was quietly closed.

Jean Hardham said many girls smoked. 'Of course you weren't allowed to smoke. I didn't but my mother thought I was smoking because my roommate smoked heavily and if she heard the Home Sister coming she threw her cigarette into my wardrobe. So my clothes did smell of cigarette smoke.'

The working environment

Writing from the perspective of her training days, Sheila Ferguson said:

> If I could be blindfolded and taken back in time to the old Children's Hospital in Carlton in 1936, then led along the covered way from the main car park to the Nurses' Home, I would immediately know exactly where I was. This was an area always permeated with a particular odour,

compounded of steam, vapours from the kitchen, floor polish and antiseptics.[11]

The Nurses' Home, adjacent to the chimney of the boiler house and laundry, dominated Rathdowne Street. Two refurbished cottages, numbers 107 and 109, once condemned, then renovated, became a warm and comfortable haven for the senior sisters. Matron Hilda Walsh, known as the Lady Superintendent, lived on the first floor of the Resident Medical Officers' quarters, a three-storey building designed in the same architectural style as the Nurses' Home. The ground floor became the hub of the administration, with offices for the Medical Superintendent and Matron, a library, a boardroom and a doctors' dining room. The Matron's private rooms in the doctors' residence had little privacy. From Ward 9, nurses could look directly down into her window where the maid was making her bed.[12]

The basement of the Princess May Medical Wards had multi-purpose functions: the X-ray Department, a massage gym for polio patients and from 1924, a canteen where nursing mothers could have a cup of tea and a scone for a sixpence, breastfeed or warm baby's bottle. Tiny service doors opened directly from the basement on to the corner of Pelham and Drummond streets at ground level for the delivery of goods and, according to nurses' folklore, the grim exit of little bundles labelled neatly for the funeral parlour.

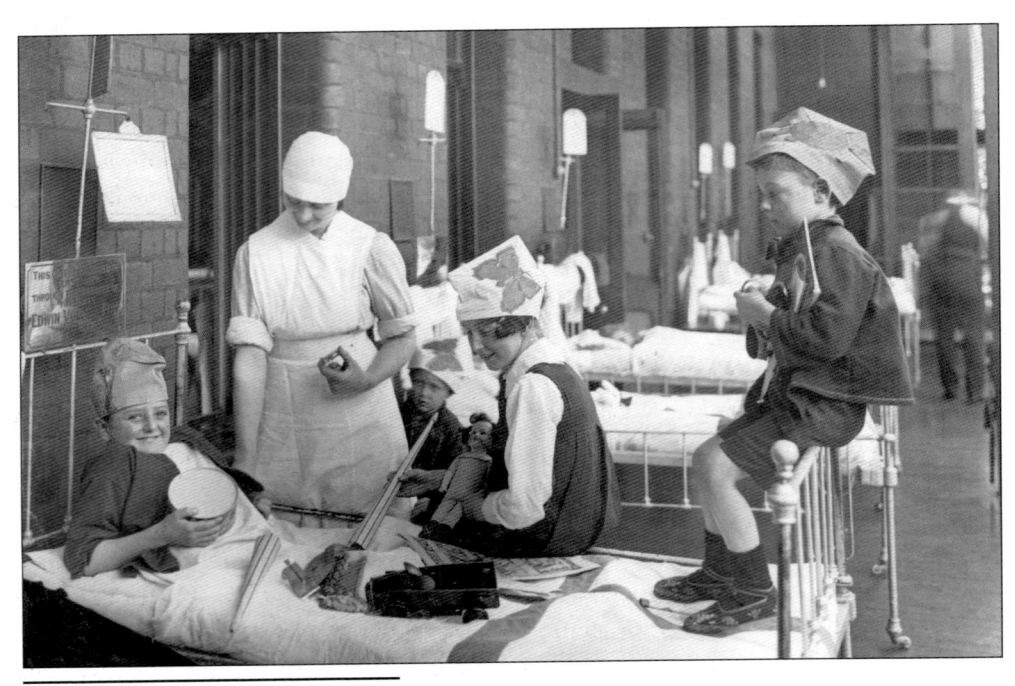

Ward 9, Surgical balcony party.
Argus, 1920s.

The Out-patients Department received a fourth floor, a Tonsil Theatre, an Ear, Nose and Throat Clinic, a gymnasium and plaster rooms. Baby Wards 12 and 14 were soon crowded and Ward 15 became the first research ward. The sterilising rooms, Isolation and Sick Nurses' Ward 16 and the small free-standing Venereal Diseases Ward 13, crowded the additional spaces.

For the public, facilities were far from comfortable, in modern terms really quite basic. At the Annual Meeting in 1938, complaints were received from disgruntled subscribers about the coldness of the Out-patients Hall. The Committee realised that it was probably very cold in winter and resolved 'that enquiries should be made to the feasibility of placing foot rests on the back of the forms for the use of people sitting in the row behind so that their feet would not have to rest on the concrete floor'.[13]

A modest building, the Pathology laboratory and mortuary on Drummond Street was a source of wonder and mystery to the nurses. Some recall checking their watches each morning when the diminutive, white-coated figure of the Pathologist, Dr Reginald Webster, emerged from his workplace, a tin shed. A creature of habit, he made his way at exactly 10.30 am past the Out-patients building, along the path beside the tennis court and the Casualty entrance, to the doctors' dining room for his morning tea and scones. A convivial chat with colleagues, no doubt, was a highlight of the lonely day at the microscope and the mortuary table.[14]

A new operating suite, the Annie Higgins Theatre, next to the already overcrowded Surgical Wards, was occasionally used as an overnight rest for parents. But complaints were received that mothers of patients in the Surgical Wards had to sleep in the bathrooms where dead babies were washed and laid out. Matron and the Medical Superintendent, Dr Robert Southby, issued a strong denial but admitted that mothers did sleep in bathrooms. 'Everything possible was done to make them comfortable and to find a parent's room.' The Committee bought six folding stretcher beds for mothers detained overnight.[15]

In the wards

Marjorie Allnatt had no idea what nursing would be like. She had a godmother who was a nurse and believed she would be physically nursing children—like Florence Nightingale—rather idealistically. But she found as a junior you were 'broken in'. You did the inkwells, the desk and all sorts of jobs. Some Sisters were gentle. Marjorie went to Sister Webster's ward—'she was an absolute dear and taught us how to feed a baby so gently'. They didn't pick baby up in those days; it was tucked up tight. There was nowhere for nurses to sit in the room, no chairs for nursing babies. They stood at the side of the cot to bottle feed. Some time later, Sister Agnes Morris allowed the nurses to hold the baby, if there was time. She recalled, 'there was a certain way of doing a round, if you were on evening duty with the Sister. Each baby would be tucked up, its hot water bottle filled and as she did this she would tell you about the baby and what was wrong with it. You couldn't do that with the older children. It was very regimented.' There was usually a Staff Nurse and a Sister but in Ward 8 Medical, Sister Liddicutt made 'life hell on earth for us'. It was not until after she finished training, in 1941–42, that Marjorie taught the nurses to hold a baby.

The nurses were taught by example by the seniors talking to you as they did their work. You went to the babies either in Ward 12 or 14 for a gentle introduction. They made sure you saw the procedures that went on in the ward. 'Of course a blood transfusion was a real event, and in the old Ward 12 you used to go into the little room and stand and stir a warmed metal pot and try not to faint.'[16] Blood was usually taken from the donor by inserting the large needle into the vein and received into a bottle containing 3.8 per cent sodium citrate solution to guard against clotting. It was stored in the refrigerator ready for use, then inverted a few times and warmed to blood heat by standing in warm water. The nurse's role was to fetch the blood from the refrigerator and place it in the warmed metal container.

Nursing was hard work; a child with rheumatic fever stayed in bed for many weeks. The nurse necessarily became the child's constant companion, feeding, sponging, bed changing, toileting and poulticing with hot-pack methyl salicylate wool binders, four-hourly observation charts and reports; the routine was that of a medical ward.

Pyloric stenosis babies required careful nursing, with sips of glucose and water every fifteen minutes to prevent dehydration—there were not the intravenous drips of today—and the baby had a subcutaneous drip in the abdomen. A spectacular projectile vomit often clinched a diagnosis and caused everyone to pay attention, from the lowliest nurse, medical student and doctor. But it was the nurse who cleaned it up!

With little help for children with pneumonia except careful nursing, maintaining the best possible position to have maximum help with breathing was a constant worry. Oxygen administered by tube or tent, with morphine and atropine ordered on occasions, were the only aids. Morphine was regarded as dangerous for children but occasionally a doctor prescribed it as a last resort in a difficult situation. The preparation of morphine was quite a procedure: the dose was checked by the doctor or senior Sister, the tablet then dissolved in a teaspoon of water boiled over a Bunsen burner and drawn up in a small syringe.

Careful sponging to keep the body cool and comfortable, and the administration of fluids, were the most usual nursing aids. 'Otherwise we had to watch the children panting for days, and mercifully, many did recover.' Kidney failure was common, following streptococcal infections, and children sometimes spent many months with increasing oedema and constant discomfort, with little or no medical treatment available, merely rest in bed. Nursing a child with ascites, or fluid in the abdominal cavity, was a challenge.[17] Children were susceptible to albuminuria; urine testing became a routine and unwelcome part of a nurse's day: the terrible smells, the boiling urine, the burnt fingers and the mess were all part of a junior's work in the pan room.

The old wards were warmed by coke fires lit at each end on alternate days. Nurses took a side, forty beds divided into twenty each. Babies were not segregated, except those with diarrhoea, who were placed in the Baby Wards. Nurses welcomed a little light relief on night duty. It was fun if the fire smoked; the fire brigade was called and the routine was broken by a chat with the young firemen on duty. With a bit of luck they stayed all night—for safety. Jean Hardham remembers how they longed for the fireman to come to break the monotony.[18]

Probationers with previous experience of children in kindergarten teaching and Mothercraft nursing in Babies' Homes had an easier transition. Jane Aicheson studied basic child psychology at Mooroolbark Kindergarten Teachers' College in the early 1930s. She preferred nursing children to adults from the point of view that 'children had no mental stress of the world'. She said: 'Adults always had the strain of what was going on at home, whereas children, if they had an operation today, may be well enough to get out of bed tomorrow, and they will.'[19] The children were subjected to much tender loving care 'rather than to get them through their illnesses with a hypodermic'. Jane was in charge of Ward 10 for about two years and remembers the primitive and run-down conditions. Nurses frequently received electric shocks from the steriliser.[20]

When Jean Hardham entered nurse training at the Children's Hospital in 1929, the transition was not nearly so strange or difficult. She went immediately into Ward 12 with babies. Although she was little more than a schoolgirl, the work was familiar. 'I could take temperatures, but had no idea how to take a pulse.' Newcomers were taught by the next most senior.[21] As an eighteen-year-old, she was worried by deaths in the Baby Wards.

> There would be, in Ward 14, about seven deaths a night or day, and they put the babies in the little [service] room on the bench together under a sheet. As people came in to visit their babies—we always laid them out beautifully with a little cotton wool around their necks—it always worried me that someone might put their hand on another baby which was under that sheet.

Hope Clark had a similar story and was far less prepared. One of her peer group had been laughed at: she had put out a seat for the Resident Doctor who asked for 'the stool'. She said: 'Learning from your own experience was the greatest difficulty before lectures began.'

There was no humour in Hope's first experience of death. Going straight into a ward without any previous knowledge was a great strain. A junior's task before seven in the morning was to take the Sister's ink bottles from her desk and wash them in the sewerage room. When confronted with three tiny dead babies under white sheets with little flowers in their hands, the two earthenware ink-bottles crashed to the tiled floor, and blue and red ink flowed down the corridor. Subsequently sent to Matron, she was threatened with expulsion for lack of self-control.[22]

The world of Hilda Walsh

A graduate of the Royal Melbourne Hospital and disciple of Jane Bell, one of Australia's pre-eminent war-time and civilian nurses, Miss Walsh first applied for the position of Matron at the Children's in 1920. However, Grace Wilson, the war hero, was chosen instead. Hilda Walsh's intervening two years were filled with private nursing, before she returned to the Children's as Matron. A contemporary described Hilda as 'a good person, a particularly brilliant bedside nurse and administrator'.[23]

Miss Walsh had no personal or working experience of children and their needs. A contemporary, Dr Howard Williams, considered her limited in her knowledge of children's nursing. Certainly, she did not have an easy way with children. Her ward rounds concerned matters of protocol, tidiness and general efficiency. Nurses loved to embellish her eccentricities. For example, she lectured wearing a tennis eye shade and could not easily make eye contact. These characteristics could have been an early foreboding of her later illness. Her need for perfect order—straightening the red crosses on the quilts, ensuring that the level of the window blinds all matched and that the castors on the beds all faced the same way regardless of the crises occurring in the wards—has also been seen in retrospect as a way of covering her pathological shyness.

Jeanette Pollock remembers that Miss Walsh said very little. An angular, tall lady with very long narrow feet, she wore the same style of uniform for twenty-six years: a drooping white organdie veil, and wire-rimmed glasses which gave her a mournful look. In the 1940s, she wore white stockings and white shoes with cross-band straps and little Louis heels with pointy toes.[24] Odd-looking and a little old-fashioned, this shy, introverted woman was the subject of much fun. She could disguise her characteristics for the first decades of her incumbency, the 1920s and 1930s, but as time went by, successive generations of young nurses and doctors overlooked her considerable qualities, dismissing her—with the other ageing staff Sisters—as simply old. This was not confined to the nursing profession. It must be remembered that during the years of World War Two the young, vital members of all the professions were called up or volunteered.

The doctors lived in their own accommodation facing Pelham Street, away from the Nurses' Home. There was strictly no socialising for them with the nurses. Exuberant young Resident Medical Officers (RMOs) played cricket in the passage on the first floor, and Matron Walsh was not amused. The constant crashing on her

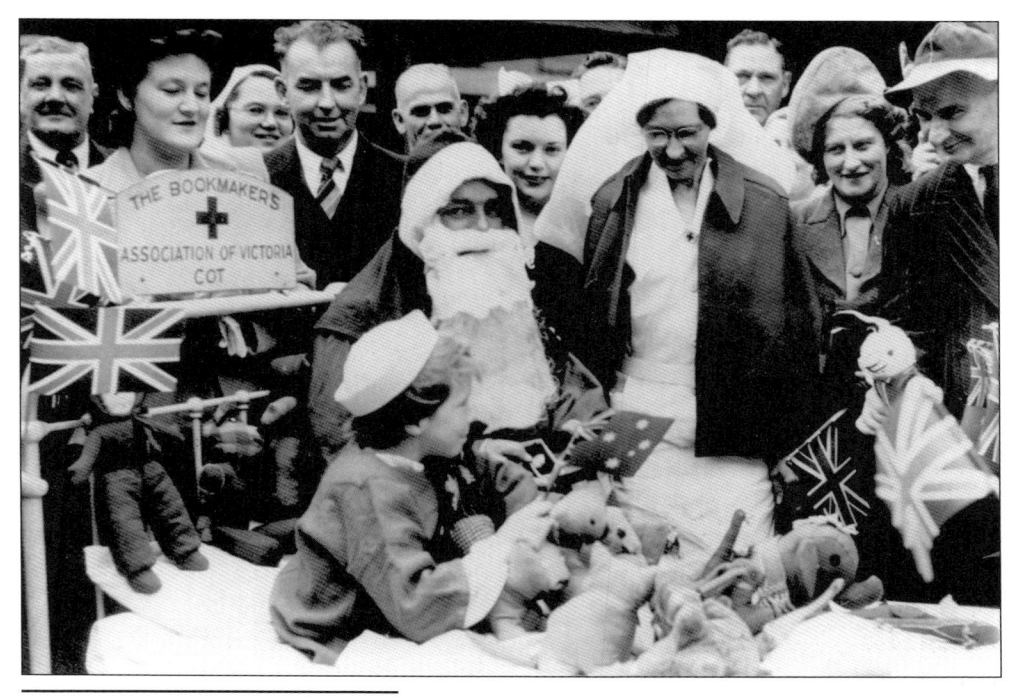

Matron Hilda Walsh, Christmas 1944, with the Bookmakers Association of Victoria.
RCHA/Cunningham Family Collection.

door was bad enough but there was worse to come: expecting a colleague, the residents threw a bucket of water over the balcony as a joke and missed, soaking a couple bringing in their sick child. 'Needless to say, that caused a big stir.' Jane Aicheson felt that the RMOs were cruel towards Matron Walsh, constantly playing tricks like 'putting salt in her teapot, which was dreadful'.[25]

Hilda Walsh's influence has been under-rated, for she was an excellent general nurse and lecturer. One of the most notable things remembered about her was that she always started lectures with the Nightingale Pledge, that the qualifications of a nurse were to be considered under the headings of 'physical, mental and moral attributes'.[26] This was common at the time and is seen in the textbooks of the day. Many nurses have said they owe everything they learned about bedside care to Miss Walsh. Generally, she had the good of the institution at heart and was—in her early days at least—a formidable presence. One of her most remarkable talents, to pick the right person for the job, was shown by her choice of Ward Sisters, Assistant Matron, Home Sister and Tutors who ran their own departments. In June 1929, the first full-time Tutor, Sister Jessie Morrison, was appointed followed by other outstanding Nurse Educators, Isabel Pilkington and Marjorie Allnatt. Other important advances occurred with the appointment of a Theatre Sister. In 1938, Sister Lyall was sent to

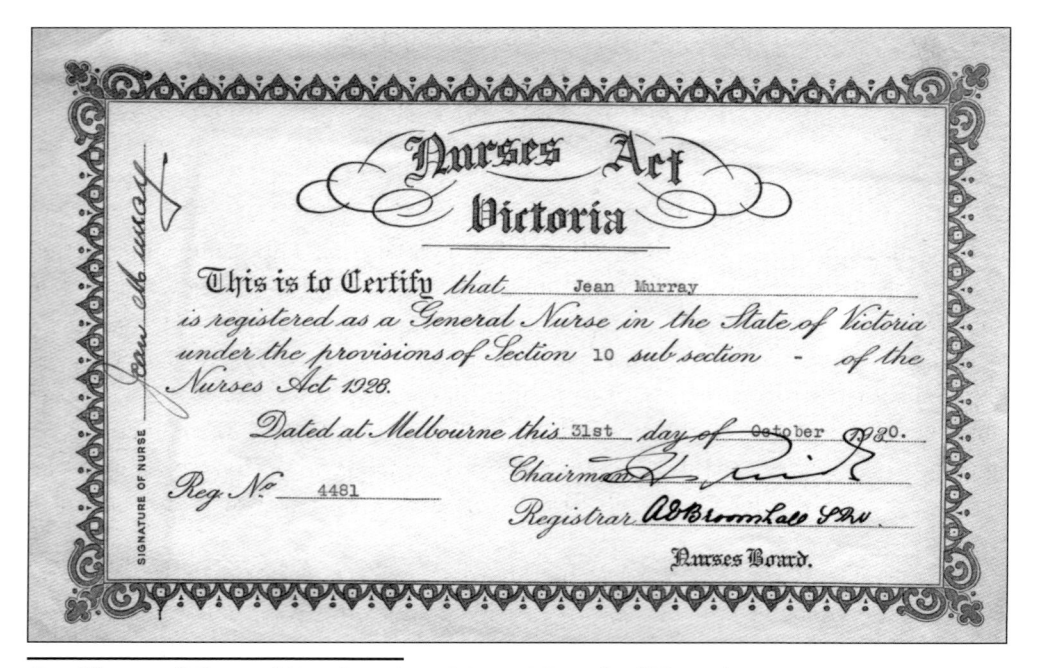

Certificate of General Registration, Nurses' Board of Victoria.
RCHA/Murray Family Collection.

Edinburgh to study dietetics to become the first Hospital Dietician and founder of the diet kitchen and infant formula food room.

For the first few years, Miss Walsh's personality suited the Committee of Management. She was never required to publish an Annual Report, but she was in weekly contact with her Committee.

With a continuously understaffed workforce, Miss Walsh carried an enormous workload, supervising the domestic side as well as the training of nurses through the heartbreak of the Great Depression and several severe epidemics. During these years tuberculosis, a legacy of the nineteenth century, was one of the most widespread, chronic and debilitating scourges. In her first years, 1922–23, the deaths of 464 children were recorded at the Children's Hospital; almost half died of gastro-enteritis or pneumonia.[27] The most serious poliomyelitis epidemics in the history of Victoria occurred in 1931, 1937 and 1938.

The 'new fad' Heliotherapy Ward was established in the 1920s; the Orthopaedic Hospital opened at Frankston in 1930 with a limited forty beds, and the 'Cripples' Ward at Hampton Rehabilitation Section was expanded to seventy beds so that the Elizabeth Kenny method could be used on children with poliomyelitis. All of these developments put huge extra burdens on the nursing administration. The loss of senior staff to World War Two was only saved by the essential 'Manpower' restrictions.[28]

Miss Walsh demanded high standards. During these years, she regularly attended and chaired the meetings of the League of Former Trainees and the Hospital Auxiliary.

Aspects of nurse education

Isabel Pilkington lived at Orbost on the Snowy River in Gippsland and reached Leaving Standard at school, which was quite unusual in the 1930s. She wanted to be a teacher. There were very limited opportunities for women in the professions but, as Isabel observed, 'nursing was available because student nurses provided an economical labour force necessary to maintain hospital services'. She believed more importance was placed on the availability of the necessary staff members than on the quality of training offered for a profession. 'Even when training was completed, the status of nursing as a profession was low. Nurses were regarded as the handmaiden of the other professions.'[29]

Isabel showed talent from the moment she entered the Nursing School and Miss Walsh, with her usual shrewd insight, allowed her to 'shadow' the Tutor Sister, Agnes Morris. Isabel eventually took on the mantle of Senior Tutor and, with Marjorie Allnatt, became the most important influence of that generation.

In 1935, a theoretical programme of lectures was developed and laid down by the then Nurses' Board. It consisted of:

First Year
- General Nursing—approximately 12 lectures given by Miss Walsh.
- Anatomy and Physiology—12 lectures given by a senior member of the Resident Medical Staff.

Second Year
- Medical Nursing, 12–16 lectures given by a Senior Honorary Medical Officer.
- Surgical Nursing, 12–16 lectures given by a Senior Honorary Surgical Officer.

Third-year nurses received four to six lectures on *materia medica*, covering special aspects of drugs, given by the Medical Superintendent or Senior Registrar, while three lectures of ophthalmic nursing were given by the Senior Honorary Eye Specialist. Bandaging, a short course, was conducted by Miss Walsh who had a special interest in this subject.

Infectious diseases, ear, nose and throat diseases and orthopaedic conditions were covered in the Medical and Surgical lectures. Some instruction was given in orthopaedic conditions covered by the staff at the Orthopaedic Hospital at Frankston (Mt Eliza), where students spent six months.

Isabel Pilkington said of that time: 'In all honesty, I confess that more emphasis was placed on how we carried out the cleaning and scrubbing of canvases from the turning frames then used than on the physical and psychological situations of the patients.'[30]

On completion of the sets of lectures, several weeks would elapse before the examination. During this period, instruction in small clinics was given by the Tutor Sister. These clinics were compulsory, and students frequently had to return from a day off or remain behind. When the results became available, they were posted on the notice board and those who failed were permitted to take the 'supplementary exam'. On some occasions they were given an extra tutorial. Isabel felt that, in retrospect, a weakness of the system was the initial entry. No Preliminary School existed and it seems that as a student nurse completed her training, a new student commenced. Notice sent to report for duty gave very little consideration as to distance to be travelled, or availability of transport. It might be that three or four arrived on the same day or during the week, or there could be a gap of several weeks before a new nurse arrived. It was the custom for new nurses to be placed in the Babies' Wards. There were two of these with about thirty patients in each.

The system of recruitment meant the Ward Sister might receive upwards of five or six new girls on the one day with an imbalance of suitable staff. Nurses did six months' probation and were then asked to 'sign on'. Another aspect of the training that worried Isabel was that a nurse, as she ascended the ladder of seniority, was expected to take more responsibility, sometimes without sufficient instruction.

The Committee made repeated efforts to bring about an amendment to the *Nurses' Registration Act 1924*, for special consideration as Certified Children's Nurses such as those in England and Wales. The *Amendment to the Act* introduced in 1928 enabled children's nurses to complete an additional three to six months at an approved adult hospital and register as trained nurses. An exchange occurred with the Women's Hospital and, after 1934, Prince Henry's. Children's Hospital nurses found the conditions at the Women's Hospital daunting. The issue of general registration was not resolved until 1939 despite many representations to successive Ministers of Health to have a special register for children's nurses. Then finally came the establishment of a six-month adult training scheme with the Melbourne Hospital and a Preliminary Training School. But those nurses who travelled overseas could not work in adult or children's hospitals or receive registration. Most found themselves working as child health nurses in England or Wales. When the most experienced and respected of nurses, Marjorie Allnatt, travelled to Britain in 1938 to widen her experience and work at Great Ormond Street Hospital, she was dismayed to be given a lowly position.

Further training

Charity Hospitals in the state of Victoria were the subject of enquiries, reports and recommendations in the 1920s and 1930s: their validity, cost-effectiveness, staffing of doctors and nurses, research facilities, the age of buildings and the need for expansion were all examined. The future of the Children's Hospital arose during a State Government sponsored visit in 1923 of Dr Malcolm MacEachern, the Canadian Superintendent of Vancouver General Hospital and Fellow of the American College of Surgeons. The Annual Report of the Children's Hospital for 1926 listed the observations and recommendations arising from this visit: there was to be a new Outpatients Department, a new X-ray Department, additional accommodation for patients, one or two more storeys, and an extension of Heliotherapy facilities. It also noted that the Hospital demonstrated the right care of the sick, as well as education of doctors, medical students, nurses, technicians, hospital personnel and others. For the times, the Hospital was considered well-organised, splendidly equipped, comfortable and attractively appointed.[31]

In 1933, with a view to providing the best possible experience for trained nurses in the Baby Wards, the Committee of Management adopted a suggestion that Sisters and Staff Nurses attend the Presbyterian Babies' Home for special infant welfare training. Three senior Sisters attended courses and, in 1934, a few trained nurses were

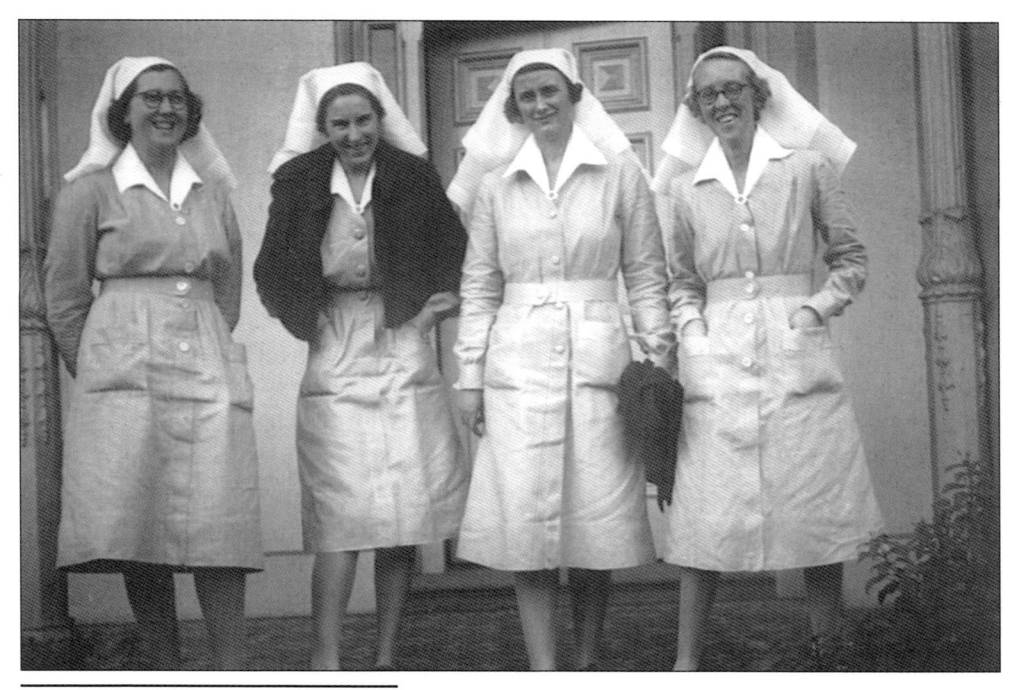

L–R: Joan Gendle, Sophie Brodie, Doris Whitfield, Kate Wilson, 1939.
RCHA/Robinson Family Collection.

> **Invalid Cookery Certificate**
>
> This is to Certify that
>
> _Jean Murray_
>
> has attended a Course of Ten Lessons in Special Invalid Cookery and has passed a written Examination in the same.
>
> Signed _Emily Noble_
> Examiner in Cookery.
>
> Melbourne, Oct 10th 1930

Invalid Cookery Certificate, Gas and Fuel Corporation.
RCHA/Murray Family Collection.

accepted under the Royal Victorian Trained Nurses' Association (later the College of Nursing) for a postgraduate paediatric course. Dr Douglas Galbraith introduced a popular and successful postgraduate orthopaedic course at Frankston Orthopaedic Hospital in 1938. None of these courses continued after the outbreak of World War Two. The paediatric course was not to resume until 1959.

In 1939, the Children's Hospital finally won registration as a general training school with the Nurses' Registration Board of Victoria and rotation was established with the Royal Melbourne Hospital. The Preliminary Training School was extended to four weeks. Study blocks were introduced and Marjorie Allnatt became the senior Tutor. Notable Ward Sisters from this period were Sophie Brodie, Margaret Adams, Joan Gendle and Kathleen Wilson. All except Margaret Adams, who left for war service, went on to distinguish themselves in the various functions of the Children's Hospital.

Although nurses' lives continued to be characterised by unrelenting hard work with poor pay, restrictions on freedom, lack of nourishing food and very long hours, the universal love and dedication to the welfare of children created an atmosphere of cohesion and friendship; the pleasures, enjoyment, companionship and tremendous feeling of goodwill far outweighed the deprivations. The attrition rate of nurses was the lowest on record; the major reason for an inability to complete training was a high rate of illness and, in some cases, death.

Learning by apprenticeship was hard but the messages were never forgotten throughout their lives: the seriousness of obligation was drummed in from the first day of training. Kathleen Wilson, the very able Tutor Sister who helped and inspired many, had the last warning: 'any fool can pass exams, but God help the community'.[32]

When war was declared in 1939, many nurses, doctors and other Hospital staff joined up. There was a great air of uncertainty; staff was completely unaware of what to expect.

Sheila Ferguson summed up those carefree days: 'We worked, laughed, cried and were let loose on the world, a caring fraternity confident of our ability to help sick people.'[33]

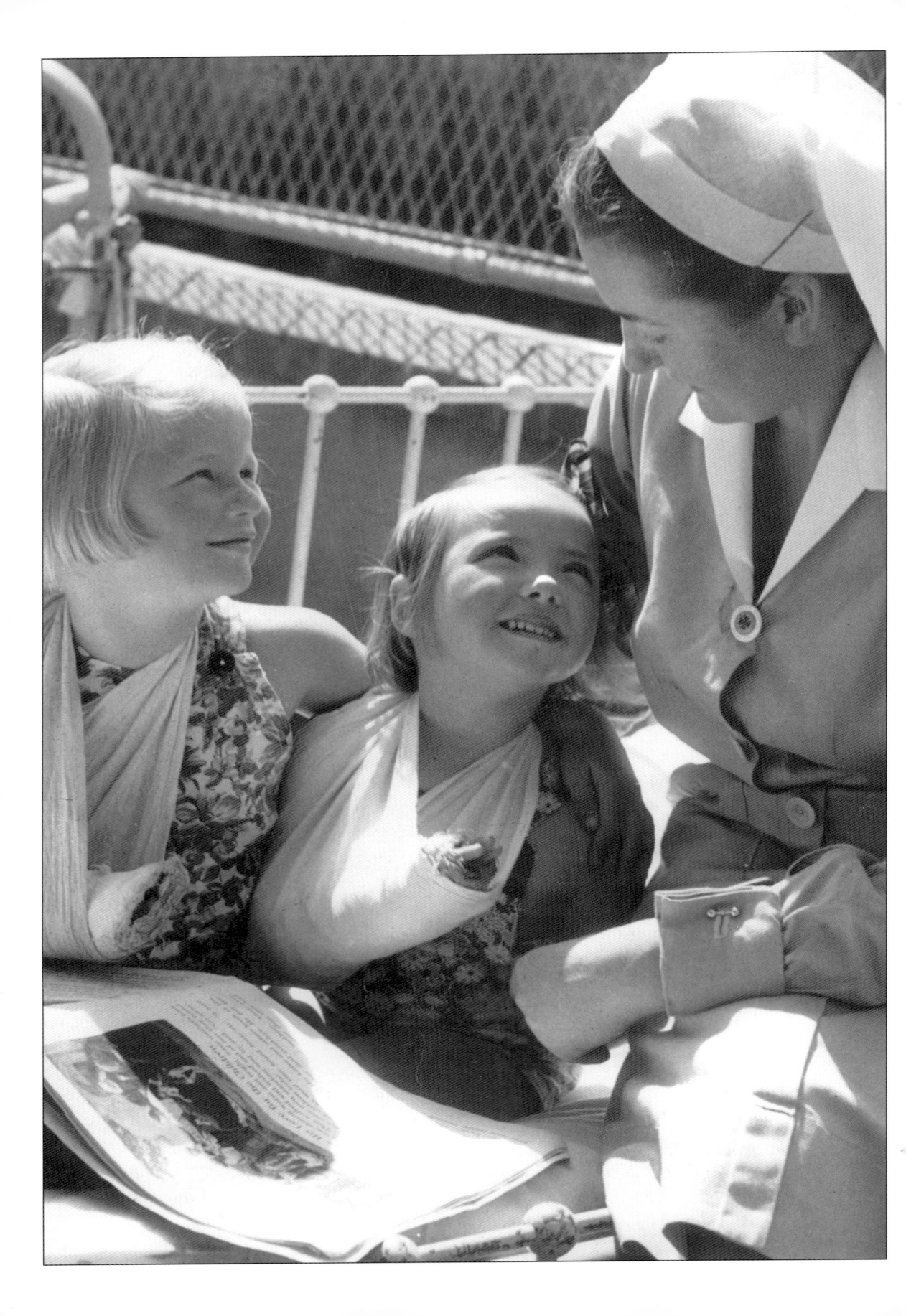

CHAPTER 8

Nursing Disabled Children
1930s–1940s

*I*n the 1930s, Children's Hospital nurses were introduced to more varied and interesting experiences. Over a decade, the Hospital had grown enormously. In 1938, with all its various branches, the number of beds had risen to 448 and the nursing staff had grown to about 250.[1]

While the Carlton site had become a jumble of old buildings criss-crossed by covered walkways with obsolete equipment and cramped accommodation, there were now several branches: a new Orthopaedic Section at Mt Eliza (known as Frankston), a Convalescent Home and ward for polio patients at Hampton, sometimes referred to as the Brighton Cottage, and the Sherbrooke Convalescent Cottage in the Dandenong Ranges. In the Annual Report for 30 June 1938 the Committee recorded that:

> This is now one of the largest Children's Hospitals in the British Empire. Moreover, in providing for the infant a few days old as well as for the adolescent who, in the Craft Hostel, whilst under medical supervision, is commencing the training which will lead to earning a living, the Hospital is covering as wide a field as any Children's Hospital in the world.

This period between the world wars was one in which the study of orthopaedics (literally, the straightening of children) came into its own and, as in all

---

Sister at the bedside, Frankston, 1940.

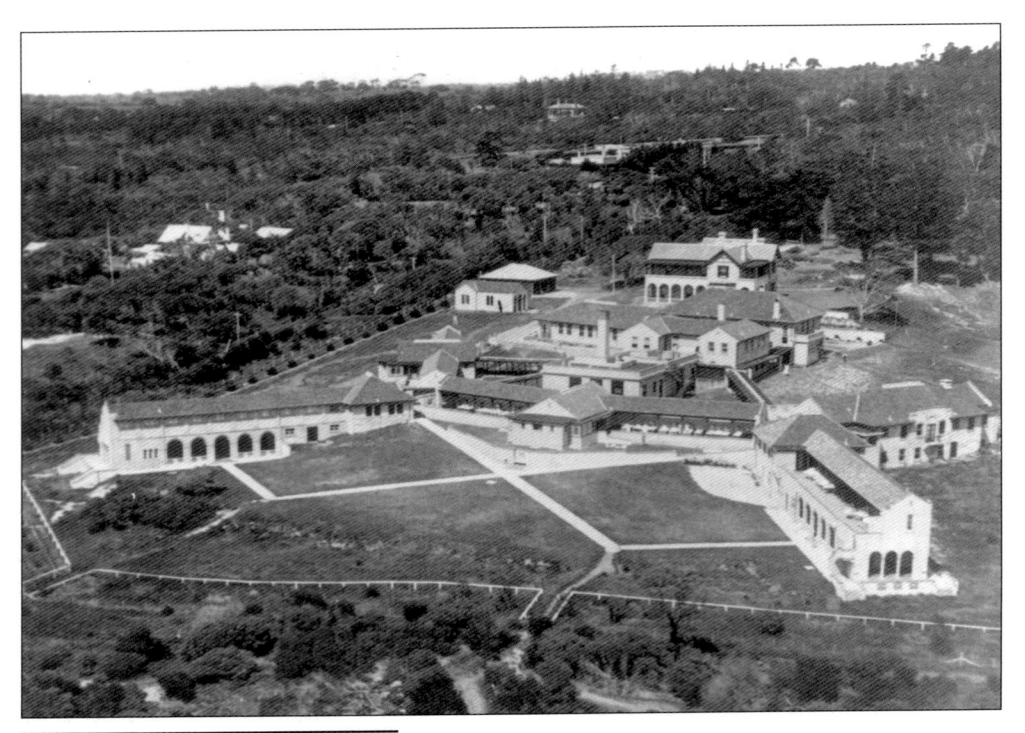

Frankston Orthopaedic Section ('Beachleigh', the old Nurses' Home in the background).
La Trobe Collection, State Library of Victoria.

other surgical disciplines, improved anaesthetics and knowledge of the technique of asepsis opened new horizons in this specialty. Since early times, children had been diagnosed with tuberculous bones at the Children's Hospital, but the epidemics of poliomyelitis in 1908, 1926, 1931 and 1937–38 focussed greater attention on the 'crippled' child. These decades spawned alternative medicine, cranks, quacks and theories.

The Frankston years

Not all the nurses spent time at Hampton and Sherbrooke, but they did have a compulsory rotation to Frankston, usually three months at the end of the first or at the beginning of their second year. Bon Winstanley began her nursing at the Children's in 1936 when she was eighteen years old. 'I was sent to the Frankston Orthopaedic Section of the Hospital from Brighton, a very different type of nursing with the children having dreadful cases of tubercular spinal conditions and osteomyelitis that had to be dressed daily.' They were mainly on frames or [in] splints, to be turned regularly. Clothing consisted of cotton triangles tied at the hips and the

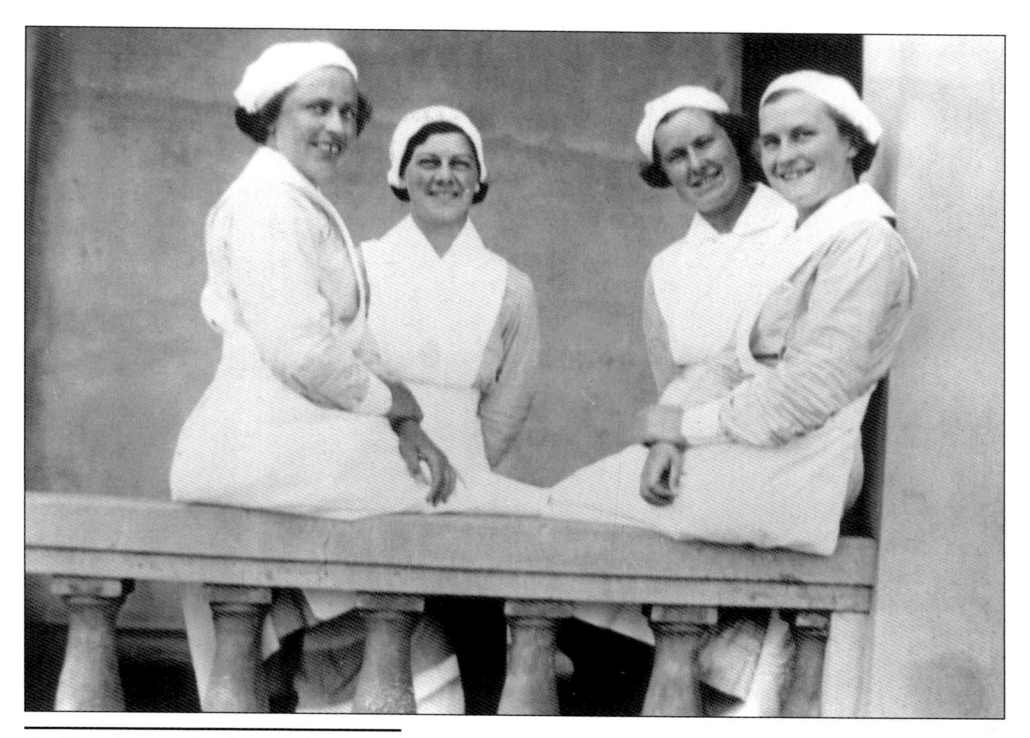

At Frankston Orthopaedic Section, Nurses' Home. *L–R:* Fay Hollow, Marjorie Vance, Beatrice Wilson, Hope Clark.
RCHA/Menzies Family Collection.

children were exposed to the sun and fresh air during suitable weather conditions. For the nurses, the close proximity of the beach was most attractive on their hours off.[2]

The Orthopaedic Hospital, sited on a twenty-two-acre property, 'Beachleigh', on the picturesque Ranleigh Estate on the Mornington Peninsula, was purpose-built. The architects emulated the European ideal of a mountain sanatorium resort for those with tuberculous dispositions, but there the similarity ended. The buildings, in the modern Spanish Mission style so popular in Melbourne in the 1920s and 1930s, had sun-drenched pavilions branching off a central administration block with breathtaking views of Port Phillip Bay. In winter, the pavilions were bitterly cold.[3]

In April 1930, the residents of Frankston and Mornington were the guests of the Hospital President, Mrs Lauchlan Mackinnon, with a view to forming a branch of the Children's Hospital Auxiliary. The *Argus* reported that the new Orthopaedic Section opened with all the most modern equipment, accommodation, electric power, heat and steam. 'The kitchens are heated from burning oil on the same principle used in the engine rooms of a battle ship and ocean liner.'[4]

Due to the depression, the Orthopaedic Section was partly opened with forty-four beds in 1930. By 1933, eighty-eight beds were fully occupied. Many of the children required very long-term care and treatment of between one and five years.

The Frankston branch provided an opportunity for nurses to move out of the high pressure of Carlton. Three months' rotation—often extended to six—was regarded by some as a holiday. First-year exams were over and, not knowing what to expect, the prospect was an adventure. Wearing full uniform, one or two nurses at a time were driven to Frankston by Fred Morgan, the hospital driver, in the small hospital ambulance. He always had a few children on board.

Mary Brodribb recalled: 'We enjoyed the fresh air and lots of sunshine with the patients, as every day their beds were wheeled into the sun. Off duty, we could go to the beach or, as some of us did, walk into Frankston (four miles) for the day.'[5] For most nurses, it was usual to spend days off swimming or sunbaking at Half Moon or Canadian Bay, or in winter, to go walking. The beach was accessible by a steep path down the cliff. As usual, where young women congregate, difficulties were encountered: 'peeping Toms' and 'flashers' on the beach. In the summer of 1936, a bathing box was built for nurses and female professional staff.[6] Most nurses enjoyed the relaxed atmosphere, the fresh air, the nourishing food in a modern new dining room, and the luxury and privacy of individual rooms in the Nurses' Home. Permission was given to hold a dance in the new dining room and the Lord Somers League offered to pay for a tennis court in the grounds, provided nurses always had first call on its use.[7]

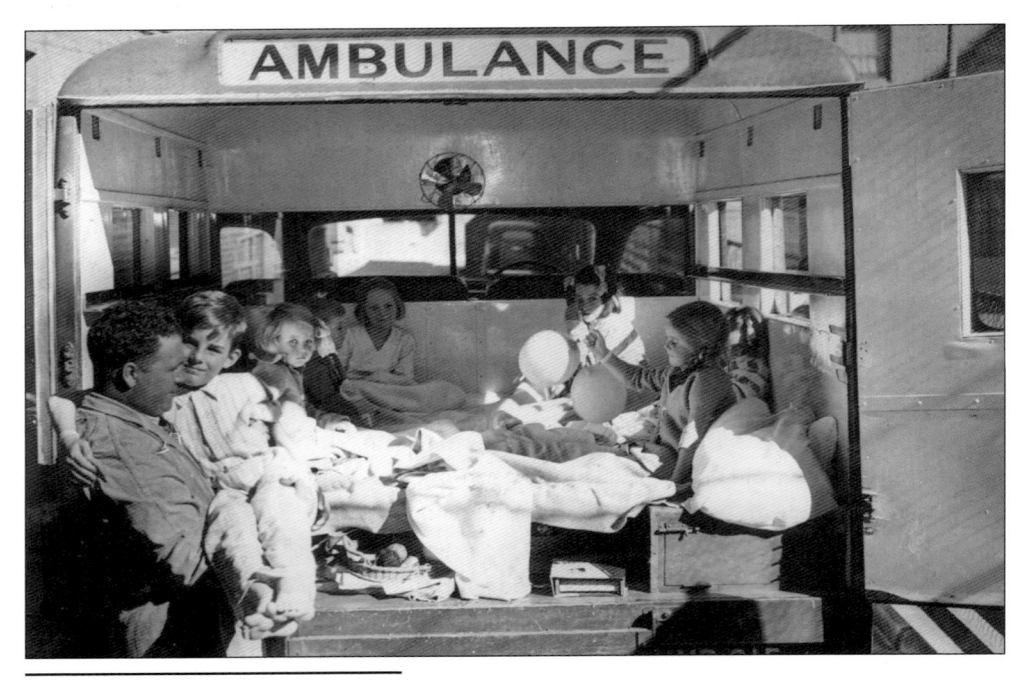

Ambulance to Frankston and Hampton, c. 1947.

Those few months were a restful interlude between the Children's at Carlton and the world of adult nursing at the Women's, Prince Henry's and, after 1939, the Royal Melbourne Hospital. Health was restored, the stresses and strains of life at Carlton were eased, and spirits were raised.

The children

Margaret Warr remembers nursing at Frankston in the late 1930s. There were about one hundred child patients, victims of tuberculous disease of the bones (particularly the hip), osteomyelitis, congenital deformities of the hips and feet, and some in recovery from poliomyelitis.[8] Each ward had about twenty children in various states of immobilisation. Some surgery was carried out in the modern operating theatre, but most operations were conducted at Carlton. The Charge Sisters generally reinforced plasters from wear and tear, a procedure carried out in the plaster room.

Children with primary and acute miliary tuberculosis, tuberculous bronchopneumonia, pleurisy, intestinal or peritoneal tuberculosis and bronchiectasis, tuberculosis of the trachea, larynx and tuberculous meningitis were not treated at Frankston. Often gravely ill, they were treated (in the late 1940s and early 1950s) with streptomycin by IM injection in conjunction with para-amino-salicylic acid (PAS).

The work at Frankston was extremely heavy; there were no lifting machines. Transferring children to trolleys, changing beds, toileting, carrying children to grassy areas for picnics, moving beds on to the balconies and generally assisting in every way, were all tasks that took a tremendous toll on nurses' physical strength. The children could be demanding, for they were not acutely sick and constantly planning tricks. Many manoeuvred their trolleys down garden paths and corridors to the alarm of the staff. Despite their immobilisation, they made complicated pulleys with string from bed to bed to send messages to each other. In some cases, unwanted food found its way down these chutes.

The fetish for fresh air, rest and continuous exposure to sunshine, known as heliotherapy was, by the standard of today, carried to extremes. A disciple of the method, Dr John Colquhoun was recruited as Medical Superintendent from Scotland in 1928. A tough, stocky man, he was reported by the *Argus* on his arrival in Australia on 5 December 1929:

> The sad effects of infantile paralysis, osteomyelitis and tuberculosis can be seen every day in every country of the world. It is by carefully planned treatment, the use of sun and fresh air combined with scientific adjustments of the joints and bones of the little sufferers, and the applications of modern methods that we hope to reduce the number of cripples.

The nurses were not usually aware of the current orthodoxies and controversies swirling around in medical circles regarding the treatment of children with disabilities, commonly called 'cripples'. They did notice the Spartan conditions: one thin red blanket in all weathers on the open pavilions was particularly upsetting when they found the small children covered in dew in the morning. But nurses were not known for making a stand on any matter. In December 1933, a brave teacher, Miss Collier, wrote a long letter to the President, Lady Latham, charging exposure to the cold. The President investigated but did not think there was any substance to the complaints. Dr Colquhoun stated 'that the absence of colds was proof that there were no ill effects from exposure which is part of the treatment of the types of cases at the Orthopaedic Section'.[9] Miss Collier was found not suitable or sympathetic to the philosophy of the institution; she left to be replaced by Miss Doble as head teacher.

Nurses also suffered from exposure. The canvas blinds were down in winter but their legs and feet became so cold and wet with driving rain, that Matron Laidlaw suggested gumboots. Finally, the Committee resolved that two pairs of rubber snow boots be purchased for each ward, for trial purposes, for the nurses.

Generally, the staff was unaware of the terror and loneliness experienced by the children. Former patients now grown to adulthood have related their experiences as children at the Frankston Orthopaedic Hospital where practices had barely changed over thirty years. Inez Ferguson remembers her time in 1960 vividly. She suffered and cried from hip pain when she was nine, and was taken to the Children's Hospital on a Friday, because that was the day her brother attended an Out-patient Clinic for a cardiac condition. She was admitted to the Orthopaedic Section of the Children's Hospital that night. Variously diagnosed as Perthes disease and arthritis but likely to be 'growing pains', her condition was never satisfactorily explained.

Her family lived at Richmond, and Inez remembers how difficult it was for her mother to visit in those days:

> She had to get the train from Richmond where we lived to the city, and then to Frankston. There was only one bus on Sunday [from the Frankston station] and I only ever saw her on Sunday—the visiting hours were between two and four, just once a week. Mum said, 'if you missed that, you just didn't get a bus. There was only one, that was it.' And if she didn't walk in that door at 2 o'clock—it wasn't like it is today where you can come and go at any time—you would be in tears because you would think: where was Mum? You would think Mum had forgotten you.

Inez's plaster was up to the middle of the armpits 'so you couldn't sit and you couldn't stand. It was a one-and-a-half plaster full on the left leg and a half on the right with a bar across.' Inez could not go to the toilet. It was the bedpan or nothing. She recalled: 'We had a little bikini, I called it. Privacy! I still have a problem to this day when I am in Hospital, because I have this mental block, I can't use the pan. If anyone's there, I just switch off. I can't remember the first experience but with me, they just rolled me over on my side and I can remember being frightened that if they pushed me too far I would roll off the bed.' Because they were only single beds, she remembers thinking 'they are going to push me too far, and it was a fair height'.[10]

She remembers the long corridor and, in the middle, the nurses' station: 'Towards the left side was for the under-teenage years and towards the right side were the older girls over thirteen. But how they got on I don't know because that is a very personal time in anybody's life.'

It is easier to understand why children of earlier decades (before antibiotics and public health strategies were introduced) endured restrictive visiting hours. Although they were bright and physically active, the isolation was in keeping with contemporary notions of separation from sources of infection. In most cases, at least one parent or relative living in the house had tuberculosis.[11]

The Medical Superintendent of the Carlton Hospital referred to the very bad conditions existing in Melbourne at that time regarding the disease. His report to the Committee was startling: a very large majority of the tubercular cases at the Orthopaedic Section was the result of direct infection from parents, whilst the whole of the twenty-four children who died from tubercular meningitis in the hospital during the 1938/39 financial year had contracted the disease from their parents.[12]

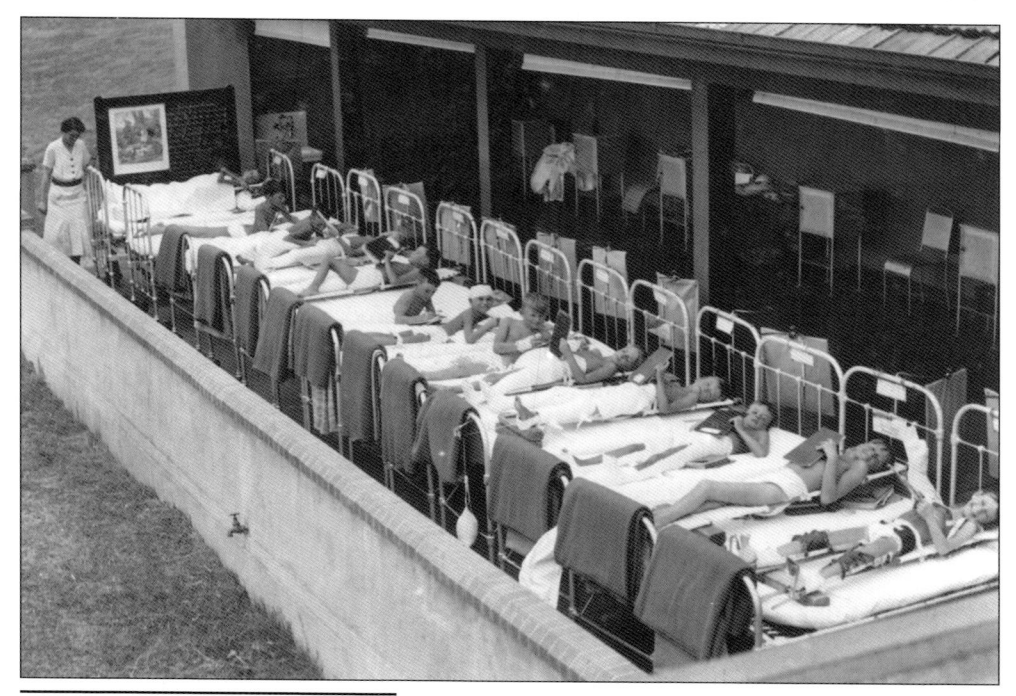

Boys in school: Frankston Orthopaedic Section, c. 1930s.

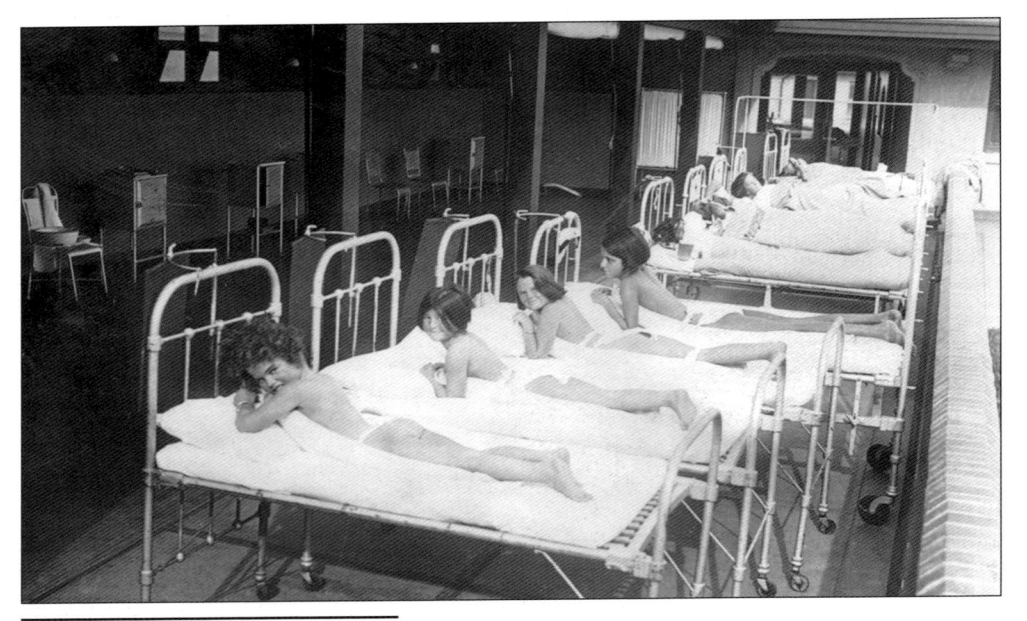

Girls segregated from the boys, enjoying the sun on the balcony. Frankston Orthopaedic Hospital, 1940s.

During the polio epidemic of 1937, Dr Galbraith relaxed the visiting rules, permitting restricted visiting of parents to Frankston as the prolonged and excessive quarantine was becoming a hardship to them. He suggested a rope barrier to be placed from post to post down the centre of the ward in order to separate visitors from patients.[13]

School helped to pass the day; the introduction of craft workers (later occupational therapy), massage for the polio patients and salt baths became routine. This was the beginning of the era of allied health specialists.

Dr Galbraith was very fussy about the segregation of boys and girls. The ages were staggered in order of the oldest to the youngest, and boys and girls were not to be on the craft hostel property together. He thoroughly disapproved of noise on the Sabbath but finally compromised: 'children were to be quiet until midday'.[14]

Nurses were kind. With no formal instruction about the psychological needs of the children, they instinctively became friendly and loving to the children. Gradually, they were aware of the practices and biases of one or two Sisters-in-Charge. The most controversial issue was the punishment of an occasionally 'naughty' child for refusing food or for cheekiness—they were put on the balcony all alone at night. The Night Nurse felt very sorry for the child and 'just tucked it [the blanket] a little more snug around the shoulders'.[15] The definition of 'naughty' was never really established. The children who lay flat on their backs on a Stryker bed or a Bradford frame had no

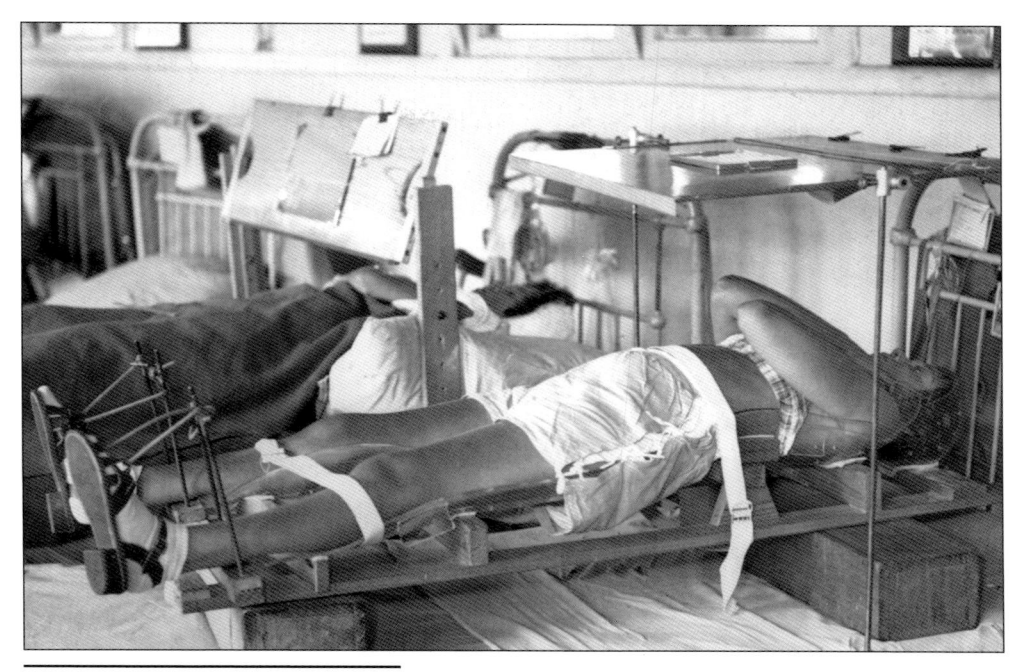

Child in Bradford frame (note the foot traction). Mid-1940s.

relief but for the attention of the nurses and the daily turn, communicating to each other by mirrors, little notes and paper darts they threw around the room. The children were completely at the mercy of those caring for them.

The unrelentingly boring food related to the nutritional practices and beliefs of the day that children should have very large amounts of calcium. When Dr J. G. Whittaker reviewed all his cases of bone and joint tuberculosis under treatment in the Hospital, he was so disappointed with the rate of healing and new bone formation that he arranged to operate only on six patients and a possible additional four, 'but to wait a while'. As several months went by, the X-ray results were impressive. Dr Whittaker had been so much impressed with the improvement shown in that period that he decided not to operate on any of them. He expressed the conviction that the increase in the supply of milk (two pints each a day) and eggs (the bone-forming materials) had been the deciding factor in bringing about the results.[16] This was not always the preferred treatment, and it was even sometimes controversial; an excessive incidence of renal calculi was a risk in children immobilised for months or years.

Kind people donated thousands of dozens of eggs; every school and Scout group, Brownies, Guides, Clubs and street stalls had egg collections. This went on for many years. Consequently, children had eggs twice a day and most hated them. Inez Ferguson tells of her experience:

There was one nurse—I remember…one night, we had tea about 5 o'clock…and then Milo or Ovaltine, something like that, and maybe half a sandwich for supper. One nurse came along and I said, what is in that sandwich and she said 'egg'.

I said, 'I don't like egg'.

'You have to eat it, you do'.

I was so determined I was not going to have it and she was determined I was…a struggle ensued. Maybe she was having a bad day. Maybe I was having a bad day. I can laugh now, looking back.

The warmer weather was welcome but Inez has another outstanding horror memory of her years at Frankston: she developed a real phobia of the huge Bogong moths and Christmas beetles which swarmed each evening and throughout the night, filling the open balcony, the wards and crawling into the beds. The children encased in plaster were not able to defend themselves from the flapping, monstrous sized pests that crawled up and over the bedposts, onto their faces and in their hair.

Her terrified calls and screams received a response: 'They won't hurt you.' Inez has remained terrified of moths in her adult life, and to this day hides in corners from the tiniest insect.[17]

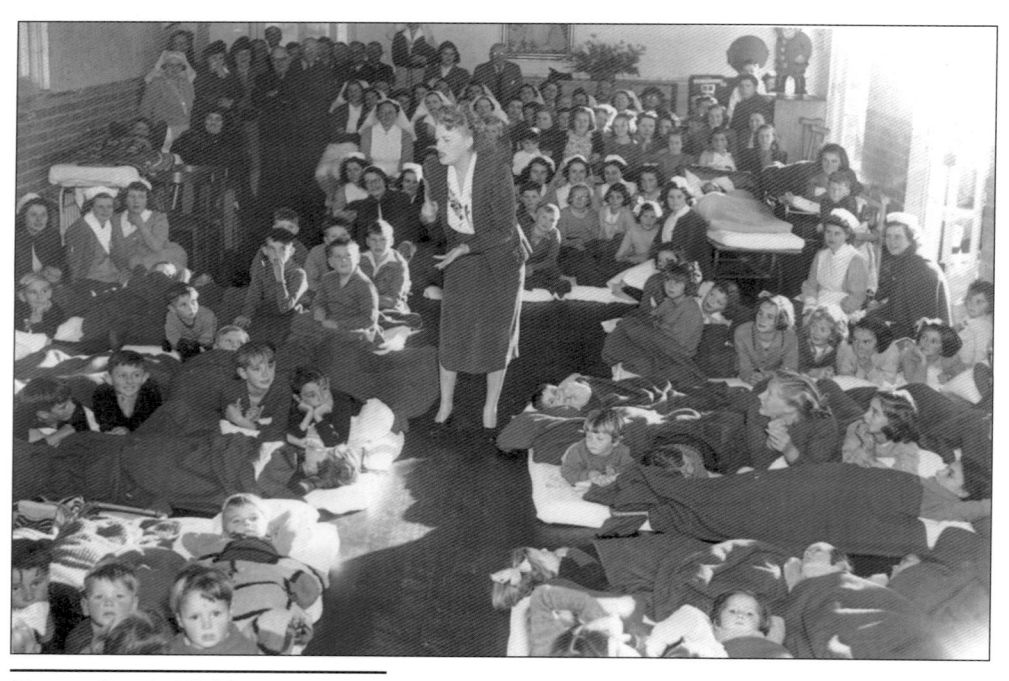

Singer Gracie Fields entertains the children at Frankston Orthopaedic Hospital, 1945.

Nursing Disabled Children

The daily routine—nursing at Frankston

The trainees worked under the direction of the Ward Sisters in Wards 1 to 6 and with Ward Assistants (nursing aides) carried out the cleaning, scrubbing canvas frames, lacing and unlacing splints, attending children on Bradford frames and Thomas splints, feeding, toileting and sponging: these were shared tasks. Nurses administered the basic medicines: para-amino-salicylic acid (PAS) isoniazid (INS), streptomycin, aperients, cough mixtures and gentian violet tablets (for threadworms).

There were few lectures. Because they were doing the menial tasks and the dirty work, nurses believed they had little status and were equated with housemaids. A major task was keeping plasters clean from urine and faeces; many children had threadworms and the girls often had urine infections.

They rarely saw members of the administration and did not know what was happening at other branches. There were no Hospital newsletters or bulletins. They relied on each other for companionship.

Peg Orford remembers there was virtually no social life: 'At Mt Eliza [Frankston] we worked thirty days with three days off. On night duty there was not a lot to do—regular checks on the children, do a round, comfort them, tuck them in.'[18] In 1940, she remembers it as an eerie place; by design each ward looked over the sea; one wing had a swimming pool, and in the moonlight it was all rather ghostly. A certain Sister always wished to stand on the balcony and look at the stars. Ward Sisters had generally been there a very long time and, in the opinion of some, 'too long'. Una Wishart hated it. 'It was heavy [work] and so smelly under those plasters'. She thought the Sisters were hard on the nurses. 'Perhaps the senior staff had their own way too long. It was despicable.'[19] She recalled: 'A Sister laid traps: she put bits of paper in tubing to test if we cleaned properly. Cleaning was a must in those days. I remember we did a lot on night duty. We were not amused!' A night duty nurse told how, in the morning, Sister would come and pick up the blotting paper and hold it up to the light to see if she had been writing letters on duty, or 'hide a bit of fluff behind the steriliser in case you did not clean there. Of course, word got around so you would be sure to do it. They set out to more or less trick you.'[20]

The physiotherapy profession was in its infancy and Dr Galbraith stated that he had commenced to train 'intelligent' nurses to take over some of the actual physiotherapy treatment. In 1938 he recommended a Certificate of Orthopaedic Nursing 'only if he could find some nurses capable of doing this!' By then a fifty-hour week was being implemented and the number of nursing assistants increased. Matron Laidlaw disapproved because of the cost.

ANNIE INA LAIDLAW, Matron of the Frankston Orthopaedic Hospital, 1930–42 and 1945–50.

Ina Laidlaw came from the Western District in Victoria and began her nursing career in 1913 at the Children's Hospital. In June 1917 she joined the Australian Army Nursing Service. At the end of the war, she resumed her civilian career and became Assistant Matron and then Matron of the Orthopaedic Hospital at Frankston. In 1942, she was head of the Royal Australian Naval Nursing Service (RANNS), appointed to the rank of Lieutenant Commander and assisted with the recruitment of qualified nurses as RANNS officers. The service began with twelve Sisters from Melbourne and twelve from Sydney and grew to a total of sixty. At the end of the war, she returned to her position at the Orthopaedic Hospital until 1950. She then took the position of Home Sister to the Queen Elizabeth Hospital for Children in London, returning to Australia as Resident Matron of the Freemasons' Homes of Victoria and retired in 1957.[21]

The Orthopaedic Certificate course began with an intake of twelve but ceased at the beginning of the war. Dr Elizabeth McComas, the first female surgeon to graduate from Liverpool University, returned to Frankston in 1939 and re-commenced the course with nurses drawn mostly from other hospitals, including the Alfred. Unfortunately, the course ceased altogether at the end of the war for lack of funding.

Hampton and infantile paralysis

The Brighton Cottage was first established in 1884 to accommodate fifteen children and was burned down in 1909. When new accommodation was found in Beach Road, Hampton, the demand was so great that the house was enlarged to twenty-five beds for children with tuberculous bone and joint disease, osteomyelitis and rheumatic heart disease. The main treatment was heliotherapy and salt baths, the therapeutic seaside holidays being popular at the time. Children were accommodated for other reasons: complete rest, sunshine and nourishing food in the aftermath of debilitating illness. In 1937, the impact of the poliomyelitis epidemic changed this focus.

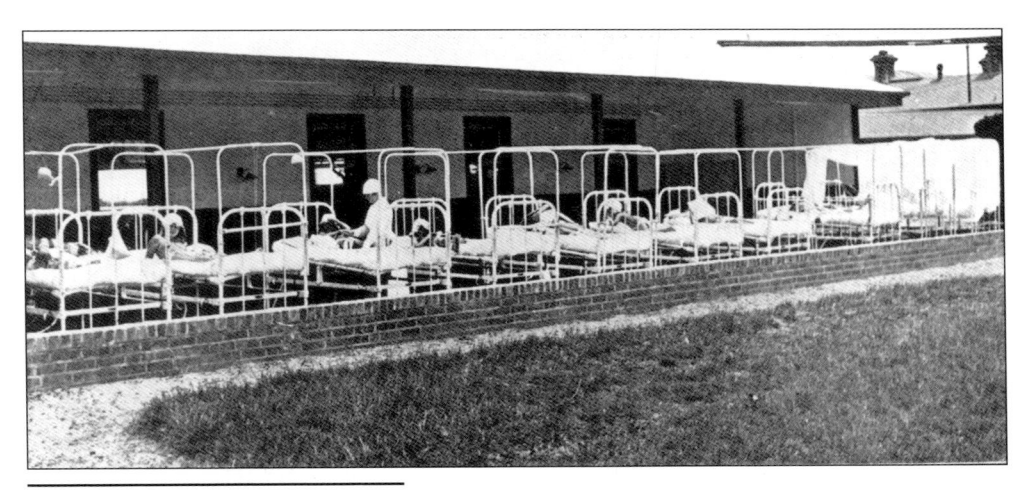

Hampton Convalescent Cottage, 1930s.

It would be difficult to exaggerate the fear of infantile paralysis in the epidemic of 1937–38. People stayed indoors, theatres and schools were closed and children were segregated on trains. Many patients were sent to the Frankston Hospital where a new ward was built for the purpose and the Committee received a grant for a new building at Hampton.

Staff members were vulnerable. Dr Jean Macnamara asked for an increase in pay for physiotherapists to compensate for the risks associated in attending infectious patients and for the isolated life they led. There was no such advocate for the nurses.

Nurse Hope Clark, six weeks from her final exams, was taken ill with extensive paralysis and nearly died. Her brother, Manning Clark, wrote of the profound impact of her illness:

> In the second half of 1937 infantile paralysis broke out in Melbourne. Of the many children stricken by the infection, most survived. The adults were not so fortunate. My mother told me my sister Hope, then a nurse at the Children's Hospital in Carlton, had caught infantile paralysis. Within a few days, complications set in…her face swelled up to the size of a soccer ball. The doctors talked of death. We were at a loss with neither medical nor surgical answers to the problem. Father and Russell were convulsed with grief…I said not a word, believing that we were all in the presence of something which we did not understand.[22]

Hope spent three years in the Infectious Diseases Ward 16 where two trained nurses were allocated to 'special' her (give one-to-one nursing on a 24-hour basis) under the supervision of Dr Jean Macnamara. She made an almost full recovery and was discharged in June 1940. Six years later, she took her final exams.

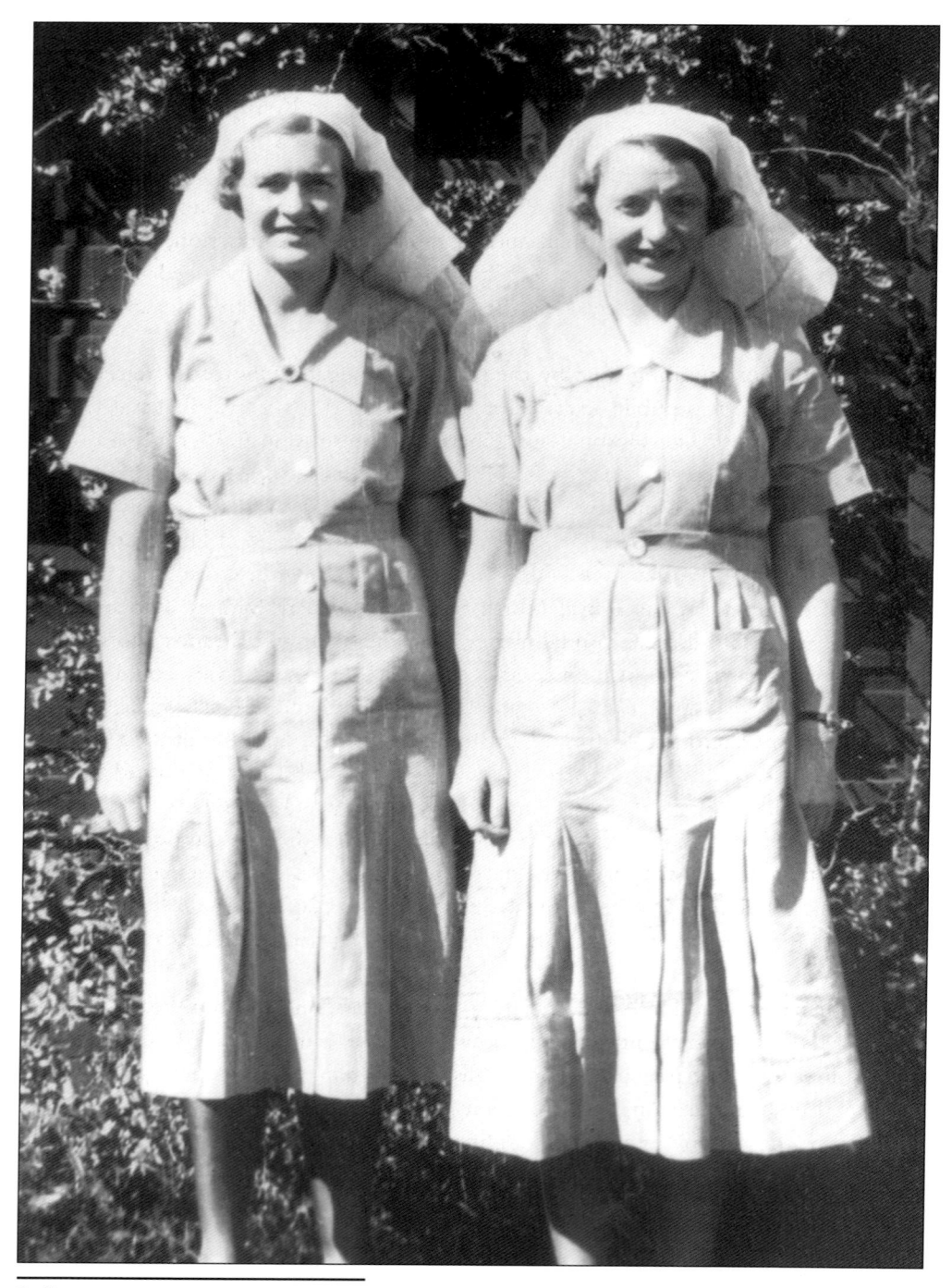

Polio nurses at Hampton. *L–R:* Thyra Thomas (née Watson) and Eleanor Moss (née Peck), 1937.
RCHA/Moss Family Collection.

Alternative treatments

Dr Jean Macnamara had a well-established system of treatment and aftercare for infantile paralysis when attention was diverted to Elizabeth Kenny.

Elizabeth Kenny (1880–1952) was born at Warialda in Queensland. An untrained bush nurse, she became famous for her unconventional and unscientific methods in the treatment of poliomyelitis, then known as infantile paralysis. Central to the controversy was the treatment and recovery of muscle function, the contradiction between long periods of immobilisation in splints and the need to provide solutions to enable patients to lead useful lives, therefore preventing deformity and crippling.

The orthodox splinting used by the medical profession was totally rejected by Kenny, but so wide was public acclaim for her method that the Hospital was forced to declare an interest. The Hospital and Charities Commission in Victoria arranged for a team to work at the Hampton Convalescent Home where the Children's Hospital had allowed twenty-two beds for children with infantile paralysis. The *Herald* of 30 November 1937 carried a headline announcing that six nurses had been elected by the Infantile Paralysis After-care Committee to study the Sister Kenny method of treatment at the Royal North Shore Hospital in Sydney. Two of these were Melbourne Children's Hospital nurses, Thyra Thomas and Eleanor Moss.

This became a problem because the Children's Hospital nurses could not be registered in New South Wales, despite having completed their training to the satisfaction of the Victorian Nurses' Board and completed six months at the Epworth Hospital.[23] Thyra and Eleanor did not go to Royal North Shore and instead trained on the job at Hampton with two Kenny nurses sent from Queensland.

Public panic was high and nobody wanted nurses in contact with polio patients. There was no accommodation for the extra nurses and, as a consequence, they were forced to board at the local hotel for a week. A couple eventually took them in as boarders where they shared a bed-sitting room, had their own kitchen and shared a bathroom.

Dr Eric Price and Dr Wilfred Forster supervised the nurses from the Children's, and the Medical Superintendent came down from the old Carlton Hospital once a week to look over the patients. Thyra recalls: 'I must admit he was not sympathetic. However, I enjoyed [learning] the treatment. It was very intense.'

Under the Kenny method no splints were applied but orthodox medical intervention prevailed when a patient with neck paralysis wore a brace at all times. A few wore night splints on hands and feet to prevent wrist and foot drop. All the beds had an upright board attached to the foot, and children were to keep their feet firmly against the foot of the bed.

For the nurses, it was not an easy job to keep children in that position. Treatment consisted of assisted slow, passive movements to all affected limbs first thing in the morning. The nurses explained at all times what they were doing: 'I am bending your knee, I am straightening your knee, now you try.' Each movement was repeated three times. Later, the child was plunged into a bath with alternative hot and cold sprays to the affected limbs.[24]

All the patients were supposed to stay in bed. When the nurses went out of the room, the children would get out of bed and run around. Some had to be fed. All were wheeled on to the veranda, weather permitting, and bed clothes were kept to a minimum. Visiting hours were similar to those of the patients in other wards.

What was most impressive was the total lack of pain and stiffness compared to the splinted patients as the affected limbs were exercised three times each day.

Unfortunately, this treatment became too expensive to maintain with its almost one-to-one nursing and was discontinued after 1939. It was an experiment for all, because Sister Kenny had treated only long-term cases of paralysis and none in the acute stage.

Thyra describes her training days:

> We had to go up to Melbourne University to Prof. Wright to look at bodies, the muscles. We hadn't learned that before we went down [to Hampton], while we were still at the Hospital. We just stood around and he, Prof. Wright, showed us the corpse in a similar way to the medical students.

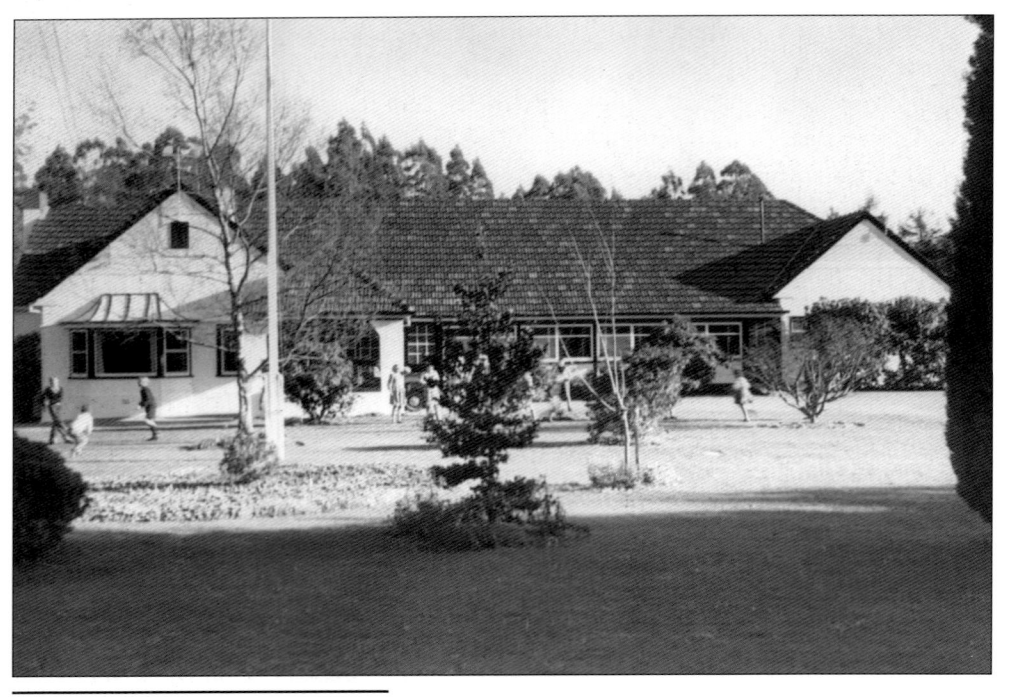

Sherbrooke Convalescent Cottage, 1938.

Thyra thought Sister Kenny was a very public-minded person, attracting a lot of attention. Well-known in Queensland, she nevertheless fought for recognition. Aggressive in her manner, she had the impression the doctors were pressured into trying her method. They were very polite. Eleanor and Thyra saw the final report of the evaluation commissioned by the Hospital Committee. This result was inconclusive, with no discernable difference.[25]

In December 1938, the Committee of Management discussed the future of the Sister Kenny Unit at Hampton; the Honorary staff requested that the Infantile Paralysis After-care Committee take over the unit but the government intervened requesting that the Kenny Unit continue. The Hospital agreed and retained it until August 1939.

Sherbrooke

The peaceful setting of 'Sherbrooke Forest' was a home away from home for many frail Melbourne children. The house, built for Mr Charles Wilson on his twenty-two-acre property, was offered to the Children's Hospital in memory of his handicapped nephew who died at the age of twenty-one. Mr Wilson continued to live next door with his two sisters.

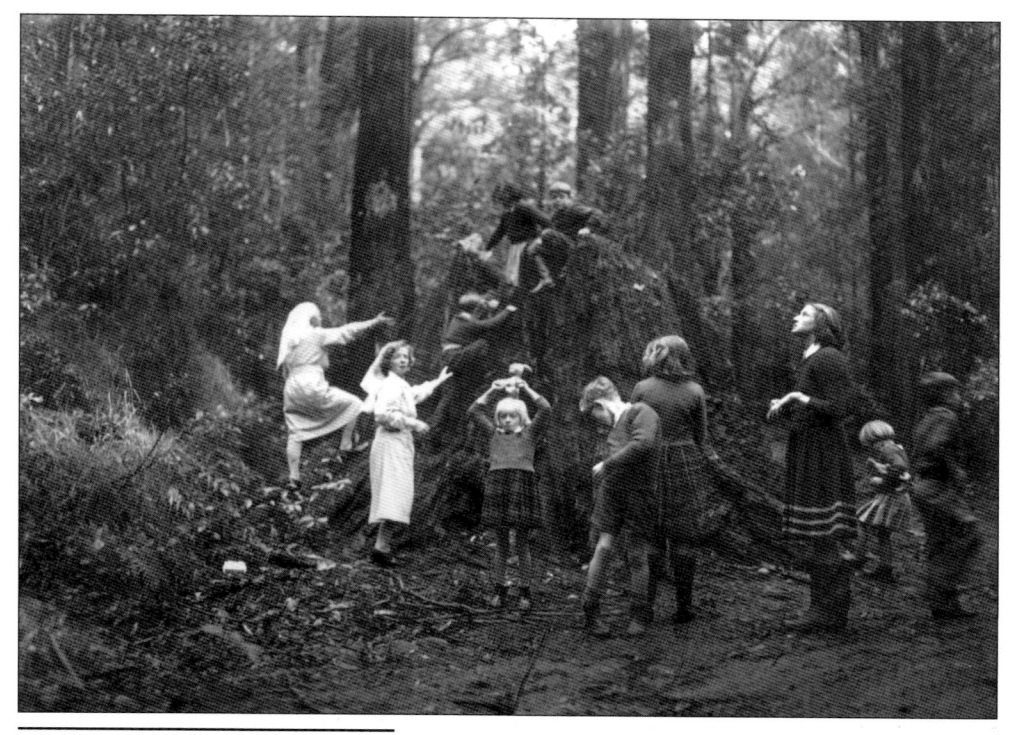

City children taking a nature walk in Sherbrooke Forest, c. 1947.

The Cottage also became a firm favourite with the Ladies' Committee. Lady Murdoch donated a radio and sandals for the children and Mrs Higgins, a football and football boots for the boys. Mrs Isabel Nicholas of 'Burnham Beeches' arranged for fresh produce to be sent over from the kitchen gardens. With publicity gained by Vice-regal patronage—Lady Huntingfield, the Governor's wife, officially opened the Cottage on 19 December 1936—future success and interest from locals were assured.

Only those children who were up and about or well enough to be up and dressed were recommended for transfer from Carlton. The children were usually recovering from chronic chest infections, rheumatic heart disease and lack of adequate nourishment. The fresh food and clean, crisp air of the Dandenongs saved many from a lifetime of illness. Before the days of antibiotics, these children had little chance of complete recovery, suffering recurrent infections. Ann Milburn, a Children's Hospital trainee and experienced bush nurse, was an excellent choice to take charge, not only for her love and understanding of children, but also as 'an admirably suitable person having regard to her housekeeping experience'.[26]

The Cottage became Ann Milburn's home and the children, her surrogate family. She gained great pleasure introducing to the bush the children from impoverished circumstances. With tender care and the companionship of the local staff, the Seamer family of Monbulk and Mick Drury, the general handyman, the Cottage became a home away from home. The average number of children there was between twelve and sixteen and all were capable of taking long walks in the forest. In the early days, Sister Milburn did care for one baby but it was found to be too disruptive and needed one-to-one care. No more babies were transferred, probably because the Committee was not able to pay for an extra staff nurse. An additional challenge was the time taken socialising disturbed children separated from their families.

Despite the air of normality about the house, the Hospital authorities still insisted the children be dressed in red flannel jackets and grey trousers on outings and entertainments. It was not unusual to see the house Sister in full uniform and veil with her conspicuous little band of red-jacketed children walking in the forest.

During the war, Sisters Hazel Belfrage, Jane Arthur, Nurse Chalmers and others were seconded from the branches at Frankston and Hampton, while Ann Milburn took the overall responsibility for the whole complex: 'Burnham Beeches', Sherbrooke and the nurses' accommodation at Marybrooke.

Very few nurses ever saw the Sherbrooke Cottage until the evacuation during the war. It closed in 1952, having outlived its usefulness. Ann Milburn was transferred to Frankston until retirement.

By 15 December 1938, all nurses except those in the Baby Wards at Carlton were working a forty-eight-hour week. The President, Lady Latham, suggested that members of the Auxiliaries should train as Voluntary Aid Detachments in case of war, as many nurses would no doubt enlist and she would prefer that the Hospital draw up war contingency plans. On 4 March 1939, twenty-four trainees began as volunteer assistant nurses in the Hospital and a course of first aid and gas precautions commenced on 8 March, the latter being limited to sixty persons.

However, life for the nurses remained comparatively peaceful. Margaret Warr, then nursing at Frankston Orthopaedic Section, summed up her memories of that time:

> A never-to-be-forgotten sight, I remember brought back to mind the fact that we were at war: an early winter's sunset with a line of naval vessels slipping down the Bay on their way to action.[27]

The authorities soon moved the children from Frankston to several spots in the Sherbrooke area, 'the babies…were at the Convalescent Cottage, the Orthopaedic children to 'Burnham Beeches', the lovely home of the Nicholas Aspro family, and the nurses lived at 'Marybrooke', a guest house taken over for the duration of the war.

ANN MILBURN trained at the Children's Hospital in the 1920s and worked with the Victorian Bush Nursing Association in the Otways before taking charge of the Children's Hospital Convalescent Cottage at Sherbrooke. She was Matron there from 1936 to 1952. Many of the children became very attached to Ann, returning to visit her as adults, particularly some of the young men who joined up, making a special trip while on leave. After her death, a memorial was established by the people of the Dandenongs at St George's Uniting Church, Monbulk, as a tribute to her work: a beautiful window incorporating Ann's name entwined with the Children's Hospital Nurses' badge.[28]

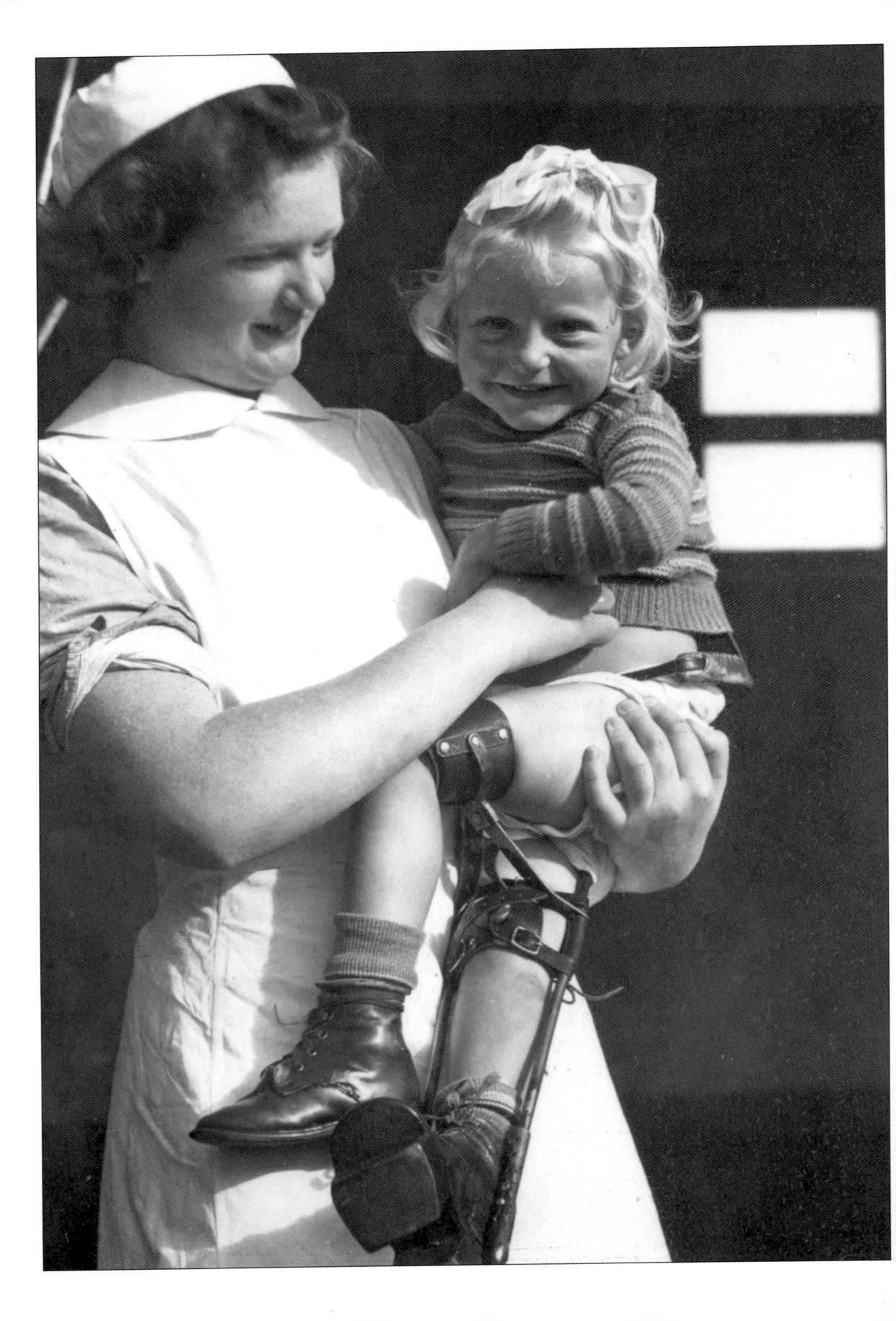

CHAPTER 9

The Years of World War Two
1939–1947

World War Two halted progress in many ways. Essential services were disrupted when nurses, doctors and other personnel joined the forces. Emergency plans were introduced in an atmosphere of anxiety and uncertainty; no one was sure what to expect.

Lady Latham first raised the issue of planning for an emergency as early as December 1938 and introduced the idea that Auxiliaries should train as assistants and Voluntary Aid Detachments (VADs). In case of war, many nurses would no doubt enlist and she preferred the Hospital provide its own rather than rely on others.[1] The newly appointed Tutor, Sister Isabel Pilkington, was asked to give First Aid lectures to a group of volunteers connected to the Committee of Management. Isabel said 'it was, in fact, a futile exercise. The women were completely unaware of what would be required. They were quite unused to, and resentful of, any discipline, [were] irregular in attendance, and of course in a situation where they had to be handled with great tact.' The exercise did not last very long: 'fortunately they found it more difficult than they had imagined…' She gave lectures to the trained staff about air-raids, a subject, she said, 'about which I knew nothing, an agonizing experience'.[2]

A Hospital Special Emergency Committee met on 4 September 1939 and decided that the bayside port area was vulnerable and that the Frankston

---

Nurse Jill Harris Stainsby with child in a Thomas splint, 1940s.
RCHA/Catto Smith Family Collection.

Orthopaedic Branch should be relocated. Lady Latham suggested Sherbrooke was suitable for relocation of the children should it become necessary.[3] This seemed rather curious as the emergency was in Europe.[4]

Despite the ageing of the Hospital and the crowded, old-fashioned and inadequate buildings, the Nursing School was progressing well. In 1938, a small trial Preliminary Training School was introduced under the direction of Sister Jessie Morrison assisted by Isabel Pilkington. Isabel had always wanted to teach and regarded this as a 'God-given opportunity'. With hindsight, she realised that she lacked wide experience and probably would have benefited from seeking more adult and other experience before embarking on this path. She remembers 'there was at this time considerable criticism that the Children's Hospital was a recognised training school' and was aware that her position was under constant scrutiny when she attended meetings of tutors from other hospitals. This put considerable pressure on her, although she believes she made a small but worthwhile contribution to the training of the student nurses 'because I was eager and dedicated, and I had that natural ability to impart my knowledge to other people'.

Isabel also paid tribute to Sister Agnes Morris, in charge of the Baby Wards (1925–50):

> She had been a superb Charge Sister…it is to her I still look in gratitude for what she taught me, not only by instruction, but also by example, never being hurried, irritated or rude. The babies were cared for superbly, the medical staff given every help and consideration and the ward administration seemed flawless.[5]

In December of that year, Joan Gendle came top of the State Final Examinations. All nurses except those in the Baby Wards worked a 48-hour week. In May 1939, the Hospital received accreditation with the Nurses' Registration Board as a general training school.[6]

In January 1940, Noel Holcombe (née Heley) was one of the first of twelve girls to start in the first four-week Preliminary Training School. On her first day, she was ushered into a three-bed room in 'Extension A' built on the Nurses' Home. This room, above the kitchen, had a constant odour of cabbage and became known as the 'Cabbage Room'. Isabel Pilkington was their Tutor: 'so considerate of girls starting their training'. Noel remembers, 'We learnt rules, how to make hospital beds and babies' cots, do correct corners and quilts with the Red Cross all in place, how to take temperatures and record these, how to feed babies, change napkins, bath and sponge children and babies.' If a thermometer was broken, it was: 'report to Matron'. They had tests at the end of each week and spent time in the wards 'watching, doing and learning under Pilks' kind eye'.[7]

The evening of 19 February 1940, the appointed time to present for training at

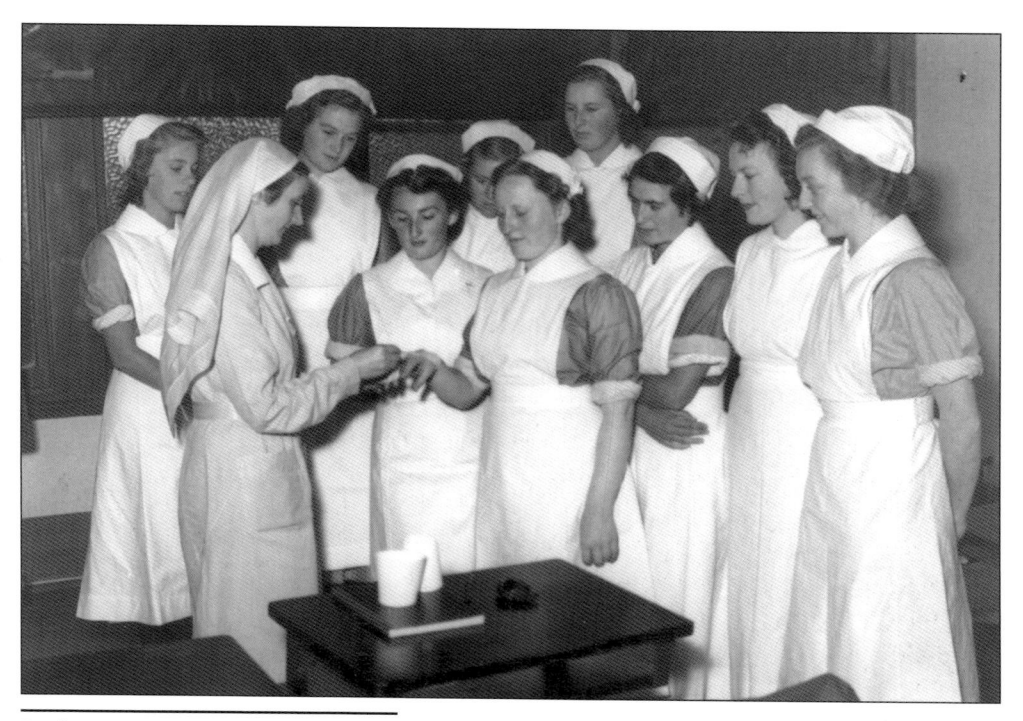

Preliminary Training School, 1946. *L–R:* Agnes Morris Tutor, Joan Terry, Barbara Catto, Barbara Schapper, Valerie Lark, Audrey Bult, Meryl Smith, Judith Heley, Joan Cheatley, Rhonda McCredie.

Sun Herald, 1946. RCHA/Heley Family Collection.

the Children's, remains vividly imprinted in Margaret Warr's mind. She arrived with her mother at the front office in Pelham Street where the Home Sister, Miss Webster, 'a really wonderful person', met her. Only four nurses assisted by Isabel Pilkington started that day. 'Day followed day and week followed week; ward moves came and went, then night duty when nurses lined up at 9 pm outside the Deputy Matron Sister Flower's office to answer your name.' The junior nurses in each ward collected the night meal for the ward from the Home Sister at the dairy.[8] She felt that they were grey, dreary times.

Country girls training at the Children's during the war were surprised to find stringencies in place by 1941: Melbourne was largely 'blacked out', food and clothing were rationed, and with little to spend, everyone made their own fun. 'When meals were insufficient, a group of friends went to the shop to share a piece of fish and a penny worth of chips.'[9] Others remembered that complimentary theatre passes were sometimes available for nurses, to *Charlie's Aunt* or Gilbert and Sullivan. 'It was always "May I have a late pass, Matron?" It was impossible to dodge [Mr] Upton or [Miss] Jarrett at the front office who signed us in.'

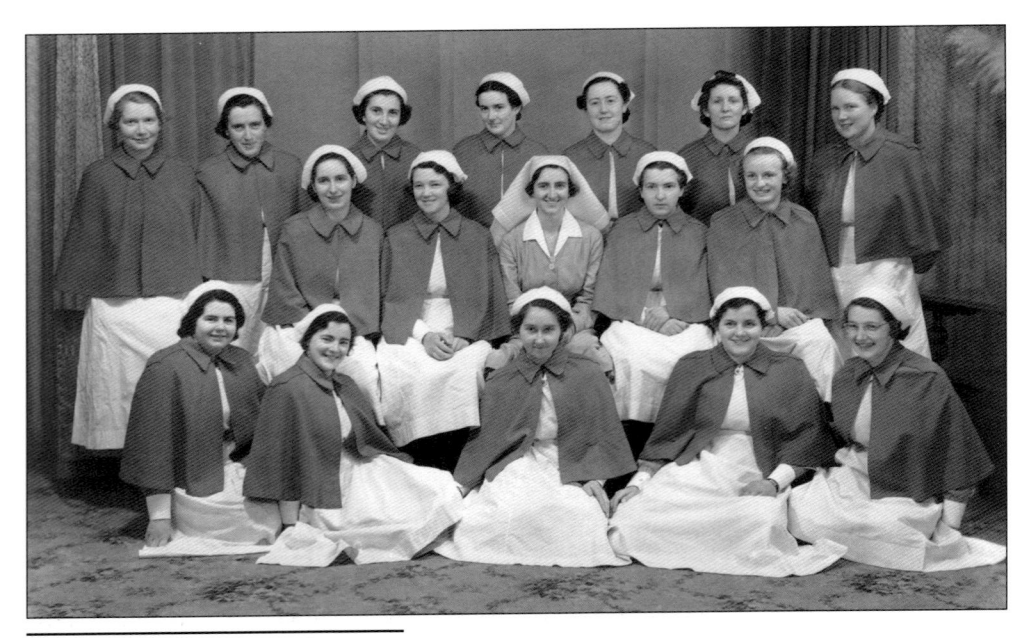

Successful finalists, July 1941.
Back L–R: Helen McMeekin, Joyce Chipperfield, Jean Hoadley, Hazel Belfrage, Gwenneth Richards, Kelly Gunn, Pat Slater.
Middle L–R: Edith Penn, Una Wishart, Isabel Pilkington (Tutor), Peggy Casey, Vivianne Daniel.
Front L–R: Anne Gordon, Edith Boyle, Marjorie Hosking, Rita Curtis, Mary Quiney.

Nurses were generally not aware that emergency precautions were in place. In retrospect, they have expressed surprise about the procedures. The ARP (Air-Raid Precautions) Sub-committee was formed on 26 January 1942. The members were: Lady Latham, Mrs J. Knox, Matron Hilda Walsh and Dr Howard Williams, who was delegated as the air-raid warden. They planned to blackout the whole Hospital, paper over the fanlights, brick in the doors, distribute necessary fire-fighting equipment on every flat roof, provide material to prevent glass shattering, and remove the glass doors in the north and east of the Out-patients Hall. An air-raid shelter was arranged for nurses on the ground floor of the Nurses' Home 'Extension B' and on the first floor, 'Extension A'. The Hospital architects, Stephenson and Turner, were called to test the feasibility of storing cast iron water tanks on the flat roof of a Baby Ward or alternatively, on the Out-patients building. They strongly advised against it as the old buildings could not take the weight. The pharmacy was to be a converted bunker, a concrete roof installed, the walls bricked up, and the Out-patients' entrance on Drummond Street sand-bagged.

The Children's was allocated for the reception of adult casualties; surgical instruments, additional blood transfusion equipment, adult size beds and copious amounts of linen were to be purchased. Matron Walsh was authorised to purchase adult gowns. Dr Williams arranged for resident staff to be blood typed and to carry identification. The nurses carried a small card. A supply of drugs, instruments and sterile dressings were to be placed in an emergency cupboard in each ward and 'to also include chocolate, barley sugar and tinned milk'. No detail was left to chance—'the cupboard was to be locked and the key to be accessible to the person in charge'.[10]

Sister Lyall, the dietician, had responsibility for catering: to arrange food and water for three days and bulk supplies for three months without deliveries, in case of air raids.

Evacuation

The Japanese bombed the American Fleet in Pearl Harbor on 7 December 1941, and shortly after the event the State Emergency Council informed the Children's Hospital that evacuation of the main Hospital should be carried out at the earliest possible date.

The Orthopaedic Section and the Convalescent Home at Hampton were to be continued, but the number of cases in each was to be reduced to the absolute minimum. The main Hospital was to be used as a first-aid post and for casualty cases in the event of attack. Frankston was to become a military hospital for the American

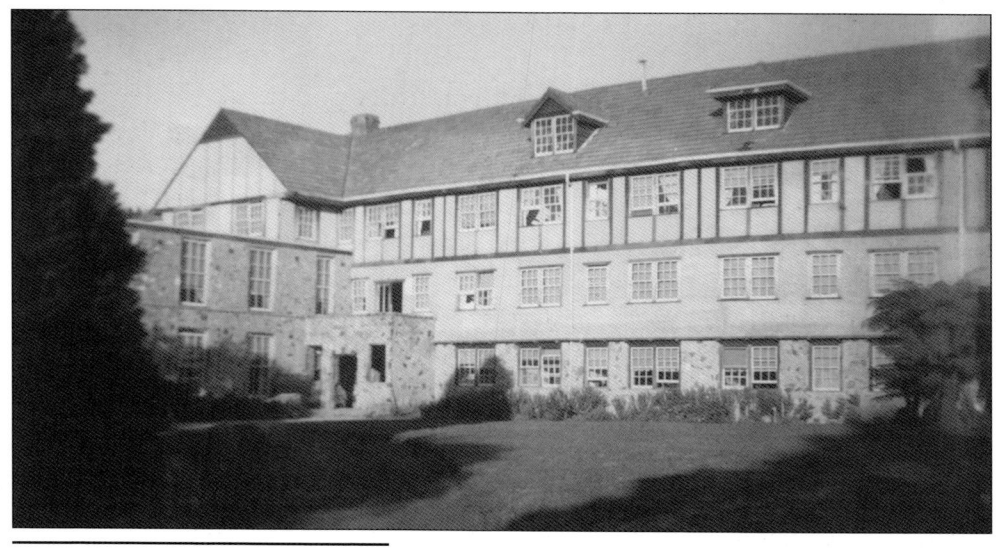

'Marybrooke' at Sherbrooke, was used as a Nurses' Home during World War Two.
RCHA/Cunningham Family Collection.

officers, Hampton for American nurses. Children too ill would be relocated, the remainder sent home.[11]

Lady Latham formally approached Isabel Nicholas, widow of Alfred Nicholas, within days of Australia's declaration of war, with the intention of borrowing 'Burnham Beeches' for conversion into an emergency wing of the Carlton Children's Hospital.[12] Not unexpectedly, there was some diffidence on the part of Mrs Nicholas.[13] The house, only three years old with newly laid-out gardens, was complete with interior fittings imported from England. Mr C. L. McVilly, Inspector of Charities and member of the State Emergency War Committee, soon influenced Mrs Nicholas. Mrs G. J. Coles, a close friend and Children's Hospital Committee member, may have also swayed her.[14]

Sherbrooke was eminently suitable for relocation purposes: the Convalescent Cottage was useful for sharing staff and facilities, the wooded mountain district offered protection from attacks by sea; it was convenient to Melbourne via Ferntree Gully Station and road bus transport and there were many additional large private mansions and guest houses to choose from should that be necessary. More than 100 children, possibly up to 150, needed accommodation. Several additional large houses had been considered, including the guest house, 'Lorna Doone', at Sassafras, and 'Bolbek' and 'Huntley Burn' at Mt Macedon. In anticipation of an immediate emergency, enquiries were made at country hospitals: Bendigo and Northern District Base Hospital.[15]

In July 1940, the Emergency Committee learned that 'Burnham Beeches' was available and, at the same time, 'Marybrooke', a private guest house within walking distance, was available for use as nurses' accommodation.

Although 'Burnham Beeches' appeared to lend itself to conversion to a hospital, the practicalities were doubtful. The architect-designed house with fresh, white painted walls, central heating, electric lift, internal and external electric lighting, modern refrigeration and water-dispensing systems required some adaptation, particularly plumbing and ventilation, a lowering of windows and widening of doors, removal of carpets and modification of bathrooms. Everything was to be carried out with prior consultation with the architect, Harry Norris. The agreement stated that 'Burnham Beeches' was lent to the Hospital at no charge and had to be left by the Hospital in the same condition as before the loan, 'fair wear and tear not excepted'.[16] Little thought was given to the tasks of the nurses in, for example, the extraordinarily difficult management of children in Thomas splints, plasters, frames, contraptions, pulleys and trolleys, as well as the handling of large beds in small spaces. The ablution, sterilisation and plaster room facilities were crowded on the ground floor.

On the morning of 12 January 1942, the first patients arrived in a fleet of ambulances and trucks from Hampton, the first Hospital branch to be completely evacuated. The exercise was completed in a day.[17] By the end of January 1942, the number of patients at the Orthopaedic Section was reduced to fifty, as twenty-seven

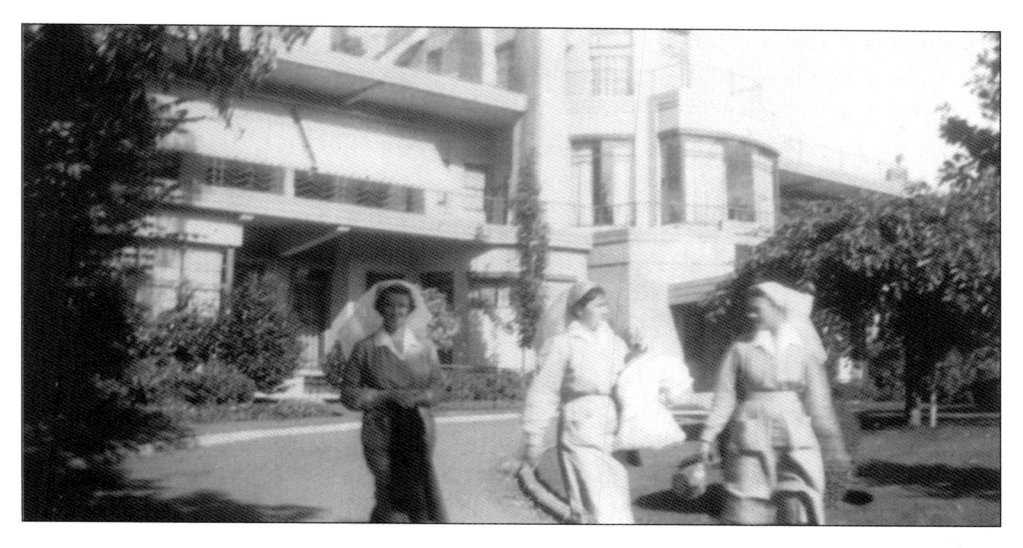

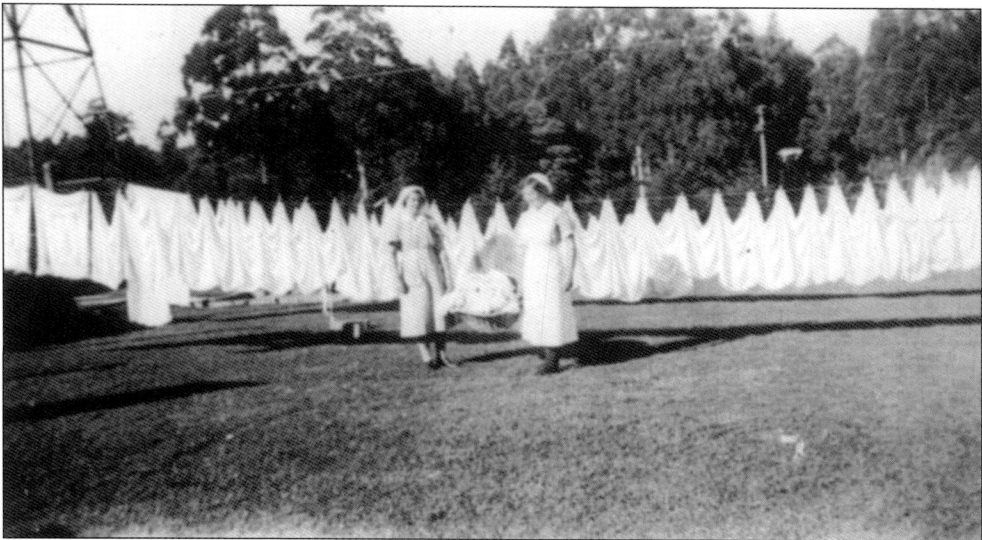

Top: 'Burnham Beeches' was occupied by children evacuated from the Carlton and Frankston Hospitals, 1942–43. Sister Una Wishart and colleagues.
Bottom: Sister Ann Gordon and Nurse Doris Chalmers hanging out the nappies at Sherbrooke Convalescent Cottage, 1941.

had been sent to Sherbrooke, twenty to 'Burnham Beeches' and seven babies with medical conditions were also accommodated at the Convalescent Cottage.

The Hospital purchased a covered-in truck for £240 to transport food, supplies and nurses between the three properties.[18] Some months later, 'Marybrooke Guest House' was adapted as a medical facility and some Carlton children were transferred there.

Meanwhile, arrangements were carried out for the evacuation of children to the Romsey–Lancefield District from Carlton. Various houses were considered for suitability to take children with rheumatic fever, heart conditions and poliomyelitis and forty-one children were transferred from Carlton to Sherbrooke. Dr Williams gratefully accepted the offer of the home of Mrs Thomas at Sherbrooke, for several diabetic children.

Nurses transferred from the branches to Sherbrooke and Sisters Huia Bristol, Jane Arthur and M. Meredith, assisted and acted as deputies for Sister Ann Milburn, who was appointed Matron for the whole complex. Sisters Hazel Belfrage, Una Wishart, Nurse Chalmers and others settled in for a long stay.

As the emergency lessened by early February 1943, the Committee decided to move patients out of 'Marybrooke' and back to Carlton. However, it was considered wise to keep 'Burnham Beeches' as an emergency hospital, particularly as many extensive alterations had taken place. The American military was slow to vacate Frankston. Fifty American nurses continued to occupy the Hampton branch and the facility was not re-opened until the end of the war.

The move from 'Burnham Beeches' was delayed until the beginning of the winter of 1943. All children left on 15 May. There was much talk of the great damage to the irreplaceable fittings and, when Lady Latham made a visit of inspection, she was appalled. Lavatory fittings had been broken, woodwork damaged, walls badly marked and china clothes hooks broken off. Una Wishart said it was truly terrible.[19] The children had been exposed to the sun on the balconies but the windows and doors were too narrow. The trolleys had knocked great chunks out of the door frames. The Hospital made good the damage but the house remained unoccupied for the rest of the war.

The Carlton hospital in the 1940s

Despite the anxieties looming in war time, Jean Maxwell Barton enjoyed her life at the Children's when she began in 1940 at the age of nineteen. Kate Wilson was the Tutor for her final year.

> We all lived in the Nurses' Home; it was added value to our training. We learnt to be tolerant of others and they of us. I enjoyed the company as a country girl; I felt safe and had plenty of relations and friends to spend days

off [with]. I have never forgotten how happy I was in the Home. Discipline never worried me; my sister Anne was there at Carlton before me. That was wonderful.

Sister Kit Webster was Home Sister, strict, fair and caring. Our sitting room and smoking room were always welcoming—beautiful flowers and fires in winter. Many hours [were] spent in these rooms laughing and talking with other staff. Meals I found satisfactory. Had to be in…at 10.30 pm (I recall a late pass—12 MN or 12.30 AM). I climbed over the fence in Rathdowne Street from the roof of a car over barbed wire, tore my clothing—very costly as clothing coupons were needed for all apparel during the war years. It wasn't worth the worry of getting caught. My first pay packet was £4/5/- after board was taken out, paid once a month…taught me to be frugal. Didn't hurt me—naturally I would have liked more.[20]

She loved the children, especially seeing them go home after long illnesses. She admired the courage shown by the children with terrible burns.

By far the most difficult aspect of the war years was a shortage of staff. Matron Walsh, the Ward Sisters and Staff Nurses were obviously under strain and this showed in their attitude towards the trainees. From the mid-1930s the Hospital had been employing nurse assistants, not always a popular move among the trained staff and the Committee of Management who thought it a waste of money. The threat also existed to the status of trainees by the creation of a second layer of untrained staff.

Early in the war years, Nancy Furnell (née Heane) had completed two years of training; Ward 14 treated babies and toddlers where 'beautiful, understanding Sister Agnes Morris was in charge. There were many admissions of children suffering from meningitis, sometimes staying three to four months—if they lived.' A long-held memory is the hum of the 'iron lungs' (respirators) in Ward 7, the children with polio, the accidents and the emergencies in the middle of the night. Nancy said:

We were so young, so much was expected of us. Night duty was twelve weeks in Ward 10, both first and second year. Each bed had a linen change, all forty-four of them! Each patient was lifted on to a trolley. Some nights the senior nurse would go to the theatre to scrub for emergency surgery and the junior of three months into training was left to care for post-op babies. I was quite terrified. Ward 16 night duty in second year with very sick diphtheria patients—the sight of the emergency tracheotomy instruments on each locker gave me the horrors. This led me to believe I'd never make it. Cutting plasters from deceased osteomyelitis patients on Ward 10 at night was horrible. Dear Sister Peck rescued me on the last occasion. How gratified I was.

Father Stuart came in from the Presbytery, the church on the corner of Pelham and Rathdowne—to anoint a girl in Ward 10. She died. He used to come over in the middle of the night and he was never forgotten. [H]e said, 'you are too young to look after these children, too much responsibility'. He sat with dying children.[21]

Father Stuart gave Nancy a photo of himself, a keepsake when he went to the war. She kept the frame on her dressing table in her room and one day she returned at lunch-time to find 'the photo face down and the next day, and the next...finally I found it my drawer. You know, it was Sister Webster, she did not like it.'

Nancy found the Nurses' Home a place where long discussions were exchanged about events of the day, the injustices meted out by the Sister-in-Charge or senior nurses who could make life unbearable at times. It was sombre; blackouts covered the windows. In the Carlton Nurses' Home, the huge baths tended to be forgotten and overflowed while the girls chatted for hours 'getting it off their chest'.

There was not much joy for nurses who worked with desperately ill, dying children: no counselling, no de-briefing. By far the most disturbing aspect was dealing with relatives and parents whose child had been injured in an accident or whose baby was dying. Beryl Sparks described 'having to lay out the dead baby and then trying to make the sluice room as accommodating as possible. We would use the best clothes and a little posy in the baby's hands for the relatives view.'[22]

Barbara Brian (née Morris) remembered 'the satisfying experiences with my dehydrated babies, giving them glucose and saline at the rate of one-and-a-half ounces hourly to prevent vomiting and thus avoiding the necessity of an IV. The constant care of prems [premature babies] and pylorics, and seeing them recover. Prems were oiled, not bathed, and wrapped in cotton wool in an ordinary crib which was lined.'

But after a few months in Ward 7, Barbara contracted typhoid fever. She remained in the Sick Nurses' Ward 16 for three months under the care of the consultant medical officer to sick nurses, Dr Grieve. Dr Cliff Sawrey, the Medical Superintendent, and Dr Elizabeth Turner assisted. Barbara's family were told she would not recover. Fortunately, she did.

Alice Charles can never forget the sad times. She recalled being on night duty with her best friend when her friend's brother, a doctor, came to the Children's Hospital in the morning to tell her that her fiancé had been killed while clearing a mine field in Bardia (North Africa). 'Our wonderful Night Sister was present...she [my friend] of course had time off. It was our first casualty and, as most of us had brothers, fathers and boyfriends overseas in the services, it brought it all home to us in reality and had a very sobering effect, one I remember to this day.'

But there were rewards: one Christmas Day on duty in the Baby Wards, Alice, who was particularly fond of a dear little girl who needed fluids, spent so much time with the child that she missed her dinner. As usual, they were short-staffed. The baby turned the corner that night and Alice was very happy. She remembers: 'no penicillin or antibiotics in those days!'[23]

Una Wishart had five brothers in the war. She was utterly heartbroken when Matron Walsh would not give her time release to see one of her brothers on leave.

The first sulphonamide drug, Prontosil, was developed in 1935 followed by other sulpha drugs, the most commonly remembered by nurses was M&B 693.[24] Used for meningitis, pneumonia, empyema, gonorrhoea, erysipelas and influenza, the usual dose of half a tablet crushed in milk was given orally to these little babies, some of them under three months, on a tiny spoon. The drug had terrible side-effects: vomiting, cyanosis, anaemia and fever. Despite the danger, particularly to babies under one year—the end result could be kidney failure—there were some spectacular successes. A baby of three months, the youngest of eleven children, was admitted from her Broadmeadows home with cerebro-meningitis and on admission to the Children's it was decided to treat her with the sulpha drug, M&B 693. She recovered, although there was evidence of some brain damage from her critical illness. Nancy Furnell was very attached to this little girl and most interested in her remarkable mother. She visited them on numerous occasions, mainly to observe her progress and to join in the day-to-day life of this well-organised family.[25]

There were glad times when a little child could go home well, but many nurses were traumatised by the death of children from uncontrollable infections and burns. Margaret Rogers (née Stockwell) nursed diphtheria patients in Ward 16 and, failing to save one little patient, became distressed.[26] Children accepted their disabilities. They showed staff and parents their courage: there was still a lot they could do. For Jean Barton the saddest time was when she nursed a seven-year-old girl with bad burns:

> She went to get her father a cup of tea; she lit the match and the head flew off into her dressing gown—she ran outside. She was due to go home after six weeks and died of secondary shock the day before. Those [were] the days before heart massage. We were heart broken! Her father was home on leave from the Army.[27]

Visitors to the Nurses' Home were strictly barred. Staying out late became an art. Sister 'Kit' Webster had eyes and ears everywhere when it came to the inspection of rooms, but sometimes turned a 'blind eye' providing a nurse could get past the front office. Otherwise it was stay out all night at your 'auntie's' place! There was no visiting between nurses and doctors, and the Nurses' Home and Doctors' Residency were strictly segregated.

Things livened up when a 'burglar' was detected in the nurses' sitting room but, after all, was found to be an American Army Officer. Peg Orford was there at

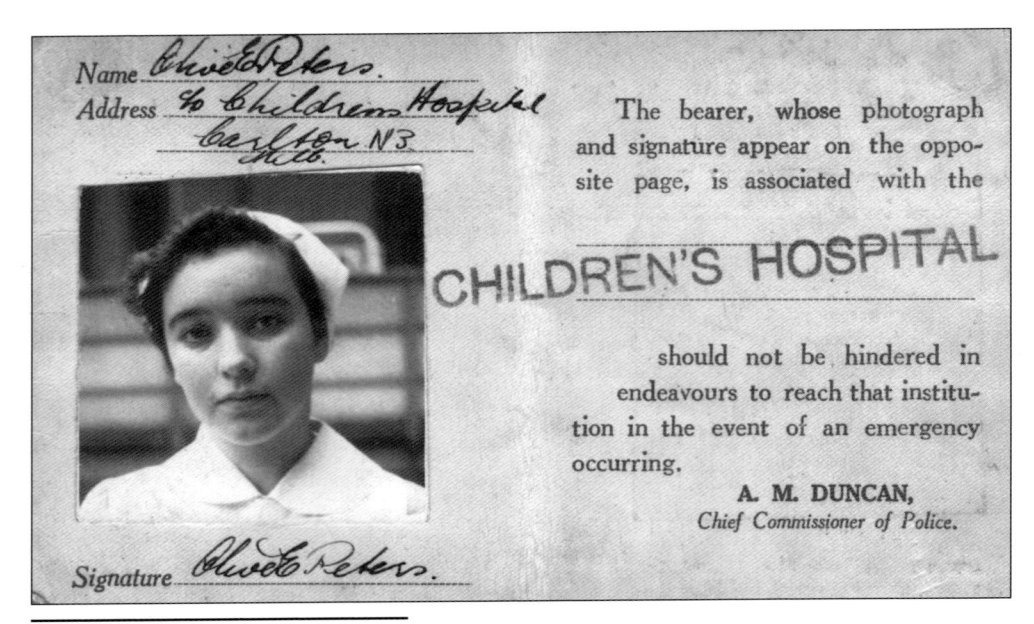

World War Two identity card, issued 16 October 1942 to Nurse Olive Peters.
Raymond Family Collection.

Christmas when 'Doctors Sawrey and Doug Stephens had a wild party and Matron Walsh called the police'. Later, when Matron sprained her ankle, she refused to see a Resident Medical Officer.[28]

Olive Raymond (née Peters) helped out on the family farm when her three brothers left for the war. She had completed her Intermediate Certificate from the Korumburra Higher Elementary School when, at eighteen, she entered the Preliminary Training School at the Children's Hospital. Within the first few months, her class was required to attend the Gas and Fuel Corporation in Flinders Street. In April 1943, she received her Invalid Cookery Certificate for attendance at ten lessons. The examiner was Miss Emily Noble.[29] For country girls reared on hearty meals and nourishing broths, this form of cookery was strange: 'barley water, strained beef tea, raw white of egg sliced with a knife and strained through a cloth'. No one ever remembered what these foods were for, and never used them in the wards. Some did vaguely remember their mothers mentioning barley water as a cure for kidney disease, or was it an old wives' tale?

Ward Sister Una Wishart recalled the terrible staff shortages: the Pantry Nurse had to scramble or boil eggs *en masse*, and put the jug of milk in the steriliser to get it hot. Invariably it would tip over and all the milk would be lost. It was a rude awakening.

Some children were sponged at night and some in the morning; the breakfasts had to be over and the mixtures done in time for Miss Walsh to do her round. Nurses

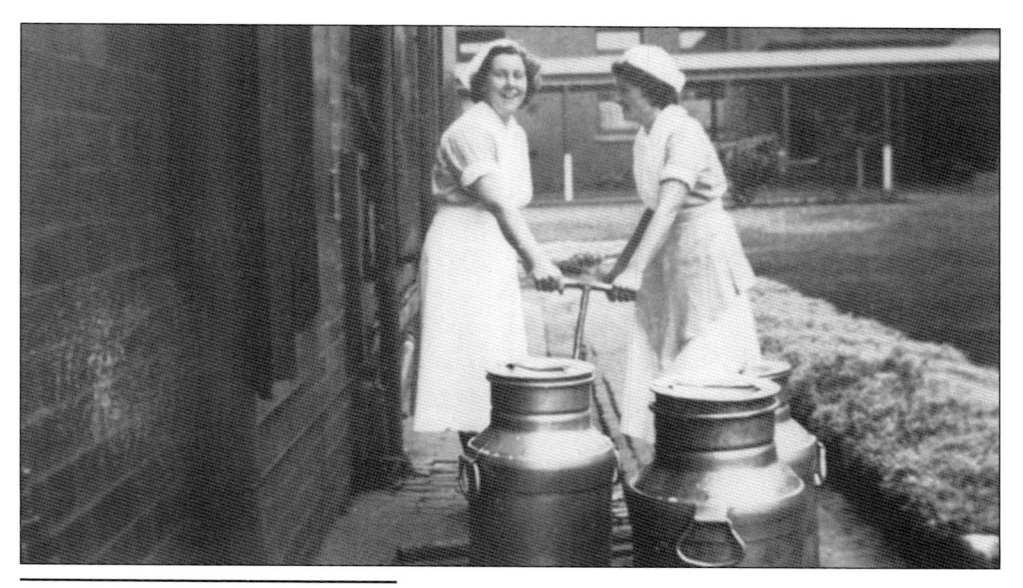

Bringing in the milk cans. Nurses Yvonne Morey and Patience Longstaff, 1943.
RCHA/Cunningham Family Collection.

swept the floors. Often the maid didn't turn up. In Wards 7 and 8 the open fires were lit on alternate days, and if the wardsmaid or man didn't turn up, the nurses took the ashes out and re-set the fire. 'Quite often in Medical I can remember being in the pantry washing up the dishes because there was no maid. You just hoped someone else was looking after the patients while you were not there. You couldn't ask the nurses, because they had many patients to look after, plus other duties.' Sometimes a new maid started, was given a room in the maids' quarters, but 'she only came in because she needed a few night's accommodation'.[30]

The most important cog in the wheel during the war was Sister Ivy Flower. Together with Sister Lyall, the dietician who ran the milk and food room, she had very full days. Her day began at 7.30 am: forwarding the cards to the kitchen, interviewing the head cook, checking the menu, ordering bulk stores of vegetables and fruit, keeping records of all stores, engaging the whole domestic staff and arranging their hours, supervising the kitchen staff of seven persons, the relief staff and the nurses' dining room and the man in the kitchen. She saw all the diets before they left the kitchen, preserved excess eggs after an egg drive, sorted the mail, checked the accounts and supervised the making of the babies' ice-cream. She also controlled the dining room staff and acted as deputy to Miss Walsh. That was all before lunch! Miss Flower was always known to put her hand to anything; she was completely unflappable and kind. In her old age she was asked what she thought of the old days in the Nurses' Home. She said 'it was good for the nurses to be able to grouse about everything, have a good talk'.[31]

IVY SILVERTHORNE FLOWER was born on 21 May 1899 in Moonee Ponds and educated at Stanmore Ladies College. She qualified in general nursing at the Children's Hospital in 1924.

Miss Flower was appointed as Staff Nurse in 1924, as Ward Sister in October 1924 and as Assistant Matron in March 1934. Three words were used to describe her: 'dedicated, conscientious and devoted'. Nurses of the 1950s recall Sister Flower as a shy, retiring Home Sister with a room on the ground floor in the Nurses' Home where she did the rosters. 'We called her 'Ivy Geranium' and felt she had been there forever. We were astounded after she died to learn that she had a life outside as a Sunday School teacher in Fitzroy.'

She retired in 1962, after forty-two years of continuous service, and died in February 1994 aged ninety-four.

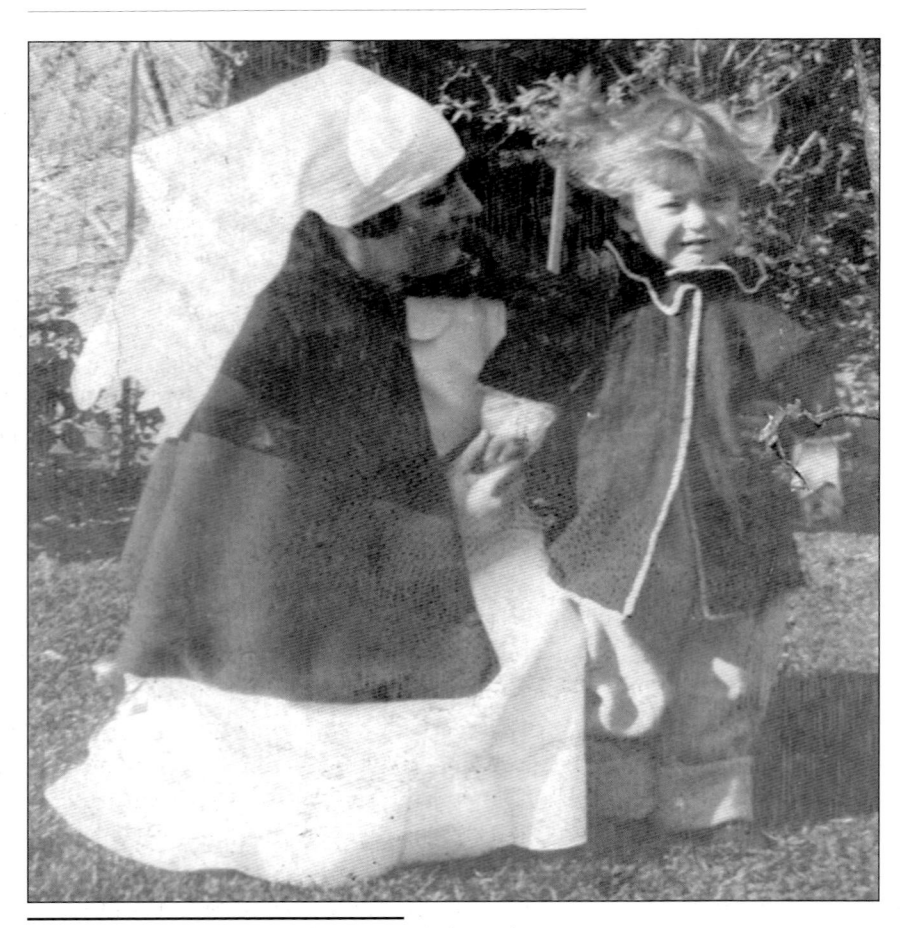

Sister Ivy Flower with child in red flannel coat. 1940s.

Nurses cooked the evening meal in the wards, always eggs for at least thirty children. The pantry nurse boiled great quantities in a huge jug in the steriliser. Night nurses signed on for duty at Sister Flower's office carrying their plate to collect their own egg and a small jelly for their supper, carrying their precious cargo back to the ward on a tin plate.[32] The meals were 'ghastly amounts of carbohydrates'. Alice Charles remembers that just before the war 'Dr Collins did something about the nurses' food. We had Weethearts on the table and more salads.' In fact, Dr Collins had long taken an interest in the diets of the children and the nurses, but unfortunately, while he was away during the war, probably due to restrictions, the dietary improvements lapsed.

Esme Nixon was older than most girls, being twenty years and six months, when she began her training in September 1943. She held a variety of jobs, included filing clerk in a government department where all employees carried 'Manpower' employment cards. Joining the Services was common for young people, but Esme's guardian was against it. Nursing was thought the ideal alternative. But nothing prepared her for work in the wards: she found an enormous shortage of domestic staff. 'We cleaned lockers, mopped floors and cooked [the children's] breakfast and tea with eggs or egg powder.'[33] A first-year nurse took turns as treatment or pantry nurse. Sometimes she brought in apples from home to make Apple Snow. This supplemented the children's bread and butter.

Peg Orford was one of the first involved in the reciprocal training of nurses with the old Melbourne Hospital during the war. Her turn came with no adult training or instruction; she was shocked by a ward full of terrible skin cases. 'The Melbourne Hospital was so old it was condemned.' She lived on noisy Swanston Street in the old Nurses' Home. On reflection, Peg believed that because her childhood was spent in the depression years in the shadow of World War One, when both her parents had been in France, she was prepared. 'We were disciplined. Training days were accepted as a job to be done.'[34]

Out-patients

On 4 April 1940, the Committee of Management decided that the Post-operative Ward in Out-patients was to be opened. This was extraordinarily difficult for the nursing administration; seven nurses were needed and some would have to live out. Miss Walsh expressed fears that 'judging from experience, a certain amount of opposition would be met from the parents [of the nurses] as it was obvious that supervision could not be exercised over them in the same way—particularly in regard to the amount of essential rest required in between periods of duty'.

Olive Raymond worked in Out-patients' theatre on day duty from 7 am. Her work sheets give us a fascinating view of her day, a mix of housemaid duties and nursing. She dressed the children going home, sat them on a bench to wait, prepared the operation bed, set the bathroom for the OP (Out-patient) nurse, set out the squares for babies, the caps, small blankets, the thermometer tray, covered the linen bin with a rug, emptied the ice-tray, made jelly for tea and set out spatulas in kidney dishes in the centre of the ward. She dusted the ward, made up histories for discharge and set them for doctor to sign before he operated, cleaned the teeth of the 'permanent boarders' and arranged the OP cards. She sat the children out, prepared the operation beds, gowns, jackets, squares, thermometer trays and atropine trays, hypodermic tray on the kidney dish. At 8.45 am she gave the atropine, made sure the child passed urine and started the steriliser. But most important was the order of children to enter for the operation: the cards had to be accurately placed (with the child's identification): circumcisions first, tonsils or adenoids or both.[35] Havoc ensued if they were mixed up.

Generally, the patients of 'Ts and As, and circs', as these operations were commonly referred to by the nurses, were seen by the doctor before going home. One of the most gruelling tasks, watching tonsil children post-operatively, engendered anxiety on the part of the nurse and commonly, a state of terror. It was here that nurses developed their keenest powers of observation: quarter-hourly pulse, respirations and blood pressure, watching for tell-tale signs of blood on the pillow. There was no IV line in those days and children were given little pain relief; morphine was taboo, and aspirin caused bleeding. The OP nurse handed out APC to the mother only when she took the child home—usually on the tram.[36] 'With the all-clear from the doctor, it was down to Miss Carruthers for discharge, back to tidy the ward, write up TPRs [temperature, pulse and respiration] and the discharge book—all the time watching the children out of anaesthetic.' That was only the morning.

Peg Orford often worked alone on night duty in the OP theatre. She remembers preparing a blood transfusion trolley, for donor and recipient, on the top floor where the Ts and As were located. 'In another ward in the building I worked in isolation with an emergency bell.'

Nurses' accommodation was apparently stretched with the opening of the new OP theatre. Without any explanation, the night duty nurses were sent to sleep for a period at St Anne's, on the corner of Victoria and Rathdowne streets, for which the Hospital paid £1 a week for each nurse. A huge grey building of three floors with attics, the former coffee palace was run by an order of French nuns. Their wide, starched head gear resembled those of the religious of the Middle Ages. Peg Orford thought it terribly creepy when you entered. 'There was no one in the building, it was dark and gloomy, the old lifts were encased in iron grills, they creaked and groaned. Everywhere you looked there were religious figures and the basement smelled of gas.' Each afternoon, nurses were called to 5 o'clock tea at the Children's Hospital dining room just up the road, despite another four-hour break before signing on at 9 pm.

Sleep was not easy at St Anne's: 'The Air Force chaps were billeted at the Exhibition Building. We just got to sleep and up they started with morning reveille and deafening band practice blowing their trumpets.' Matron Walsh reported to the Committee that she had no choice: rooms in 'B' wing of the Nurses' Home were needed to billet emergency air-raid wardens and other staff.[37]

In the classroom

The standard textbook, *Lectures for Nurses* by Gwen Burbidge, a small book with a pale blue cover, was simple by the standards of today. Divided into (1) Notes on Preliminary Training for Nurses, lectures on general nursing, hygiene, anatomy, physiology and bandaging, and (2) for the Seniors, General Nursing, the text was very basic. In second year, a small red book, *Aids to Materia Medica for Nurses* by Amy E. A. Squibbs, was kept by every nurse, if she could afford it.

The book was useful for familiarisation with ward procedures. It told how to set the lower and upper shelves of trays with the correct instruments, and how to remember the complicated set-up for lumbar puncture, abdominal paracentesis, thoracic aspiration, female bladder washouts and catheterisation of a male patient. This latter procedure, although usually performed by the doctor, was expected to be known by every nurse. The stock examination questions dealt with venesection, blood transfusion and continuous intravenous infusion, and various positions required for pelvic examination and post surgery: Fowler, Semi-Fowler, prone, flat or recumbent, Sim's or lithotomy.

An alternative textbook commonly used during the war years was *Anatomy and Physiology for Nurses* by Evelyn Pierce. *The Medical Nursing Dictionary* had an up-to-date edition with the inclusion 'what to do with war time gases' and comprehensive first-aid treatment procedures.

Treatment of bedsores and general care of the skin were an important component of junior lectures. People stayed in Hospital for much longer than they do today, and instructions invariably included techniques for removal of slough and stimulation of healing by packing the cavity with gauze wrung out in 'red solution': ether in saline, monsol or eusol. Bed baths were common: the gutter bath for typhoid was a contraption of canvas slung up to the bed posts. Ambulatory patients could have a vapour bath or a hot air bath.

These texts, excellent as they were, taught little or nothing about children. More advanced and interested nurses acquired their own set of Caxton's *Modern Professional Nursing* incorporating chapters on the 'Management of the Child in Health and Disease', 'Medicine and Surgery of Infancy' and 'Childhood and the Era of Social Medicine'.[38]

The greatest loss to the Nursing School occurred when Isabel Pilkington decided 'to move on' in 1942. Ahead of her time, she led a movement to break down the rigid hierarchy, common to all large public hospitals of the time. She tried to make the nurses feel more valued and respected. One constructive achievement was the support of Dr Collins. He took a keen interest in the nurses' education and helped Isabel produce the 'Traybook' before he left for England in 1939. This was the forerunner of the much expanded 'Procedure Book', which was typed, duplicated and distributed with what seemed to be only minimal interest from Miss Walsh. Isabel also arranged with Dr Collins a series of demonstrations of procedures, for example, running drainage tubes into buckets.

Isabel thought the appointment of Miss Kathleen (Kate) Wilson as the new Tutor Sister was a bold and brilliant decision. With support from Dr Howard Williams, a vacant ward became a Tutorial Department.[39]

Dr Collins' relationship with staff was not always smooth. Less than satisfied with the diets of the children and their nurses, his differences with Sister Lyall, the Edinburgh-trained dietician, were not easily resolved. She simply had too much to do. Her duties included conferring on a daily basis with the Honoraries and Almoners about children's various dietary problems, arranging financial assistance for parents of children on special diets and juggling shortages in the food room. For example, babies' feeding bottles were in very short supply and older babies were often fed from large tomato sauce bottles.

Before he resigned to go to England to pursue postgraduate studies in 1939, Dr Collins' advice was sought by the Committee of Management on many matters. Among these he advocated 'educational propaganda' in the form of notices in the Out-patients Hall to educate parents on correct diet, the general care of children and the prevention of common infections such as impetigo and injuries.[40]

War service

Australian nurses were mobilised for the Army from the civilian community and the Army Nursing Service Reserve. By 1940, almost one-third of Australia's trained nurses from a total of about 13,000 volunteered; in all, 3,477 nurses served in the Australian Army Nursing Service (AANS) between 1939 and 1947.[41]

The AANS was attached to the staff of the Director General of Medical Services, and administered by the Matron-in-Chief, Grace Margaret Wilson, formerly Matron of the Children's and Alfred Hospitals. Miss Wilson was evacuated from North Africa because of ill health in May 1941 (she was then sixty-two), and Annie M. Sage, Matron-in-Chief, AANS, CM and AIF, was appointed for the remainder of the war.[42] It is not known how many Children's Hospital nurses served in the AANS. The Hospital Minutes of 29 February 1940 record that Sister Logan was the first to leave to join the 2nd AIF, and on 14 May 1940, Sister Betty Westland (née Jeffrey) sailed to England on the *Stratheden* via Colombo, Capetown and Freetown escorted by *HMS Australia*.

On arrival, Betty was stationed in Surrey at Godalming, the 600-bed Army Hospital. Trenches had not been dug and the nurses would stay in bed and hope for the best during air-raids. In May 1941, Betty left England for the Middle East and slept in a life jacket for ten days at sea. Stationed at Alexandria in a modern Greek hospital of 200 beds, she gained a lot of experience with burns patients injured on a ship. After returning to Australia, Betty was next posted to Aitape in New Guinea, 'the end of the world' as far as she was concerned, and remained for twenty-two months. There she witnessed terrible hardships endured by the soldiers who contracted scrub typhus and malaria.[43]

The Royal Australian Navy Nursing Service (RANNS) was established in April 1942. Miss Ina Laidlaw, recruited from her position as Matron at the Frankston Orthopaedic Hospital, became the Principal Matron of the RANNS stationed at Flinders Naval Depot for the duration of the war. The number of servicewomen never exceeded sixty members, serving throughout Australia, New Guinea, Darwin and in the Naval wing of the Prince of Wales Hospital in Sydney. Miss Laidlaw remained at the Flinders Base until 1945. She resumed her post at the Frankston Orthopaedic Hospital in 1945 and resigned in 1950 to go to England.

The Victorian Nurses' Registration Board encouraged enlistment, with the incentive that all members of the AANS would remain registered without cost during the term of war service.[44] However, only a few trained nurses left the Children's Hospital; some were not inclined, while others were retained by the Directorate of Manpower to remain in essential services. Una Wishart and Marjorie Tomlinson 'were longing to go' and thought Matron Hilda Walsh could have been more influential. But she was also under the Directorate to retain staff and to stay at the Hospital herself as she was not old enough for retirement.[45] To sign up, nurses had to be British subjects, domiciled in Australia, and aged between twenty-five and thirty-five. Matrons had to be under forty. The age requirements were later extended to twenty-one and forty to forty-five in special circumstances.[46]

Jean Hardham was very experienced when war was declared. Her postgraduate work included infant welfare in the Plunket system at the Truby King Hospital in Dunedin. Because she had trained at the Children's Hospital, she was required to do a fourth year of general nursing to

Jean Hardham, AANS (Australian Army Nursing Service), 1941.

RCHA/Hardham Collection.

work in New Zealand. This she accomplished at the Auckland Hospital with examination.

On her return to Melbourne, Jean was called up and enlisted with the AANS. She was sent to the Army Camp at Darley, near Bacchus Marsh, and allocated to Ambulance Sea Transport. In April 1941, she boarded the *Queen Mary* at Jervis Bay bound for the Middle East with 15,000 troops, the 2/25th Field Regiment, a Queensland Unit and the 2/2nd Pioneer Battalion (Victorian). They were escorted by the *Isle de France* and the *Mauritania* and sailed with the *Queen Elizabeth* and the *Aquitania*, proceeding via Trincomalee to Port Tawfiq in the Suez Canal. On board there were fifteen nurses under the supervision of Matron Anne Jewell AANS, two doctors and a physiotherapist. This level of staffing was seen as sufficient, as the troops were fit and well. But the troops 'went down like flies' in the heat and there were cases of pneumonia, mumps and other infectious diseases. With no antibiotics, aspirin was the main medication. Jean said, 'It was a very makeshift hospital but they were well cared for. We had to watch the basins [slopping over] going through the Bight; it was quite difficult.'

From Port Tawfiq, the nurses went to Kantara to the 2/2nd AGH (Australian General Hospital). In Egypt, they were put on the train and, in typical Army style, became lost. The nurses stayed in the Gaza Ridge for three months before the authorities caught up with them and put them up in tents with the 1st AGH. Every second night they were allocated to go up the Allenby Bridge by train to bring back the wounded, then into hospital and on to Kantara. Suddenly the Army found the nurses again but by that time there was a lot of typhoid. One of the nurses became very ill and the others mildly so. They concealed this, knowing they would otherwise be left behind, and eventually were allocated to the *Queen Elizabeth* being used as a prisoner of war ship to transport Italians and Germans to Australia.

The Japanese were already in the war and progressing down the Malay Peninsula when Jean was called to sail to Singapore to take troops to Ambon. Singapore fell and she departed on the Tasmanian apple ship *Zealandia*, a little ship full of civilians including six new babies and six soldiers, all stretcher cases. The ship's carpenter made cradles from apple boxes and wedged the babies in the narrow alley ways. The ship eventually arrived in Darwin, ten days overdue.

Jean was next posted to the *Centaur* but her place was taken by Margaret Adams, who desperately wanted to go. Jean has never ceased to be grateful about being pulled out of the fateful trip.[47]

Margaret Adams was educated at Presbyterian Ladies College (PLC) and trained at the Children's Hospital, 1932–35. She was working at the Hospital when she enlisted as a volunteer with the AANS. She was not in the original team of nurses but was later posted to the hospital ship, *Centaur*. Her burning ambition won the day; it is believed her father was in the Department of the Navy and she was able to take the place of Jean Hardham. The ship was torpedoed by the Japanese submarine 1-177

Margaret Adams, 1941.
RCHA/Adams Family Collection.

about twenty-three miles off Cape Moreton, off the south coast of Queensland, on 14 May 1943. The incident happened at 4.10 am in fine clear weather conditions. The ship, brightly lit, painted white with the Red Cross fully displayed according to the Geneva Convention, sank instantly. On board were 332 people of whom 212 were Australian Army medical and field ambulance personnel; eleven Army nurses and eighteen doctors perished in the shark infested waters. The one nurse to survive was Ellen Savage.

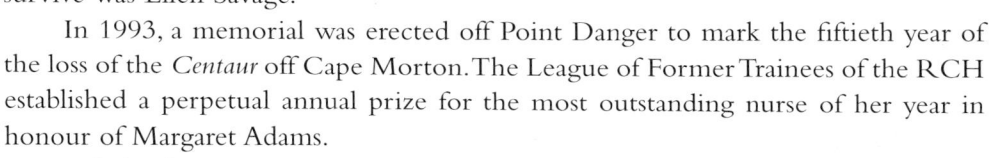

In 1993, a memorial was erected off Point Danger to mark the fiftieth year of the loss of the *Centaur* off Cape Morton. The League of Former Trainees of the RCH established a perpetual annual prize for the most outstanding nurse of her year in honour of Margaret Adams.

Isabel Pilkington recalled her memories of Margaret Adams:

> I was associated with her as a work mate but not a close personal friend. I did, however, have the privilege of visiting her home. The occasion was a Sunday evening—after joining her family at a large well-furnished table we washed the dishes, then all attended the local Presbyterian Church prior to returning to the Hospital. This was the natural pattern of life at that time.
>
> I recall her parents as splendid people living in comfortable middle-class conditions. The atmosphere was so far removed from the modern lifestyle, I can only suggest that the Margaret Adams we knew was a natural product of her environment. She being a Presbyterian and I coming from a long Anglican tradition would share light-hearted jokes about the relative values of each form of worship—one such argument centred on whether it was better to take up the collection before or after the sermon.
>
> Margaret was big in stature and comfortable in her daily associations. To see her beautifully fresh and tidy in her uniform of the day, earnest in her endeavours, brisk in her movements, capable and conscientious in carrying out her duties, while she endowed all she met with her particular warmth, her whole demeanour was one of warmth and happiness. This was as she saw it, the natural way to live. She was the essence of a splendid Australian, a true product of her time and a capable and conscientious nurse.[48]

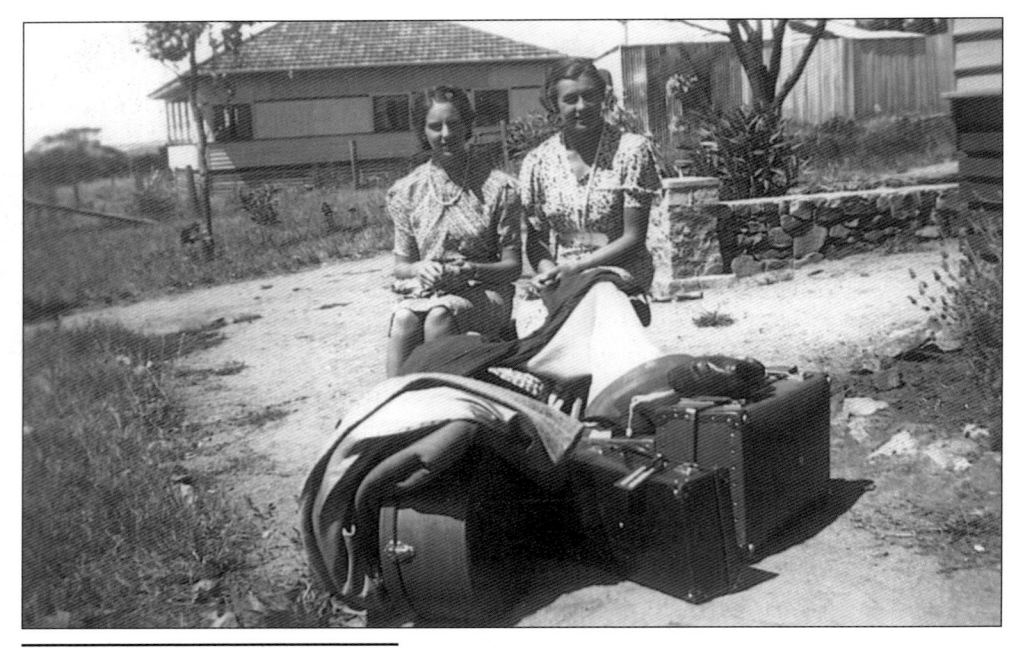

The best of friends: Sophie Brodie and Margaret Adams waiting for the bus at Frankston in more peaceful days before World War Two.
RCHA/Robinson Family Collection.

When Isabel presented the Margaret Adams Memorial prize, she felt this quotation was apt: 'Those who carry torches pass them on to others. It seemed to me that the passing on was an effortless result of the influence exercised by such torch carriers. That is how I remember Margaret—she still remains a lovely and living memory.'

When asked the difference between a nurse and an Army Sister, Sheila Brown, who entered the AANS as a very experienced nurse, said: 'two shillings a week and Sister's uniforms made by a tailor'. She was posted to Egypt and Palestine for two years and from there to New Guinea with the 2/7th AGH, where she met her future husband, Sir Geoffrey Newman Morris.[49]

Sheila Brown grew up in a large family in Kew and was educated at Ruyton. She entered the Children's Hospital in 1929 and this was to prove a very happy time in her life. Up until her death in 2003, she still had the cup and saucer taken with her when starting as a nurse.

Sheila told many amusing anecdotes about training days: nurses made afternoon tea for doctors' rounds and one very nervous girl forgot to add the tea and someone had hot water. In theatre she remembered a temperamental surgeon who threw an instrument at a nurse. Sheila insisted it be boiled for the full three minutes, much to the annoyance of the surgeon.

Margaret Rogers (née Stockwell), AANS, 1944.
Oil portrait by Geoffrey Mainwaring.
Australian War Memorial Canberra. ART 22148

Sheila married in Melbourne in 1945 and had three children. She is remembered for opening the RCH Nurses' Conference in the centenary year, 1970.

Margaret Rogers still treasures letters from 'the boys', those prisoner of war amputees whom she nursed home from Singapore in 1945.[50]

Margaret's first posting was to a Camp Hospital at Broadmeadows, then to the Middle East. She sailed on the *Queen Mary* from Sydney for the Middle East via Fremantle, Trincomalee and Port Suez. She was stationed at the 2/2nd Australian General hospital, but it was six weeks before she was able to join the hospital, suffering from illness at Gaza. The hospital moved to Borneo, and when Singapore fell, the ship returned to Australia where Margaret spent three years on the Atherton Tablelands. There the hospital catered for more than 1,200 patients. The services were being trained for jungle warfare and many casualties were brought in from New Guinea. When the war ended, Margaret was posted to Singapore with the 2/14th AGH to repatriate the prisoners of war. It was, as Margaret recalls, 'a very moving experience'. Her last few months were spent at Bonegilla where the majority of patients were suffering from tuberculosis.

While working in the officers' ward at Atherton, Margaret's portrait was painted by the War Artist, Geoffrey Mainwaring, and today it hangs in the Australian War Museum.[51]

KATHLEEN MENZIES (née Gardner) RCH 1933–37, AANS 1941–45, 1st Netherlands.

Kate Menzies, whose mother was Irene Gardner, a Children's Hospital nurse (1907–11), trained at the Children's from 1933 to 1937 including six months at the Epworth Hospital. After completing midwifery at the Women's Hospital and a year of private nursing in Queensland, she returned to Melbourne and joined the AANS on 7 July 1941. Following six months at the Heidelberg Repatriation Hospital, she was posted to the Netherlands 1st Hospital Ship *Oranje* sailing in late January 1942 to the Middle East, Africa and New Zealand. Being a cruise ship, the journey out was comparatively luxurious; the return, however, was extremely strenuous with a full load of patients. After working twelve-hour shifts, Kate and her eleven nursing friends finally left the *Oranje* in Sydney in August 1942 before being assigned to the *Centaur*.⁵² However, during a route march, Kate's heart condition showed up and prevented her from going. She never saw her friends again. The *Centaur* was torpedoed off the Queensland coast on 14 May 1943, as mentioned above.

Kate met her husband, James Menzies, at the Heidelberg Repatriation Hospital and they were married at St Columb's in Hawthorn at the end of the war. They applied for a Soldier Settlement Block in Mortlake and built a successful and happy life in the Western District. Kate's only daughter, Janet Leckie, trained at the Children's during 1963–67.⁵³

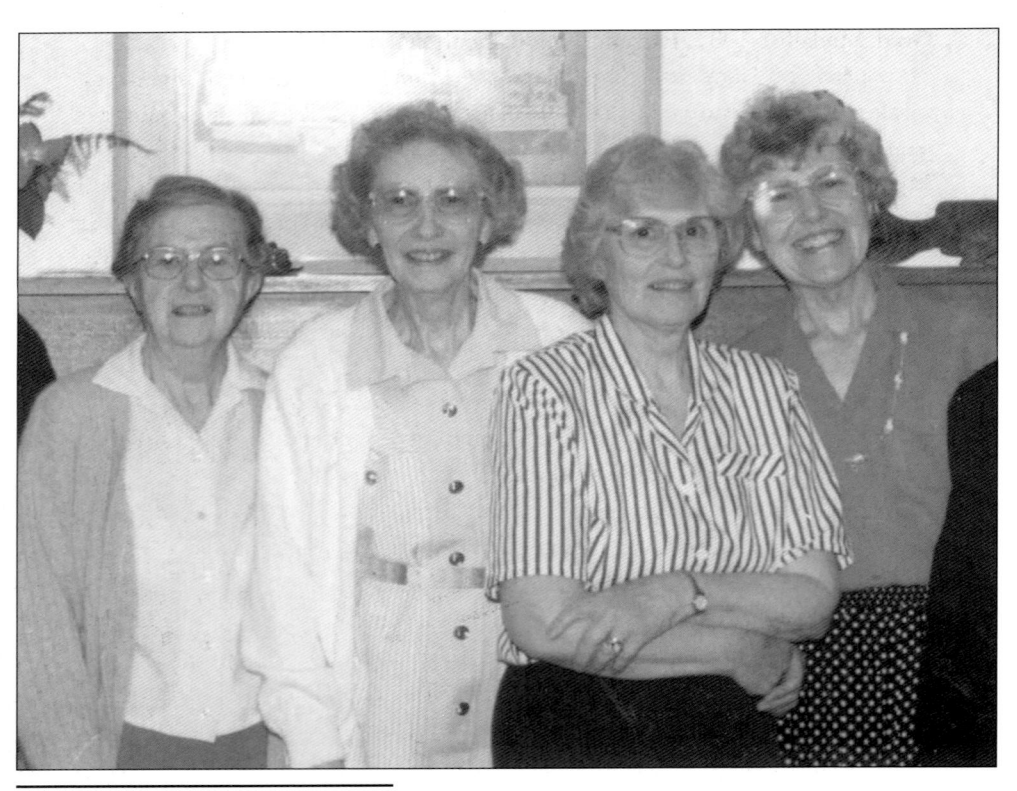

Mackenzie sisters Dr Helen, Catherine, Lucy and Sheila.
Mackenzie Family Collection.

The Years of World War Two

LUCY LANE (née Mackenzie) RAAFNS, 1942–45

Lucy is one of three sisters who trained at the Children's—Lucy, Catherine and Sheila. A fourth sister, Helen, was a doctor. Lucy was a frontline nurse during World War Two treating the wounded of the Australian Army at various points in New Guinea as they fought the advancing Japanese. Her job with thousands of others was air evacuation, dealing with injuries and tropical infections. As one of the 'air evac' nurses, she travelled to the forward areas on transport planes with cargo or troops. There they would be met by ambulances and stretchers from casualty clearing stations, getting soldiers away on aircraft to go home or to a base.[54]

About twenty-eight Children's Hospital nurses are known to have joined the RAAF Nursing Service.[55] One of those was Lucy Lane.

CATHERINE MACKENZIE, MBE RCH 1934–37, Dr Jeffreys Wood Gold Medallist 1937, Florence Nightingale Medal 1978.

Sister of Lucy and Sheila (all RCH nurses), Catherine lived and worked as a missionary nurse in Korea. Born in Korea of missionary parents and educated in Korea and Presbyterian Ladies College in Melbourne, Catherine was unable to return to Korea because of the war and taught midwifery for several years at the Queen Victoria Hospital. In 1945 she went with her sister, Dr Helen Mackenzie, to Yunnan in south-western China and, after a year of language school, established a hospital in an old Taoist temple under the auspices of the Church of Christ in China.

But it is for her work at the Il Sin Women's Hospital in Pusan, South Korea, which she began in a kindergarten building with her sister Helen, that she will be remembered. This grew to be the largest and busiest obstetric and gynaecological unit in the country.

The aim was to train Koreans as nurses and doctors in this field. In her first six months, she trained five nurses who would become the principal teachers. A larger building was erected in 1954 with the help of the American Army. Catherine spent each morning at the hospital, each afternoon at the lecture room and every two or three nights on call for emergencies and deliveries She also authored the first midwifery textbook in Korean, now in its third edition.

Catherine was awarded the MBE in 1962 and in the same year cited by the Prime Minister of Korea for her contribution to human rights for her work in Korea. She was awarded the Florence Nightingale Medal in 1978 after being nominated by the Korean Nurses' association. The International Committee of the Red Cross awards the Florence Nightingale Medal every two years to nurses and volunteer aides who have demonstrated extraordinary courage to help the wounded, as well as civilian victims of armed conflict or disaster in times of war or peace.

At a gathering of about 150 members of the League of Former Trainees at St George's Hall in Carlton in 1953, the Lady Superintendent Lucy De Neeve, mentioned the extraordinary work carried out by Catherine Mackenzie in Korea and pledged the members to assist in any way they could.[56]

Catherine Mackenzie died in Melbourne in February 2005.[57]

Nursing at the end of the war

Towards the end of the war, recruitment of hospital nurses did receive a boost, no doubt as a result of the notions of service in war time. A new generation of eager school girls stayed to Leaving standard and were really looking for something to do with their lives. Judith Lanyon returned to her school, Methodist Ladies College, to do a pre-nursing course and some Leaving subjects until she was eighteen. Her parents were happy for her to go nursing; in contrast to an earlier generation, they considered this a great way for their daughter to leave home.

Judith's Tutor at the Children's was Sister Agnes Morris (RCH 1924–48), who conducted classes of nine subjects. They were all relatively unsophisticated: how to carbolise and make up cots and beds with perfect corners, the Red Cross in the very centre with quilt hems facing the right way. 'We had high ideals. I can't remember much about lectures during training except what to put on trays. Final exams were very nerve-racking, especially the practical.'

Nurses had mixed feelings about parental visiting for these desperately ill children. Judith said: 'Looking back…parents were only allowed in once a fortnight, later curtailed to once a month, sometimes six weeks, because they [Hospital senior staff] thought there would be fewer crying children.' It was believed in those days that children settled best without the parents around. In an emergency there was little parents could do, and ward routine could be disrupted. Sheila Krysz (née Mackenzie RCH 1941–44) knew of a mother who loved her son dearly, and who was later reproached by him as an adult: 'You never worried about me when I was in Hospital. You never came to see me!' His father had visited because he was a minister, so he had the entrée, but no one had explained that his mother had not been allowed in. He had kept that resentment all those years.[58]

However, Judith Lanyon did experience an emergency when visitors were present:

A ten or eleven-year-old boy was admitted on a Sunday morning having inhaled a peanut to be removed the next day.

> It was a visiting afternoon, the ward full of people. We were cleaning instruments. All of a sudden, the boy could not breathe; the peanut had moved. I raced off to find a doctor who came but wouldn't run! Bon Ami was cleaned off a scalpel and screens rushed around the bed. The Resident—with shaking hands—performed a tracheotomy and miraculously got in below the peanut and the boy, whose colour was nearly black by this time, with a great gasp of air, turned pink and recovered!

Judith's six months at the Melbourne Hospital were traumatic and lonely. She never really felt at home there. The single bedrooms in the Charles Conibere Nurses' Home were not conducive to meeting up with friends. 'I was fairly terrified at what I might have to do [on the wards].'

Esme Nixon described those years at the new Melbourne Hospital:

> At that time the new Melbourne Hospital was only being finished and, after the attack on Pearl Harbor, the Yanks arrived in town. The war shifted north, so when the Yanks left I was sent from the Children's to the new Melbourne Hospital [and] from there…to the old wooden wards of the World War One Repatriation Hospital, Caulfield. It was cold on night duty so we wrapped layers of newspaper under our uniforms to keep us warm—always full uniform with red cape—never a cardigan.

Introduction of penicillin

Judith Lanyon remembers when penicillin was introduced:

> Giving three-hourly injections to little babies was awful. Their little arms were all bruised and so very sore. But think how things were in those days. It was supposed to be for the best. One patient I remember was a very sick little girl, nine or ten years old. The medical specialist could not find out what was wrong with her; they did many tests without result. Finally they

called in the ENT (Ear, Nose and Throat) specialist, Mr Hennessy. He saw she had a mastoid. Immediately she went to theatre and was quickly on the mend. It was very satisfying to see her well again.[59]

Marjorie Hosking (née Tomlinson) really enjoyed her training at the Children's. She trained in 1937–40, remained as a Staff Nurse and Sister then married after the war. Every ward was very special. She loved the Babies, Premature Babies, Medical, Surgical, theatre…the variety.

Out-patients was, of course, another world; it made her grow up during the war, women coping with families while husbands were away. 'When children recovered, it was wonderful. Babies with broncho-pneumonia coughing their little lungs out. If they recovered, what a reward!'

Marjorie was always very distressed when babies had gastroenteritis:

> …terrible green stools and vomiting continuously. Then magic: I think it was Dr Bill MacDonald [who] discovered that electrolytes added to the IV drip was the answer. But without a doubt the highlight was the discovery of penicillin. I was on night duty with Mona Fox…we had such a lot of children admitted with streptococcal meningitis and nothing to treat them. So many deaths, it was terrible. World War Two was on—the Americans had taken over the [new] Melbourne Hospital for a base. They had penicillin. Dr Elizabeth Turner and a young Resident went to the Melbourne and asked the Army Medicos could they buy some. The doctors gave them some, but only a small amount. Every day a large American Army car with officers brought some over to the RCH. I was off night duty and sent to Ward 16 where we had some very sick children. Nurse Mona Fox had developed this infection and was critically ill. Penicillin was used on all, and all recovered. There was a boy in Ward 9 with blood poisoning [Allan Goates]. He recovered too.[60]

Esme Nixon witnessed one of the very first penicillin injections being administered on a very young baby boy, with a less happy outcome. The parents were elderly and he, 'the only child, only son'. She 'specialled' the child, who rallied then declined. 'We [Esme and the doctor] fought for three days to save his life, then he died. The parents comforted me because they knew how we'd done our best.'[61]

DR ELIZABETH TURNER 1914–99
Dr Elizabeth Turner is revered by Children's Hospital nurses as a paediatrician of wonderful kindness and particular skills with premature babies. She was the first and only female Medical Superintendent in the history of the Hospital. On 12 March 1944, she became the first doctor to administer penicillin to a child in Australia. Nurse Margery Beavis and Ward Sister Eleanor Peck witnessed the event. Dr Turner was also the first doctor to carry out an exchange transfusion for Rh incompatibility on a neonate in Victoria, in 1951.

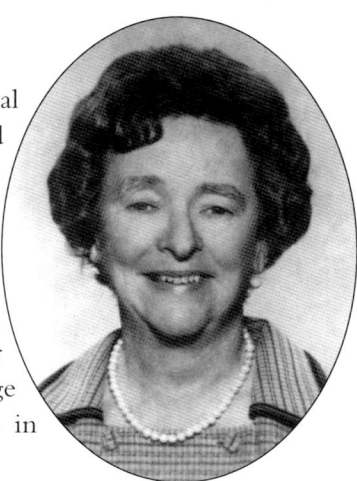

The end of the war
The war years had not prevented the Christmas spirit. The big old wards were always transformed into fairyland, a happy time. So many of the staff were clever and gave their special time to decorating the wards for the children: there were Snow White, the Seven Dwarfs, Pinocchio, Little Red Riding Hood and so many more. What an air of gaiety there was, even in the early days of the war as Peg Orford remembered: 'We went to the Vic Market at 3 am with trolleys and bought beautiful flowers for the wards. We had a lot of fun. The Resident doctors over-imbibed, turned their fire hose on to Matron's door. Water everywhere. Never heard how they got on.'[62]

Peace was declared while Esme Nixon was at the Melbourne Hospital: after coming off duty at 9 pm she changed clothes and, with some Melbourne Hospital nurses, joined in a Eureka Youth March with the Flag where 'we were carried in the crowd down Elizabeth Street much quicker. All the bells were ringing and people were joining in "Down the Lambeth Walk" and "The Conga"'.[63]

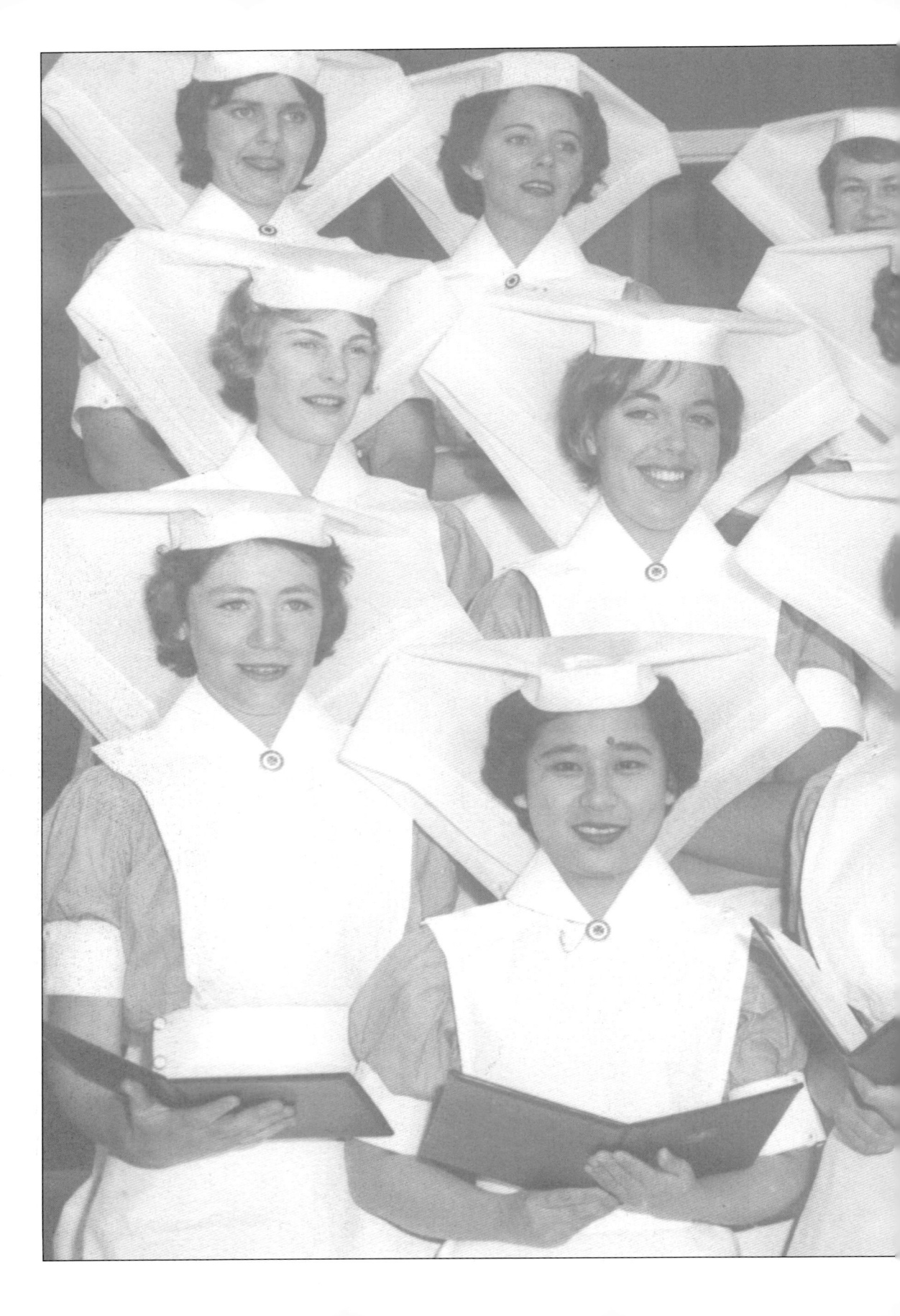

Part 4

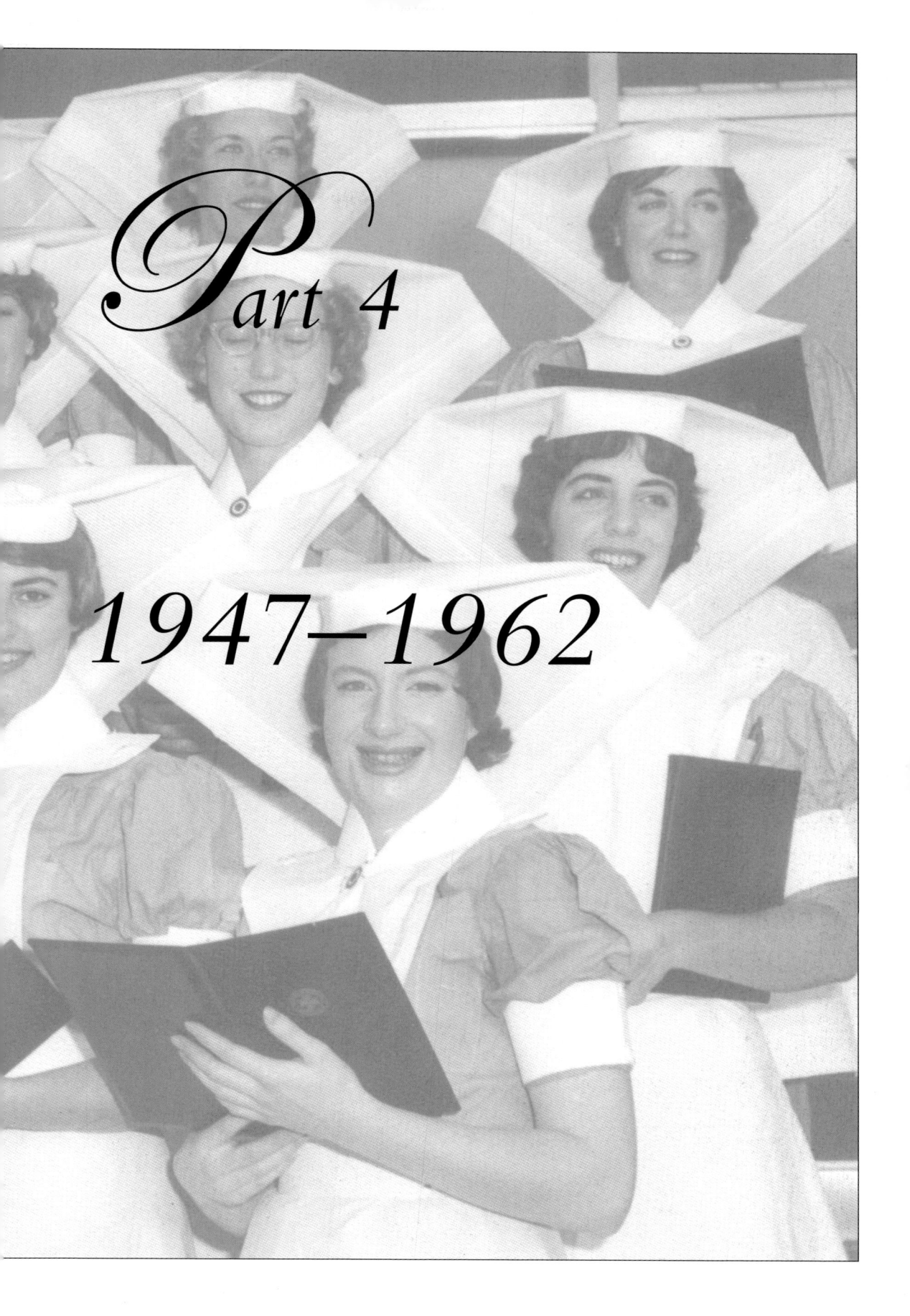

1947–1962

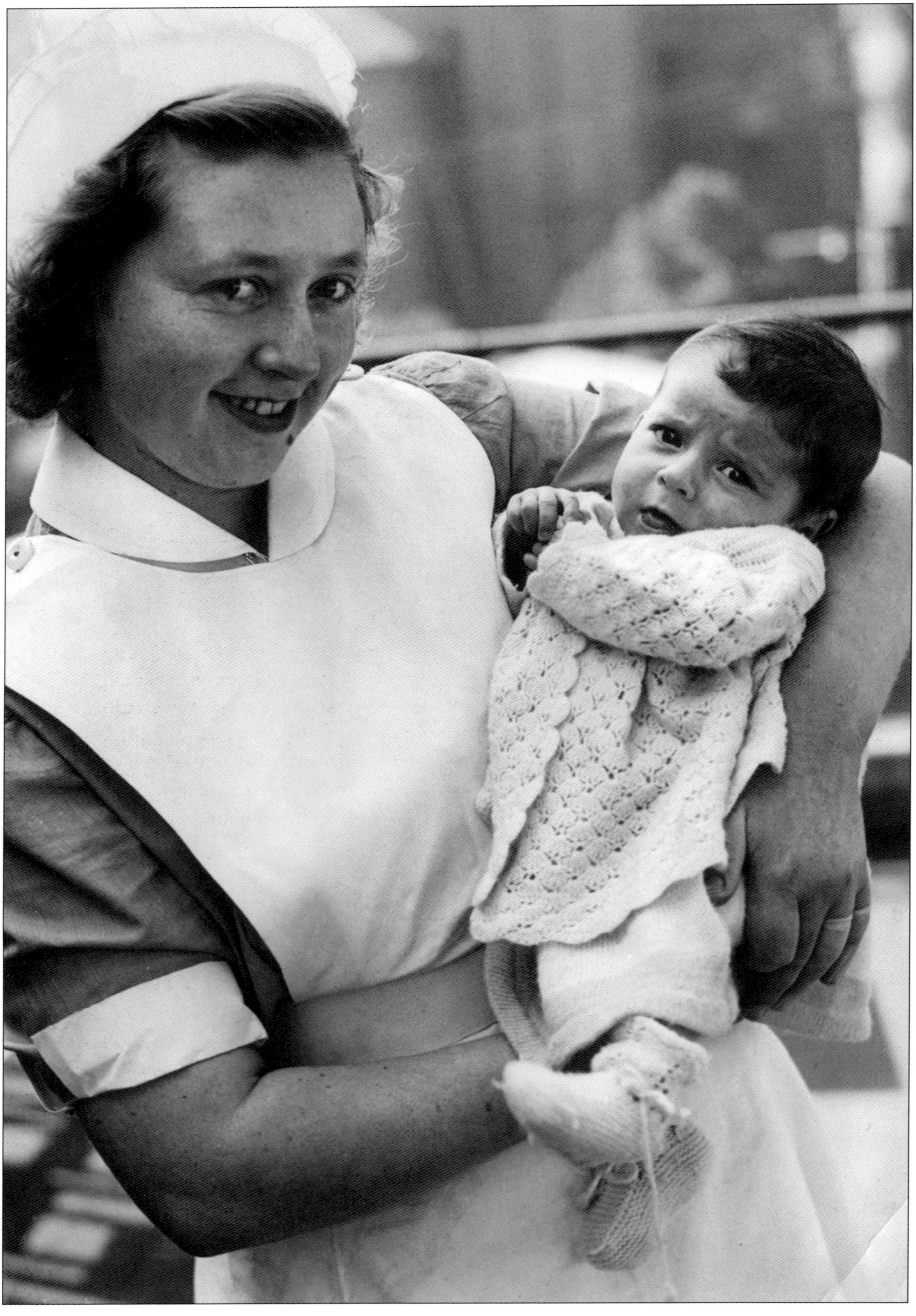

CHAPTER 10

A New Era

1947–1962

We are on the threshold of a wonderful era in the world of medicine.

Dr Elizabeth Turner, *Age,* 14 July 1945

Within a few years of war's end, therapeutic and technical advances considered little short of miraculous were making an impact on the health of children. Antibiotics and the widespread use of vaccines to control the infectious diseases of early childhood eliminated many and made others curable. In the 1950s, the convalescent homes at Sherbrooke and Hampton were closed. Improved anaesthetic techniques paved the way for dramatic progress in specialist surgery to correct many congenital abnormalities. Children stayed in hospital for shorter periods and rehabilitation improved for those suffering the aftermath of poliomyelitis, tuberculosis and other diseases.

A chronic shortage of building materials and labour delayed plans for a new Children's Hospital. It was eighteen years before hospital services for children were centralised into the new Royal Children's Hospital at Parkville. In the intervening years, the staff of the Hospital bore an increasing workload in crowded, obsolete buildings lacking reasonable facilities.

In the 1950s, working conditions for nurses remained static—a rigid female hierarchy of Matron (Lady Superintendent), Ward Sisters, staff nurses, trainees and probationers—while uniforms, caps and badges continued to denote rank. Ward

---

Nurse Nancy Hurst and baby in Ward 12.
Age September 1949.

assistants and nursing aides became a familiar adjunct to the nursing staff. The attrition rate in trainee nurses was high.

The first stage of the Children's Hospital building programme, a Nurses' Home, was completed at Parkville in 1958, providing accommodation and modern tutorial facilities for four hundred nurses. The Home remained central to vital peer support, friendship, camaraderie and companionship until the 1970s, when nurses began to live out.

A new era

Matron Walsh resigned in March 1947 after twenty-five years' service, 'to make way for a younger woman'. When interviewed by the *Age*, she expressed her heart-felt view that 'there should be more standardised and comprehensive nurse training; that nurses should not have to return to the hospital for tutorials and lectures on days off'. She believed that the 'government of the nursing profession should be in the hands of the nurses'.[1] At her farewell party arranged by the nurses in their sitting room and attended by many guests, she showed a softer side to her nature, almost apologetic, when giving her farewell speech. She explained that the shortage of nurses prevented her from introducing change.[2]

Dame Elisabeth Murdoch (then Lady Murdoch) remembers Miss Walsh as a splendid woman but old-fashioned and strict: 'I think I was amazed when I understood the [nurses'] conditions…and I had great admiration for her through all her time there in trying to improve their conditions and as to what was needed for their development.'[3]

Any of a number of extremely capable women at the Children's could have succeeded to the role of Matron. Notably, Sophie Brodie,[4] the Deputy Matron at Frankston, and the tutors Kate Wilson,[5] Agnes Morris and Marjorie Allnatt[6] were all experienced, intelligent, well-educated and widely respected nurse educators. The longest serving staff member, Ivy Flower, had been Deputy Matron since 1934.

Rather than choose any one of these women, the Committee of Management cast a wider net, advertising throughout Australia, New Zealand and the United Kingdom for a suitable person to lead the Hospital. Dame Elisabeth Murdoch did not recall why the Committee recruited from overseas, but remembered that 'Maie (Lady) Casey was on the Committee at that time and she knew Lady Reading. She got in touch with her to see Mrs [Lucy] Sechiari…we did go to a lot of trouble to make sure she was up to the job and we thought that maybe after the war and after all the difficulties, we had to have a very strong and modern person. She was loved by many people but I am sure she shocked a lot of people when she came.' Dame Elisabeth remembers that 'the Committee were right behind Mrs Sechiari, although they may have been amazed and astonished at the change in what we knew as a matron. A radical change—but I think the nursing staff liked her very much.'[7]

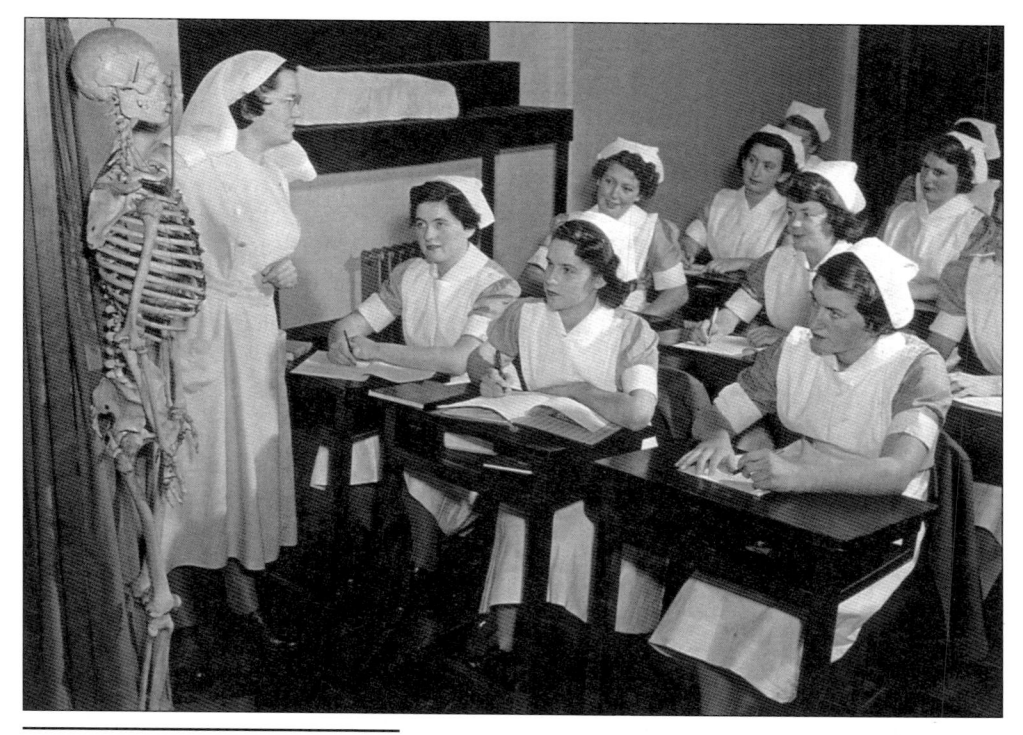

Sister Allnatt, Tutor, Preliminary Training School, 1952.
L–R: Margot Semmens, Elizabeth Strickland, Jean McDonald, Jennifer Nicholas, Marge Thomson, Joan Shepherd, Margaret Mair, Nan Hunt, Bev Heriot.
Out of sight: Pearl Massey, Betty Hulls, Wilma Macauley.
RCHA/Strickland Family Collection.

In November 1947, Mrs Lucy Sechiari became the sixth Lady Superintendent of the Children's Hospital and was a major influence in the advancement of the educational and professional standing of nursing at the Hospital in the post-war years.

LUCY WALMSLEY SECHIARI DE NEEVE
Lucy Walmsley Sechiari De Neeve was born on 25 October 1906 at Darwen in Lancashire, England, the daughter of an auctioneer. She entered Royal Liverpool Children's Hospital at the age of twenty to commence her nurse training and received her certificate in 1929. Four years later she began general training at University College Hospital, London. Her interest in paediatrics led to positions of Home Sister and Theatre Sister at the Princess Elizabeth of York Hospital for Children in London.

During World War Two, Lucy Sechiari was active at the Ministry of Pensions Hospital, Roehampton, and at Stoke Mandeville, Buckinghamshire, where she organised plastic surgery theatres. As a member of the British expatriate community while serving three years in India in Queen Alexandra's Imperial Military Nursing Service (QAIMNS), she became a Red Cross organiser. These wartime associations at the British base outside Bombay (present day Mumbai) earned her the nickname 'Poona' by close friends.

On discharge from the QAIMNS in February 1947, Mrs Sechiari applied for the position of Lady Superintendent of the Children's Hospital in Melbourne. Prior to leaving for Melbourne she gained more experience at the Lord Mayor Treloar's Orthopaedic Hospital for children at Alton in Hampshire and returned to the Queen Elizabeth Hospital for Sick Children (formerly the Princess Elizabeth).[8]

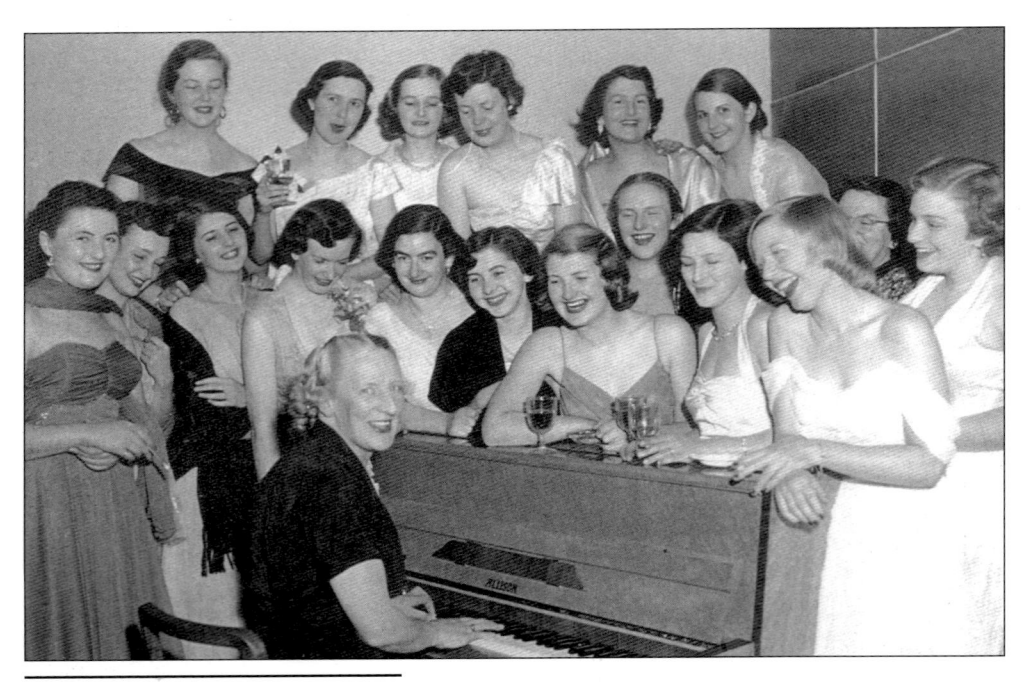

A 1950s graduation party with Lady Superintendent Lucy De Neeve.
Back L–R: Sally Gillespie, Myrtle Benton, Norma Ross, Elizabeth Thompson, Betty Hulls, Janet Jackson, Margaret Mair.
Front L–R: Anne Kendall, Elizabeth Strickland, Judy Ahearn, Diane Macleod, Bev Heriot, Mary McCallum, Elizabeth Corrigan, Jill Waterhouse, Marjorie Allnatt, Judy Thompson.
RCHA/Strickland Family Collection.

A New Era

Lucy Sechiari's appointment was controversial from the beginning. She chose to travel to Australia via a leisurely six-week cruise rather than the quicker but arduous flight out as requested by Lady Latham, the Hospital President.

As she left no memoirs, we have to rely on others to inform us of her progress in Melbourne. In November 1948, the *Age* ran a retrospective review of her first year:

> Almost a year ago Mrs Sechiari stepped ashore from the *Stratheden* into Melbourne's seething Cup-eve crowds. A fortnight later she began her duties as new Matron of the Children's Hospital. Blonde, blue eyed Matron Sechiari paused for a few minutes in her busy day to survey her year in Melbourne and to sum up her impressions of our hospital: our people and our country.
>
> Things she is happy about are: our Hospital Auxiliaries—something quite new, in her experience. England has nothing like them. She hopes the scheme of National medicine will not sound the death knell. The Hospital is the happiest she has ever worked in. Its nursing course compares favourably with similar courses in England.

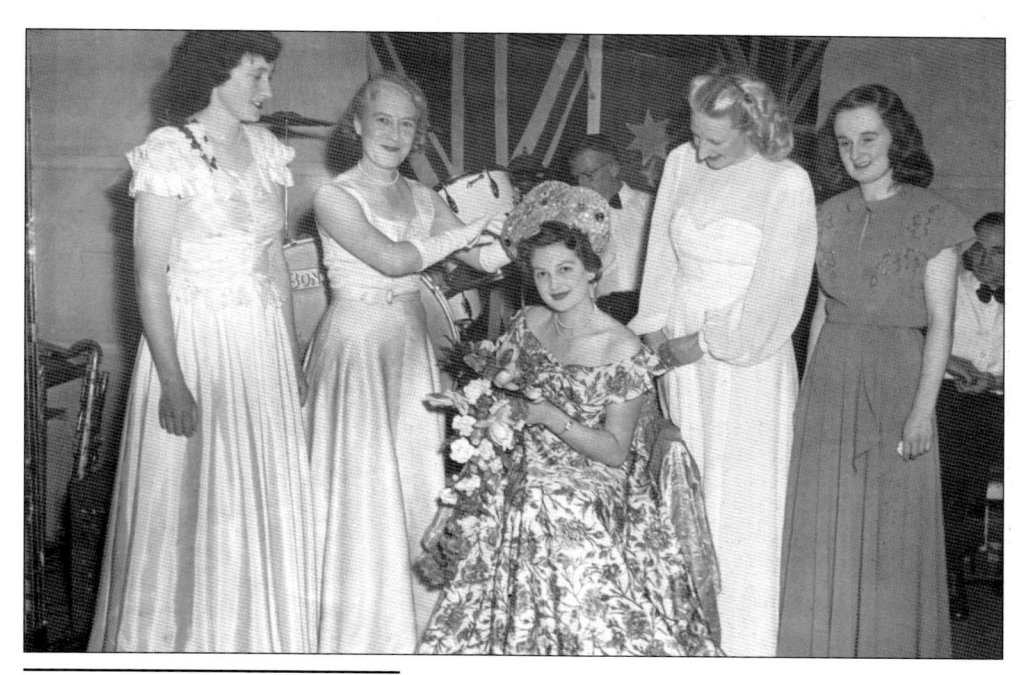

Queen of the Children's Hospital Fundraising: Barbara Catto, 1948.
L–R: Joan Hatswell, Maie (Lady) Casey, Barbara Catto, Lucy Sechiari, Barbara Hampson.
RCHA/Wilcox Family Collection.

On the debit side, Mrs Sechiari is hampered by old buildings and inefficient accommodation. 'Not even a kitten could be swung in the cramped nurses' quarters.' She has approved innovations [such as] preliminary training 1–2 months, and does not approve of starch and [has] swept it out... She said she is 'not quite sane where children's nursing is concerned. It is almost a fetish with her to get the children best possible care and training for her young nurses and for the best conditions to work in and to get children well.'

Dame Patricia Mackinnon had just been appointed to the Committee when Mrs Sechiari first arrived in Melbourne and remembers that time when they almost started together. The Committee did not see a great deal of her in those days because she was only required to attend their meetings once a month and did not stay very long. Dame Patricia said she knew her more socially, in a way, than in the Hospital, because she was a very gregarious and social person herself. She had a little house in the grounds of the old Carlton Hospital known as Matron's Flat. She entertained with Sunday lunch parties and invited members of the Committee as well as members of the senior medical staff, visiting doctors or visiting nurses. Dame Patricia said they were 'very delightful little parties. However, we always knew there was deep concern about the nurses, in the back of her mind all the time.'[9]

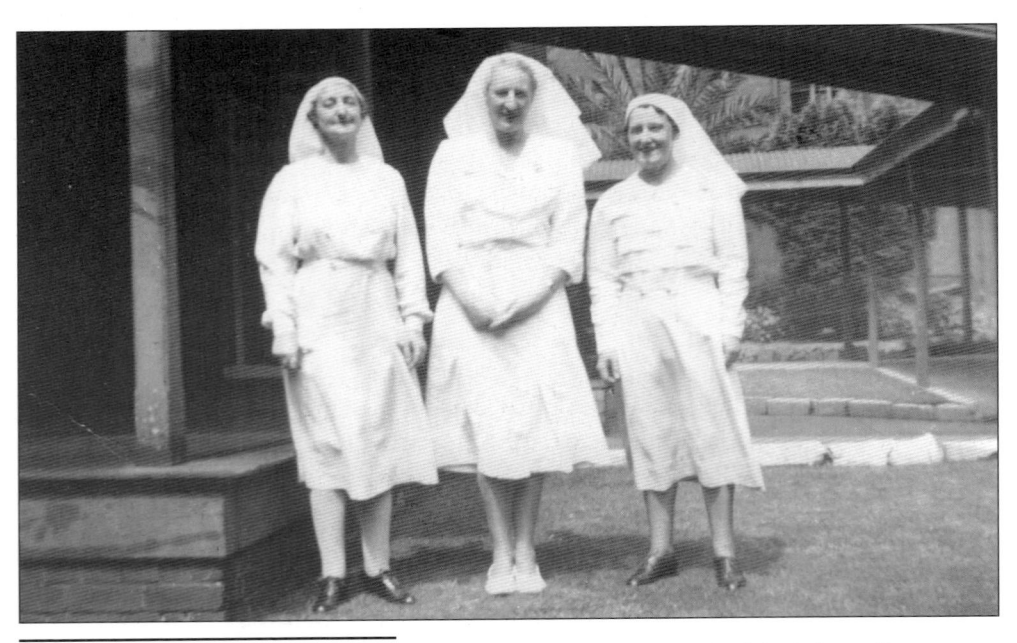

Sister Katherine 'Kit' Webster (Home Sister), Matron Lucy Sechiari (later De Neeve) and Sister Ivy Flower (Assistant Matron), 1949.
RCHA/Brain Collection.

The self-contained flat centrally adjacent to the Nurses' Home was serviced by a personal maid who attended to Mrs Sechiari's every need. This became her permanent home for almost five years, and was decorated in her own inimitable style. Unfortunately, the location lacked privacy. The comings and goings of her private life were visible from every angle of the Hospital. When she re-married in 1952, she and her husband, Mr Anton De Neeve, moved to their own home in Rathdowne Street, Carlton. Nevertheless, the Committee of Management decreed she retain the flat for use during working days and for entertaining as befitted the important position she held in the Hospital.

Lucy Sechiari was very different from previous matrons in her personality and approach to staff. When she lived in her flat in the early days, she was invariably sitting up in bed with a cup of tea when the amused Night Sister handed over her report at 7 am.[10] At Christmas, her hospitality extended to the senior Ward Sisters who were flattered to be invited for drinks—more often than not, pink champagne.

All those who met Lucy Sechiari recall being struck by her appearance: 'she dressed in a soft, pintucked ivory silk blouse and straight matching skirt nipped in with a silver buckled belt. Her starched veil appeared enormous, a contrast to the droopy organdie worn by the older administration staff. Cream shoes and stockings completed her outfit.'[11] Junior nurses thought her charismatic. There are many memories: 'She flowed into the dining room all in white, quite a vision because she was so very regal. She arrived attended by a retinue [of Sisters] in blue, probably only four—but it seemed a lot—and we all stood until she started to eat.'[12]

She bought a small car that enabled her to make regular trips to the Hospital annexes in the Dandenong Ranges and Hampton and Frankston. Those invited to travel with her described her terrible driving, for she tended to be distracted. One day she waved out the window, appearing to give a signal, when suddenly a motorcycle policeman grasped her hand. To her passenger's amusement, she was not giving a signal at all, she was waffling around![13]

Improvements

For a woman who left war-time Britain for a bright new life in a promising country, Mrs Sechiari was extremely disappointed to find many sections of the Hospital in a bad state of repair. Huge, old-fashioned wards and out-dated equipment seemed a replica of Hackney Children's Hospital in the East End of London.[14]

Diana Ramsey described the difficulties in the old operating theatre at Carlton after the war. As deputy to Sister Dorothy 'Dottie' Saunders who reigned over the theatre for many years, 'an inspiration to all who worked under her', she witnessed a memorable event:

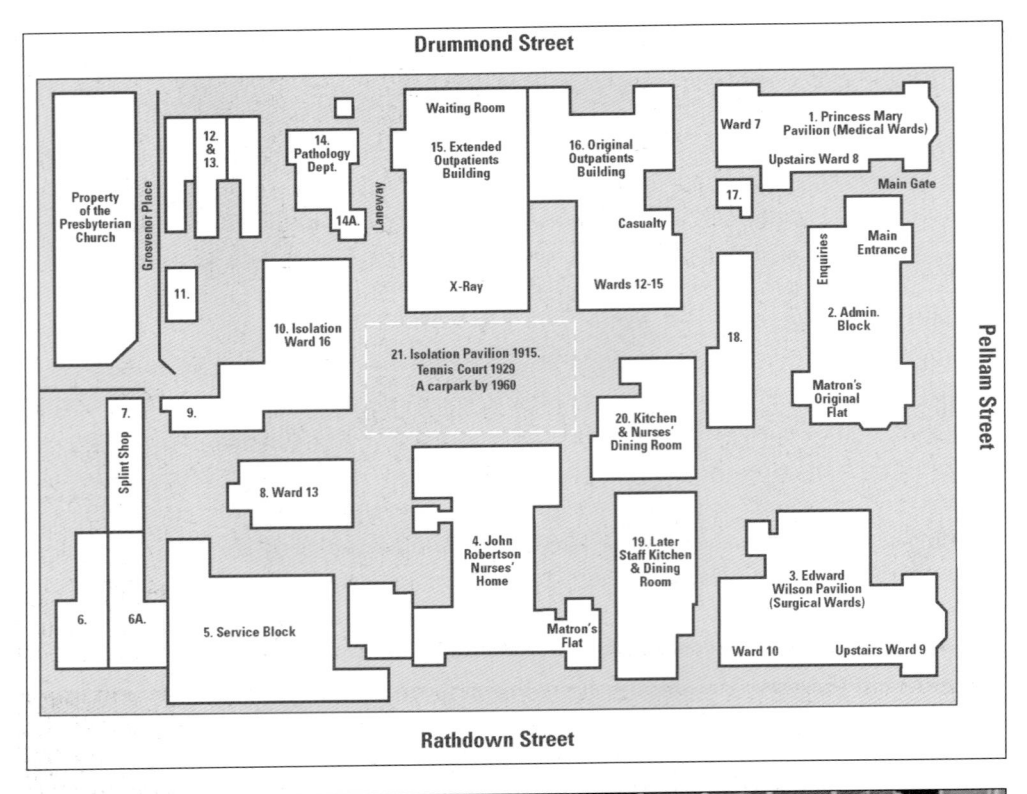

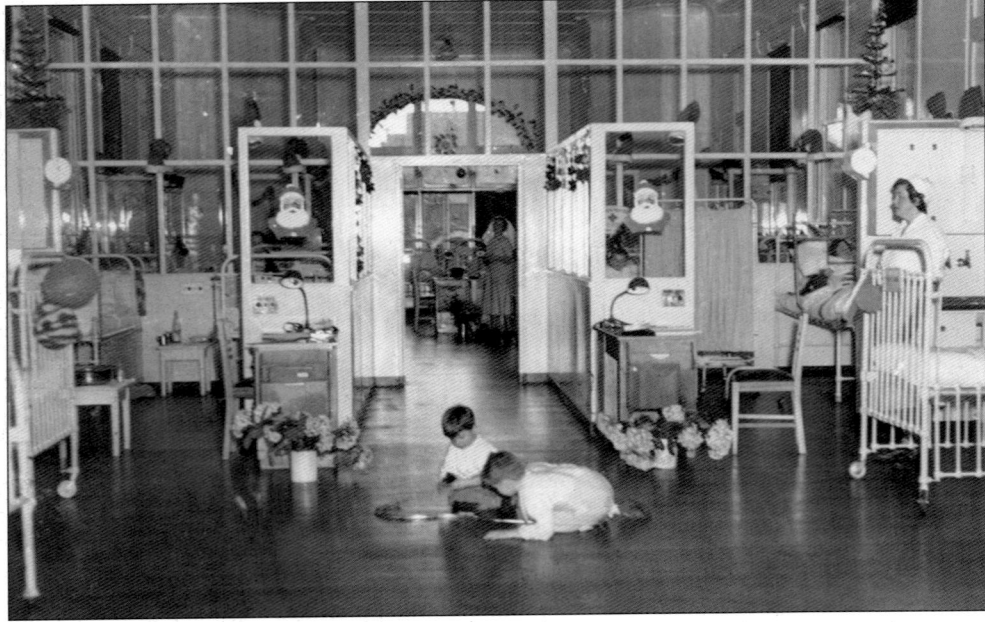

Top: Historic Ground Plan, Carlton Hospital, 1950s.
Bottom: Medical Ward, Christmas, 1950.

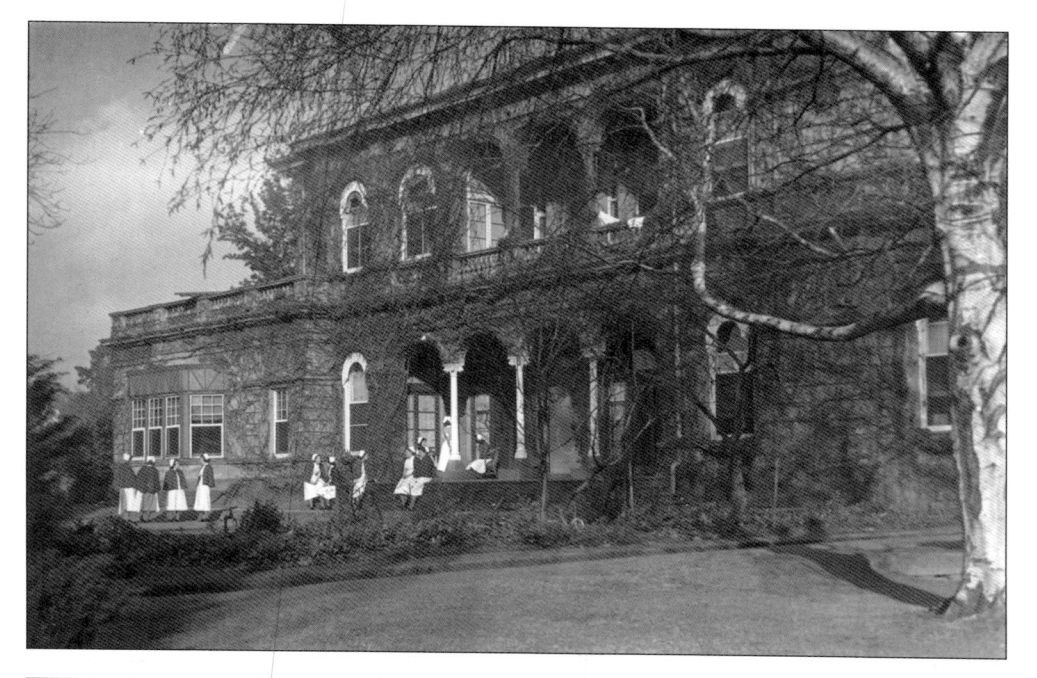

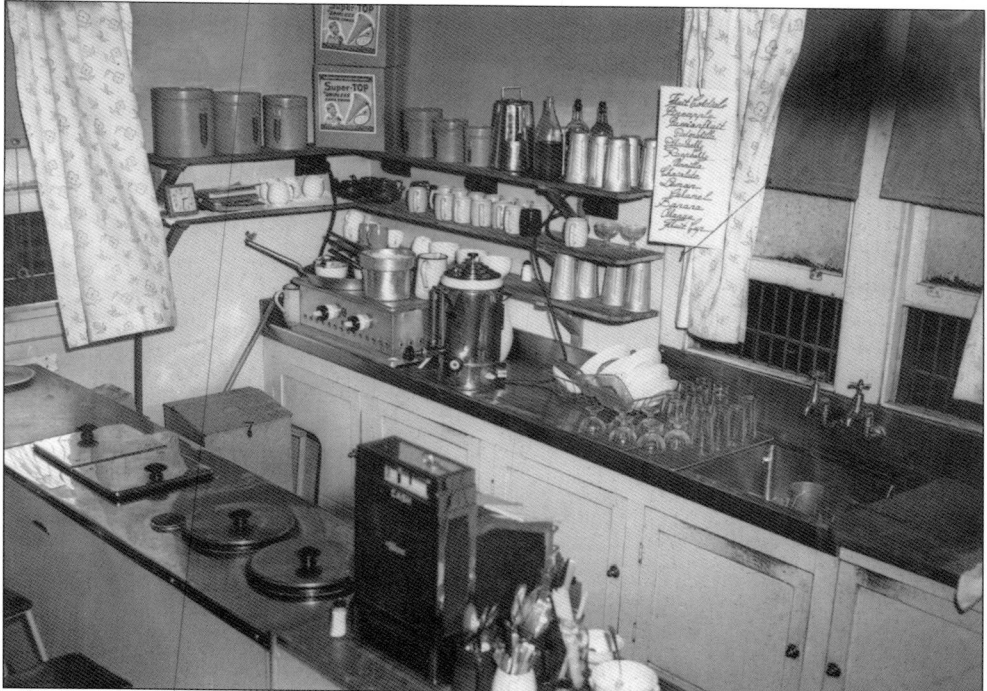

Top: Heathfield, Kenley Court, Toorak. Night Nurses' Home with accommodation for the Preliminary Training School.
Bottom: Carlton Nurses' Home canteen under the stairs.

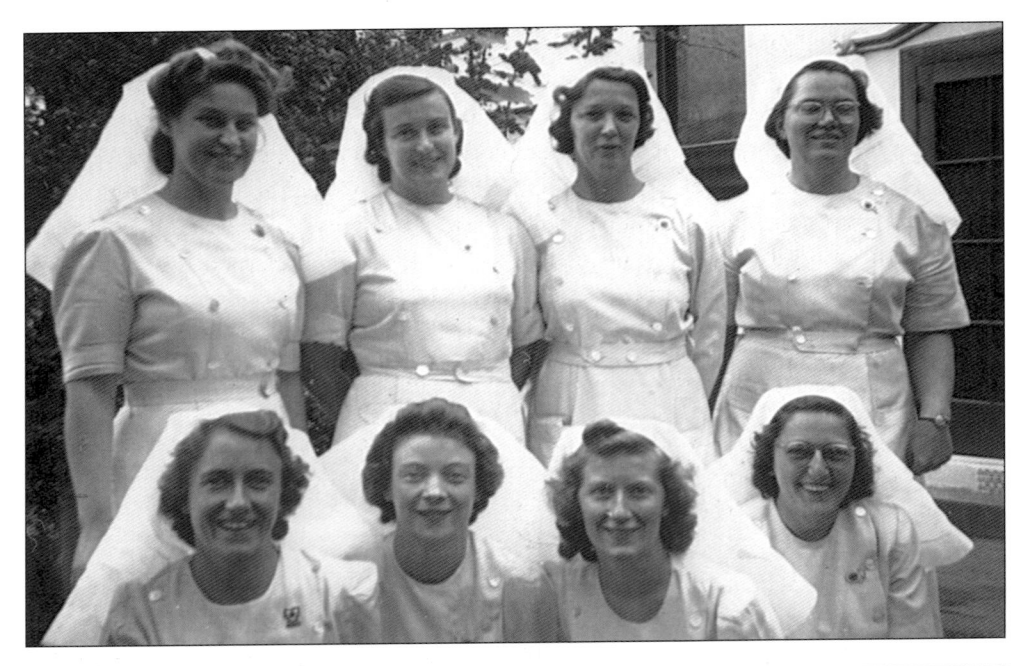

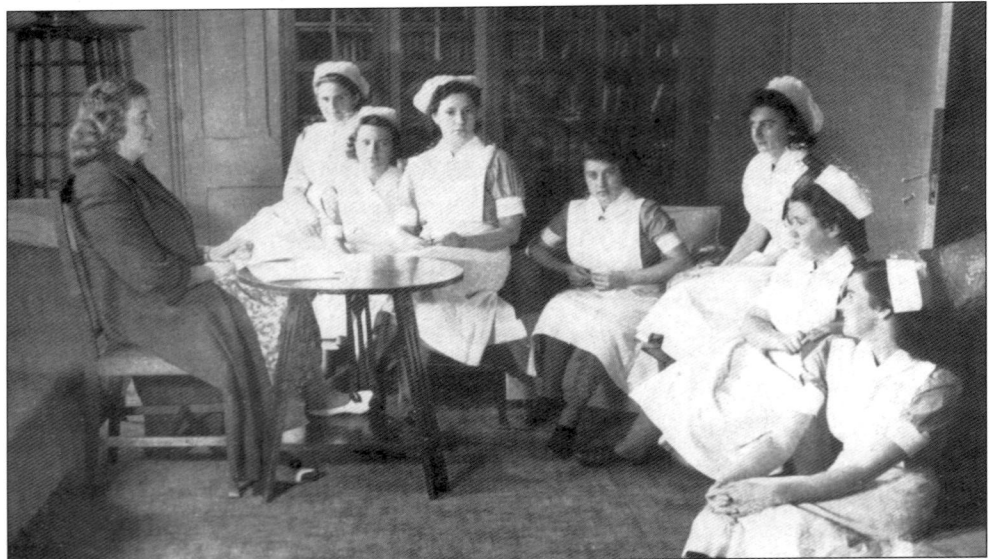

Top: Ward Sisters, 1949.
Back L–R: Nancy Castellan, Una Wishart, Marjorie Allnatt.
Front L–R: Margaret Drake, (unknown).
Curwen Walker Family Collection.
Bottom: A meeting of the Executive of the Nurses' Council in the nurses' sitting room, Carlton, 1949. Adele Brain, second right.
RCHA/Cunningham Family Collection.

A New Era

I was appointed to 'scrub' for the first, or certainly one of the first, tracheo oesophageal atresia [operations] to be performed in the very old theatre by Mr Russell Howard. He was assisted by several young Residents and Registrars, not to forget the anaesthetist. After detailed preparation, Mr Howard, with scalpel in hand, asked the X-ray technician to begin photographing. The technician obliged and, with that, the entire theatre was thrown into darkness, no power at all. Mr Howard clasped his hands together above his chest and sat down calmly waiting for order to return. We, the staff, sprang into action to see what emergency lighting we could gather from the wards below. This was carried out very efficiently and within about half an hour, the operation proceeded. I was delighted as a new Theatre Sister to be responsible for this major operation. I think I must have done well because one of the young Residents was impressed enough to ask me to marry him![15]

Elizabeth Sadlier had a personal experience of old equipment. When her time of training was completed in 1949, the Hospital offered her a 'farewell gift': a tonsillectomy. She had a great deal of time off work with a sore throat, including twelve months while at the Melbourne Hospital. A positive pathological specimen of gastric contents revealed tuberculosis. 'When the time came to leave the operating theatre, the lift to Ward 9 was out of order, and Dr Nathaniel Myers carried me down the fire escape to the sick bay.' She met him several years later; he remembered the incident and commented: 'and you were heavy too'.[16]

In 1949–50, structural alterations were made to the wards and the Casualty, Out-patients and admission areas to improve efficiency in the Hospital and lessen congestion. Largely due to the influence of Dr Vernon Collins and Dr Howard Williams, large wards were divided into two twenty-bed units and partitioned into smaller units with four babies and six children, ten in all. One Sister supervised four separate nursing teams to simulate a more intimate, homely atmosphere. Unfortunately, the plan fell short of the ideal. The cubicles were not provided with bathrooms and nurses continued to carry children who were well enough to be bathed through the long ward to the service area. Heavy nappy buckets and bed-pans added to the nurses' tasks and they were run off their feet.

Dr (later Professor) Vernon L. Collins, 1950s.

Mrs Sechiari agreed with Dr Collins, the Medical Superintendent, that children would be more stable if they had the same personal nurses around them in the early morning, day and evening, but this was difficult to achieve. The Hospital was not able to employ more nurses because of a shortage of accommodation. When the forty-hour week was introduced in 1948, the Hospital rented several houses to ease the problem: 'Park Court' flats in Parkville and 'Poolman House', Domain Road, South Yarra, were obtained for trained staff.[17] 'Heathfield' in Kooyong Road, Toorak, became a wonderful retreat for night staff and a pleasant introduction for those in the Preliminary Training School, while seniors lived at 'Marembe' in Gatehouse Street, Parkville. Mrs Sechiari expressed the view that the trained staff was able to lead a more normal life in this more pleasant accommodation and, to some extent, could forget the worries and responsibilities of the Hospital when off duty. This had been a difficult thing to do when living in the middle of Hospital activities.

Unfortunately, the main Nurses' Home was very cramped and trainees continued to work a forty-eight-hour week in broken shifts. Nurses' living conditions did receive due attention. For example, the Nurses' Home had become very shabby during the war; it was re-painted and refurbished with new curtains, beds and mattresses. Mrs Sechiari negotiated with Mrs Edgar Rouse of the Nurses' Committee on the matter of fitting up a hairdressing 'shampoo room' in the Nurses' Home. A visitors' room and a snack bar were also sources of satisfaction for some time.

The uniforms were re-designed, becoming more 'English'. The draconian black stockings were replaced by the softer grey lisle and nurses ceased to be identified as 'black legs' by patients and staff at the (Royal) Melbourne Hospital. That first hot summer, the uniform sleeves were shortened, the time-wasting wrist cuffs abolished and apron cross-over straps eliminated. Instead, there were awkward buttons with shanks and safety pins. Beginners had no belts, but a purple belt was worn after six months if the probationer was accepted. A pass in the junior exams at the end of first year earned a white belt. A frilled organdie cap, known as 'frills', was enormously important in promotion to seniority, a goal second only to the veil.

Unfortunately, the starched collar remained a horror on a hot Melbourne day. Senior Sisters welcomed the first changes introduced to their uniforms since the 1920s: the drab, fawn Holland was replaced with soft, blue Lystav dresses with short sleeves, a double row of buttons and a belt. Staff nurses wore the same version in primrose yellow.

Mrs Sechiari encouraged her nurses to speak out. Trained staff commenced meetings each Wednesday fortnight where opinions were expressed, complaints voiced and suggestions made for the improvement of the work and conditions in the Hospital. Some of these meetings became lectures at which members of the Medical and other departments were invited to speak. Mrs Sechiari elevated the status of trainees, referring to them as 'students'. The Student Nurses' Council was re-formed and meetings held every six weeks in the nurses' sitting room. The Lady Superintendent, the Medical Director and members of the trained staff attended as guests by invitation only. The Student Council gained influence and in 1954: fourth-year students were given a double row of cap frills.[18]

As with any new management, there was some resistance to Mrs Sechiari's innovations and to her style. This came largely from a group of Senior Sisters and persisted for many years. One of her strengths was the ability to gather around a strong group of women who became her supporters, some to the exclusion of others. In a Hospital with a tradition of working in a close multi-disciplinary way, particularly in the care of very difficult medical cases, this could sometimes become a 'closed shop'. Cliques were formed in the dining room and in off-duty hours. Mrs Sechiari allowed senior staff to have their way and this sometimes appeared to exclude others.[19] However, she was very encouraging to all those with initiative and open to employing good staff who were not trained by the Children's Hospital.

In 1946, Medical Ward 7, with forty children, came under the charge of Sister Nancy Castellan. An Austin Hospital trainee with a double certificate, she experienced among the Children's Hospital-trained nurses a feeling of superiority over those trained elsewhere. Nancy said, 'I was not really accepted. They liked their own trainees. Very few Children's trainees had extra certificates at that stage; their horizons were quite narrow. A few had Mothercraft Certificates, for example, Elizabeth Fearon, Sister-in-Charge, Ward 7.'

Nancy came from a very large family, the only girl of eleven children and, although she lived in at the Hospital, she did not mix easily. Her shyness was often misunderstood, creating fear in junior nurses. Later on, she was required at home; her father was ill with Parkinson's disease. She said, 'that distanced me from them [the staff]. There was very little socialisation. I overheard Senior Sisters saying, "two gone, one to go", meaning outside staff who, in their perception, did not belong.' She felt that although the Hospital was crowded and old, it was not too bad. 'I liked Lucy and I think she had problems too [being accepted].'[20]

Nancy believed that hers was a happy ward, although some former trainees have less fond memories. She remembers the Ward 7 Honoraries: Doctors Howard Williams, Mostyn Powell, Stanley Williams, Vernon Collins and Elizabeth Turner. The Lady Superintendent was a visible presence on the daily ward rounds but had very few meetings with the Ward Sister.

Another notable long-serving member of staff welcomed by Mrs Sechiari was Elizabeth Coombes, who trained at the King Edward VII Hospital at Windsor in England in November 1943. Following midwifery training at the Simpson Memorial Pavilion in Edinburgh, Elizabeth's work experience took her to the most impoverished slum housing of that city, the Grass Market, where women had no mattresses, sinks or running water, the basics of human existence, in the old upper storeys. She worked on the district with the famous Maggie Miles, the author of the well-known midwifery book used in the UK and Australia. At the Children's, Elizabeth did not exactly experience discrimination but she was very lonely. Her first Christmas at the Children's—she did not know anybody and came on duty at 1 pm, missing the morning festivities—was saved by an invitation by Dr R. Graham Orr, the eye specialist who noticed her UK badge and her lonely look. He asked if she had anywhere to go and invited her home for dinner.[21]

Elizabeth was Night Sister for eighteen months and lived in the house provided by the Hospital in Domain Road, South Yarra. She described it as 'lovely accommodation'. Her reputation was established with her appointment as the Casualty Sister. She found Lucy Sechiari 'marvellous and always willing to listen to ideas for improvements'.

In the 1950s, a new approach to children in Hospital began to emerge. Its focus was on creating a homely atmosphere, training a nurse to take the place of the mother for the duration of a child's stay. It also sought to keep the breast-feeding mothers and babies together, to ensure parents were well-informed and to reduce cross-infection.

Medical nursing

Accessed by a series of ramps, stairs and old lifts, the Medical Wards 7 and 8 accommodated as many as forty children each, sometimes more, all of them with conditions requiring intensive nursing. Diseases such as meningitis, eczema, rheumatic fever and nephritis (Bright's disease) were well represented. Babies with Pink disease were the most miserable with their chronic crying, red hands and runny noses, soft floppy arms and legs and an inability to be comforted. Irritable and photophobic (unable to stand the light), they were some of the most challenging patients in the ward. No medical cure was available, as the cause, mercury in teething powders, had not yet been confirmed. Jean Cussen remembered nursing a child with this disease. She also had another with myasthenia gravis: 'There was an electric suction apparatus in Ward 9, Surgical: you had to run down the ramp from Ward 7, across to the lift in Surgical to get it and run back. I think it was the only apparatus between two or three wards when the child choked and I needed to get it.'[22]

Diabetic children had to be monitored. The Ward Sister usually gave the insulin while the junior, on the alert for 'hypos', fetched the glucose drink if necessary. Their special food came from the food room, carefully weighed into small portions.

Juniors spent a lot of time in Ward 14 where they learned to feed and change babies very quickly. 'As a junior, feeding and cleaning was what you did. As a senior, in the morning we had to oil and weigh the "premies". They were like skinned rabbits, with no sub-cutaneous fat and thin skin. They were nursed in little wire basket cots with hot water bags and woollen clothing for warmth. Oxygen was piped into their cots. This changed markedly with the introduction of humidicribs.'[23]

A New Era

The other duty in the morning for seniors and second-years was to 'do' the eczema babies. This meant taking off the wrist and ankle restraint, splints and bandages, oiling them, then applying zinc and coal tar ointment, sometimes gentian violet and trying to stop them from scratching when the splints were off. These babies rubbed their heads, backs and whatever they could move because of the itch. They were frequently dosed with chloral hydrate. The introduction of cortisone changed all that.

Sometimes a nurse was asked to carry out a difficult and delicate procedure on these tiny babies: Audrey Grant (née Laugher) said one of her proudest moments was when she was asked to demonstrate an infant catheterisation to a group of nurses. The Ward Sister was impressed when she catheterised a neonate. 'Much to my relief, all went well.'

Ward 12 was the gastro ward and a beginner's 'first post', where she learnt barrier nursing. Separate gowns were worn to handle each baby and when the feeding and changing was completed, the nurse placed the gown in a calico bag tied to the end of the cot. Babies never saw a nurse without a mask, and were therefore unable to process the features of those tending them, merely registering eye to eye and relying on the tone of the voice. A great deal of washing of the nurses' hands followed by a rinse in Zephiran was mandatory between each baby. Failure to wash the hands was an offence.

One of the saddest events in the 1950s was the arrival of migrant babies with salmonella, straight off the migrant ships. Bound in blankets to 'keep safe from harm', as was the parents' way on a boiling hot day, some babies were unwrapped to be found dead from dehydration. It seemed so sad that these people who were escaping from their own country to start a new life arrived with a dead baby. Nine-month-old twins Andre and Alexandre Schilov arrived with their parents at Station Pier suffering extreme dysentery. Each had about eighteen intravenous injections to keep them alive and they were re-hydrated with electrolytes, quite experimental at the time. Their mother, a well-educated woman, was given a job in the Hospital laundry to be near her babies—a humane attempt at parent involvement. The family was very well looked after by the Hospital Almoner, who found them a house nearby with 'a garden and flowers'. The twins survived to adulthood.[24]

A routine part of admission was to check the child's head for pediculi, treat it with acetic acid and wrap it with a triangle bandage of calico until it was clean. The poor child was very conspicuous but was allowed to have the headpiece removed on Christmas day. A fireman visiting for the festivities was seen to put his shiny brass helmet on one of the nitty children's head for fun, much to the amusement of the nurses.

Admission required a lot of time; nurses talked at length to the parents to take as many particulars as possible because, once a child was admitted, the parents were not permitted to return for six weeks.

The Medical Wards had a certain atmosphere and smell: the methyl salicylate of bandages and blanket beds on children with rheumatic fever; the urine testing racks and test tubes in the hot service rooms; the sluice where pans were emptied and nappies were scrubbed; the zinc cream and baby powder. The work in the long wards was tiring in the long summer months.

A test for nurses was the sterile drainage procedure for children with kidney disease; Southey's drainage tubes were inserted into the lower legs of a nephritic child while the nurses kept the child quiet and comfortable as the procedure progressed. All the while, they took great care with sterility, ensuring that the escaping fluid was collected correctly in the receptacle, usually with a bucket, and that the cannulas were kept in position with sterile strapping while the patient was sitting up with legs hanging down, or sitting in Fowler's position with a cradle placed over the legs. Oedema from kidney disease commonly affecting children was leaked slowly, not only from the lower legs and ankles but sometimes by peritoneal dialysis.[25]

Children with miliary tuberculosis were nursed on the open balconies of Wards 7 and 8, facing Drummond Street, where canvas blinds shielded them from the western sun. Panting with heat and high temperatures, they required constant cooling sponges, back rubs and mouth toilets. One of the first procedures junior nurses learned off by heart was the preparation of a mouth-wash tray commonly used for unconscious children and those with high fevers: forceps, cotton swabs, bowls to contain the lotion, glycerine and borax and some pleasant mouthwash such as the pink-coloured glycothymoline. The nurse always explained what she was about to do, talking gently to the child if they were conscious, to gain their confidence.

The patient's comfort was always first: the frequent gentle turn from side to side, the back rub and a fresh clean gown, a crisp cool sheet to comfort and sooth. Often the children in the Research Ward 15 could not bear to be touched; for those with nephroblastoma, the gentlest movement was agony. The nurses were aware and observant. A frontier not conquered in the 1950s was childhood leukaemia. Judith Butt experienced the heartbreak of watching a child die in her arms: there were no visitors, no comfort in the dark, quiet ward; the Night Sister was far away and 'I felt so helpless as the child bled from every orifice. I howled and howled.'[26]

A great innovation was the employment of 'Pinkies' or ward assistants, many of them migrant women, who fed and dressed children who were up and about. They kept the utility rooms tidy, sorted the linen and assisted in the kitchen and bathroom. The nurses came to admire these women who had families of their own and brought their life experiences, customs and skills into the wards. They were kind and gentle. Sometimes in the evening or at 5 o'clock tea—if there was time—they cooked delicious, light pancakes in the ward kitchen for the children and the nurses. Most importantly, they interpreted for doctors and nurses; very often they were called to the Out-patients and Casualty departments.

Ward 17

Ward 17 was the Tonsils Ward. Children were admitted early in the morning for theatre that day. The children were carried back and forth along the corridor by an orderly, as most of them were small. Seeing them wake up with the shock of such painful throats was awful. Nurses felt children were deceived by well-meaning parents with stories that they would wake up to ice-cream and jelly and little of the reality. They had to be watched very carefully for bleeding and those that were doubtful cases were transferred to Surgical Ward. Many a nurse spent an anxious night watching for signs on the pillow. Small amounts of aspirin—'Morph and Asp', a pink mixture—was allowed but sometimes there could be a tendency to bleed. Occasionally, if post-op bleeding could not be stopped, the child was whisked back to theatre. Mothers commonly left the hospital with their child clutching their bottle of medicine for pain relief issued by the pharmacy.

Ward 16

Down the path at the end of the tennis court was Ward 16 for the infectious children. Although most with common infectious diseases such as chicken pox were cared for at home, there was not a high rate of immunisation in the 1950s and therefore the odd cases of diphtheria were still seen: the disease most often confused with this was

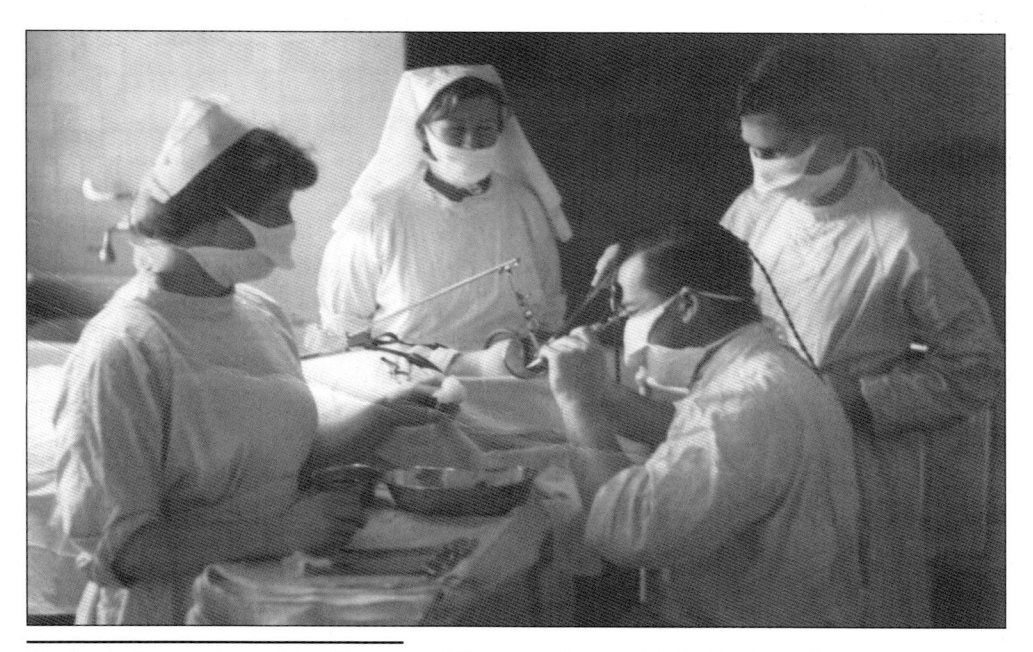

Carlton Out-patients Tonsillectomy Theatre. Nurses Adele Brain and Mary Van Leewin.

Telfer Family Collection.

laryngeal tracheo-bronchitis. The smell of diphtheria was quite unique; many doctors became adept at diagnosis by the smell alone.[27]

Commonly, the child presented in Casualty on a cold foggy night, distressed and unable to breathe, a distraught mother and siblings in tow. The nurses in Ward 16 were always required to keep the treatment room set up for the tracheotomy (now known as tracheostomy) procedure, a tray also ready on the bedside locker, where a steam tent was available for croupy children. The Casualty Medical Officer could be heard shouting from the path as he ran from Casualty where he had literally picked up the child: 'Tracheotomy, tracheotomy.' Seconds later they arrived at Ward 16. Of all the dramas a nurse could experience, the tracheostomy would be the greatest. The procedure was only the beginning of the story, as many an anxious hour was spent at the bedside with the Registrar hovering. The tension around these children was quite high. Very rapid preparation was required; there was no time for anaesthetic, local or general. The decision to make a high or low incision was the most tortuous the Resident could make in his career at the Children's. The high operation was the most usual.

The patient was laid on their back, with the shoulders supported by a sandbag and the front of the neck on the stretch. There were various sizes of tracheotomy tubes, but all were made on the principle of an inner tube longer than the outer, fitting into a wide flange to keep it in position. The doctor incised the trachea from below upwards and, after much spluttering and coughing and suction applied quickly to remove membrane and mucous, the tube was inserted. The nurse took care that the tapes were tied firmly around the neck to keep the tube in position and, if necessary, restrained the child from pulling everything out. The after-treatment consisted of keeping the child very quiet, a few pieces of gauze over the tube. Each child required a special 'trachie nurse' who became adept at keeping the airway free of mucous by suction and cleaning the inner tube.

Kate Harden, the Ward Sister in 14, remembers the changes in medical conditions occurring during those years:

> Meningitis in Ward 14, gastric drips for months on end…meningitis was treated quickly with antibiotics [intrathecally following lumbar puncture under the most sterile of conditions]. The incidence of osteomyelitis became a thing of the past. The days of the Senior Nurse in Casualty giving the children with syphilis their gold [powder of penicillin] injection, that went. Diphtheria—the pattern changed. We no longer saw children with post-measles pneumonia. Infections from burrowing lice in the hair disappeared. In Ward 14, neonatal surgical procedures improved; electrolytes came into being. In the last few years of my time, leukaemia, cardiac and renal problems became very big [in research]. Infections changed.[28]

The spirochaete of syphilis was one of the most susceptible organisms to penicillin; the use of this antibiotic in high dosage became the first line in treatment superseding the sulphonamides of the 1930s. Penicillin was most commonly given in the wards by the 'treatment nurse', usually a third-year, who had responsibility for mixing the yellow powder with sterile water and administration of the dose: 100,000 units per kilogram of body weight divided into three-hourly injections night and day spread over fourteen days. Nurses were traumatised by the number of intramuscular injections they had to give. Barbara Smith (née Catto) said, 'we couldn't do it now':

> Poor little babies and children cried when they saw you coming with the tray because they knew it was a 'needle'. Their poor little arms were like pincushions. Sometimes there was nowhere to go: you had trouble finding a place, their arms were so sore. Many children were so malnourished and sick, we worried about the needle hitting the bone.[29]

Not all babies survived. Enid Ingpen had her most awful experience when: 'just out on the wards I held a baby…for the Senior Nurse to give a penicillin injection and the baby died in my arms. I had not at that time been exposed to death.'[30]

Kate Harden was in charge of Ward 14 in 1953 when the first exchange transfusion took place. An erythroblastosis (Rh–) baby was transferred from the Women's Hospital and two second-year nurses were able to witness Dr Elizabeth Turner carry out this historic event: Elizabeth Gifford-Burgess and Margaret Mitchell. Dr Rae Matthews, Dr Lionel E. G. Sloan (known to staff as LEG Sloan) and Nurses Doris Milliken and Heather Telfer were present in the late 1950s in the tiny ward with few facilities. Wall radiators warmed the room where babies were nursed in wire bassinets, the beginning of modern neonatal nursing.

Some experiences were very satisfying. In 1952, Elizabeth Hocking (née Strickland) 'specialled' a little girl with tetanus in Ward 7 of the old Princess May building. In the little end room, the respirator chugged away where the bay window faced north on Pelham Street to St George's School. The darkened, padded room muffled the sounds of the passing traffic. But the shouts from the playground and the ringing of the school bell were enough to send the patient into spasm. Sedative drugs were required: chloral hydrate and anaesthetic by rectum. Tetanus antitoxin was administered subcutaneously or intramuscularly for a week. When the jaw was locked, rectal feeding was necessary.

A tetanus patient has stiffness of the neck and lower jaw and that very soon spreads to the muscles of the back, causing the patient to twist into all kinds of positions at the slightest provocation. The commonest is the arching of the back so that only the back of the head and the tips of the heels are in contact with the bed (opisthotonos). The patient's temperature could be extremely high and the muscles become hard and board-like. For some, death was common in a week. For those

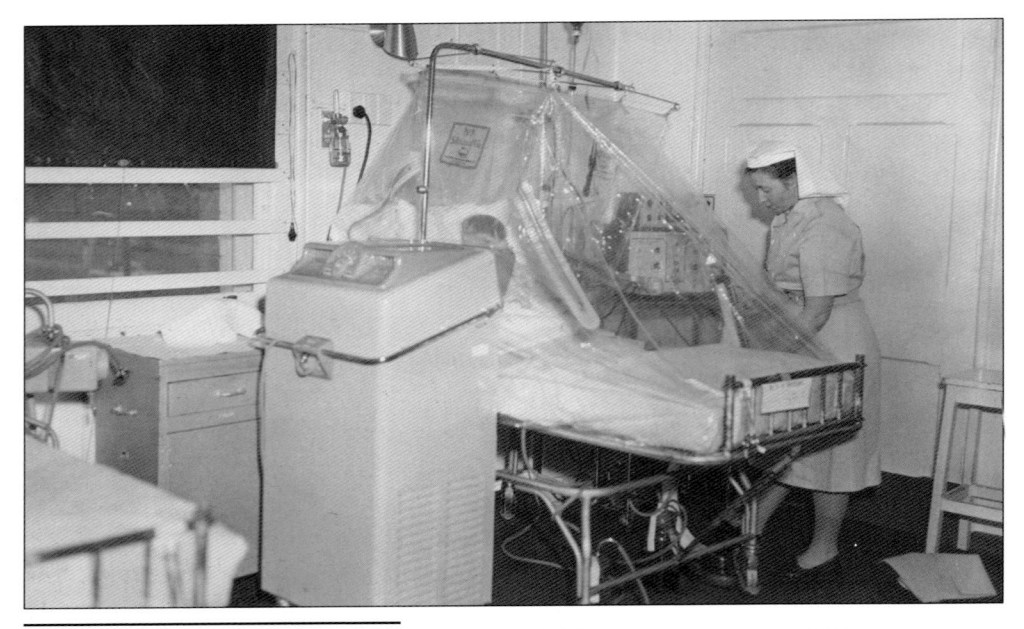

Charge Sister Nancy Hurst, Ward 9 with a child in an oxygen tent, 1953.

receiving tetanus serum in good time, the attack was mild. Nursing procedures were sometimes carried out while the patient was under the effect of the anaesthetic.

Elizabeth's patient was more fortunate, but after weeks of very special nursing care, the major part of recovery, her lovely hair became matted. 'In desperation I cut it fairly short—then I was terrified, as I hadn't asked permission. Fortunately, her mother was really pleased with the hair cut. I breathed a sigh of relief.'[31]

Surgical nursing

One of the most common procedures monitored by the nurses before the days of digital equipment was the intravenous drip (the IV). Checking eight drops per minute of glucose and saline usually fell to the lot of the junior nurse, and it is difficult to imagine how they accomplished the work in wards of forty children where up to twenty 'surgical babies' had to be fed. TPR (temperature, pulse and respiration) were quarter-hourly observations and the recording of fluid balance sheets was a routine pre- and post-operative task.

The Annual Report for 1952 notes that the Hospital had a record number of 8,041 in-patients and that it treated 133,572 out-patients. The Surgical Wards, 9 and 10, were the busiest, with the fastest turnover. Nancy Hardy was Sister-in-Charge of Ward 9 in the 1950s with forty babies and children and two Surgical beds for sick nurses at the end of the ward.

A duty list was made out each day according to seniority: the juniors, responsible for an area, usually scrubbed bed-pans although this became less frequent when the ward assistants 'Pinkies' were employed. The juniors sponged the patients, the Senior Nurse working with the junior. The Seniors took the very difficult cases. Nancy Hardy (née Hurst) recalled:

> The ward was terribly busy. We had at times, on admission day, a turnover of twenty-two children out of forty—eleven in and eleven out. We had carded cases, and 'immeds', these were accident cases. Sometimes they came from Casualty so ill they arrived at the door on a trolley, no phone call. They just appeared. There was no triage in those days. Very primitive. Car accidents, children who had been kicked in the head by a horse. We used to have burns, although they went down to Ward 10 when that unit started.[32]

In the event of an admission of a child with a fracture, a Resident Doctor was sent for, alerted by phone. There was no emergency system. The nurses did not apply airways and waited for the doctor with the trolley ready. The big black oxygen cylinders wheeled in were 'awful, awful things'.

Cardiac surgery was in its early days. Of all the doctors, Nate Myers was one in whom Nancy Hardy had great faith. He slept by the bed of the first child operated on for patent ductus. Thereafter, he was seen in the ward at all hours staying until a child was stable and out of danger. Nancy said, 'He was sometimes rude and I suppose I used to fight with him—but he was the one I turned to. Russell Howard [the Honorary Surgeon] was ex-Army and had to have everything quiet. If there was a noise, he would shout "God in heaven" and we removed the offending child to the bathroom.'

There were no facilities for parents. They simply stood or sat in the corridor. Sister Hurst rearranged the little area where the oxygen cylinders were kept; a couple of chairs and a kettle for the parents, a quiet place and a little comfort.

She remembers that 'some of the operations were horrific and chloral and potassium bromide was the effective routine medication used to settle the child, 2.5 or 5 mls measured on a spoon. It was bitter, the child spluttered and gagged, but it worked.' Nurses were not permitted to sit on the bed to comfort the child.

One of the more confronting nursing tasks was the post-operative care for babies undergoing correction of cleft lip and palate. George Gunter and John Barnett were performing this surgery in the 1950s but the most prominent in that area of plastic surgery at the time was Alan Wakefield, who succeeded Benjamin Rank. Feared by nurses in the operating theatre for his impatience, his comments and tendency to drop instruments not to his liking, he nevertheless earned the greatest admiration for his meticulous work. He was known to remove sutures and start again when not satisfied; the result told the story, and the gratitude of the parents was unbounded.[33]

The baby was usually operated on at six to twelve weeks for the correction of the lip with intra-nasal ether anaesthetic. Arriving back in the ward with tongue traction secured by a fixed suture, its lip was held with a metal Logan bow.[34] Rectal saline and oxygen, given for a few hours, were removed when feeding recommenced.

The night nurse responsible for the post-operative care in the bare, soul-less Annie Higgins Room at the end of Ward 9 had only the view over the Exhibition Gardens, a ghostly distraction in the lonely night. The parents were not present.

For a successful outcome, the baby was prevented from crying. Two or three drops of Tinct Opii, or chloral and potassium bromide, were repeated at intervals. Morphine was sometimes prescribed and given by hypodermic syringe in the first twelve hours 'for accurate dose and prompt action'. The task devolved on the Staff Nurse or the Ward Sister who dissolved the tablet by swishing it in a teaspoon of water over the Bunsen burner.

Airway obstruction or choking was the nurse's constant fear. Observation of the baby's colour and gurgling sounds was constant, while small drops of water were dripped by pipette directly into the mouth until, a few hours later, the baby could tolerate expressed breast milk. Any nurse who had this daunting task will remember the tiny baby nursed flat with its little arms splinted to the side of the cot with bandages, essential to avoid the injury that would come from pulling at the suture line. To prevent the baby's lip from rubbing on the pillow, tiny sandbags were sometimes placed for a few hours at each side of the head: perfect stillness was mandatory to allow the suture line to settle. The baby recovered remarkably well, the tongue suture was removed in twelve hours and mothers could breast-feed within a day or two.[35]

The cleft palate was not usually repaired until the baby was at least eighteen months old.

The chronic lack of staff meant that everything in Surgical Wards had to be done on the run. A night duty junior had the responsibility for 'Surgical babies', which meant feeding and changing as many as twenty without assistance, a job dreaded by juniors who raced up and down the stairs—the lifts were too slow—between Wards 9 and 10 all night until 7 am. The feeding bottles were collected from the food room in a large metal container and carried or dragged over to the Surgical Wards by the nurse. When there were many babies, it was very heavy. For the wards in the same building as the food room, the bottles arrived on trolleys.[36]

Fortunately, the evening staff—if there was a lull—gave the feeds a start. Many enjoyed the drama and tension of Surgical Wards, especially evening emergencies. Intensive Care Units were unheard of; the nurse had to be prepared for anything, always checking the resuscitation trolley, having an IV ready, waiting for Casualty to ring. Finding an empty bed could be a problem. There was always a sense of satisfaction to get off duty late at night after coping with all kinds of trauma, a possible appendicitis or a strangulated hernia.[37]

Despite the use of antibiotics, some children suffered devastating complications and tended to stay in Hospital for many weeks. The sickest and most urgent cases were children in Surgical Wards. An appendix diagnosed too late progressed to peritonitis, pelvic abscess and empyema with drainage tubes and intravenous feeding. The anaesthetics at that time left children weak and sick and they took a long time to recover.

Nurses remember the children with haunted, sunken eyes looking eagerly to the narrow glass panelled doors in Surgical Wards waiting for their mother, only to be disappointed once again because of restricted visiting hours. The child who could not understand English was a poignant sight, prompting some nurses to begin a life-time study of the language and culture they were dealing with. Some parents paced up and down outside the Hospital, particularly the fathers who came by after work to catch a glimpse of their child through the balcony louvre windows in Pelham Street.

Once the Surgical children were on the mend, their spirits lifted and some even played tricks on the nurses, throwing food out of the window, hiding toys and books, anything to break the boredom. Being strung up in traction was a burden. Many were quickly moved on to Aftercare at Hampton or sent home.

A vivid memory of the old Surgical Wards was the hydrocephalic babies, some with heads as big as their bodies. With awful pressure sores on gigantic misshapen heads, they were nursed on frames so that there was a minimum of lifting when they needed changing. Their high-pitched cries were a haunting reminder of the helplessness of those caring for them. Mr Reg Hooper began to insert shunts in the 1950s, but for many children, it was too late.

Burns

Those who worked in the Children's Hospital in the 1950s can never forget the burns and scalds, the distinct smell, and the heartbreaking experience. Children were nursed in the main Surgical Ward with a bed cradle strung with electric lights for warmth.

Despite the great progress in burns treatment during the war, as well as recently introduced antibiotics, the poor outcome of infection remained a major problem. The most serious cases arrived at the Children's.

Burns cases commonly came from the nearby crowded houses of Carlton. Two little girls had been playing near the copper in the backyard washhouse when their long dresses brushed in the ashes and caught alight. They lived about three weeks, never lost consciousness and were talking to the nurses minutes before they died. Another small child climbed on a chair and fell into a copper of boiling water, while yet another sat on a meat pie which had just been taken out of the oven and placed on the floor.

In the 1950s, these children were transferred to Mr Murray Clarke's unit in Ward 10, the start of the modern Burns Therapy Unit. The children's pain was tragic. Deep wounds were irrigated under anaesthetic, followed by daily saline baths and tulle gras dressings. These daunting tasks were carried out by the Staff Nurse or Sister-in-Charge, assisted by the Senior Nurse who was responsible for the treatment room. Children were coaxed to drink high-protein fluids. Nurses thought these were 'gluggy and horrible tasting, a thick mess' but essential because the children usually ate nothing. Many nurses found the prospect of the treatments daunting, the adjustment difficult and occasionally asked to be moved on. Or they left nursing altogether.[38] It was not until the 1970s that pain control for children was improved.

The food room

Most expected to be in the food room or in the infant formula room for at least three months in their second year, and it was commonly regarded as a good placement as the Sister-in-Charge was 'human'. The facility was much praised as modern in its day, boasting stainless steel boilers, benches, sterilisers and refrigerated storage. Sister Lyall, the first dietician, was succeeded by Sister Mavis Honey, then Sister Quiney and Grace Rogers in the 1950s, and most remember 'Gracie' as a kind person.

The food room was more enjoyable than the wards. There were opportunities to eat sweetened condensed milk (commonly given to sick babies, strength 1–8). On night duty, caramel could be made by boiling up the condensed milk and sometimes it made a terrible mess. Ice-cream and bananas were a luxury.

Duties of the night staff included filling the big urns with cow's milk and bringing them to the boil to enable the day staff to begin making the formulas when they came on duty. Most of the babies were on cow's milk diluted with water and lactose added (A1, 2, 3, 4, 5), The 'B' formulas were made with powdered milk and, if the lumps were not beaten out, the teats would clog up, much to the ire of the nurses feeding the babies. A dreaded formula was that with lactic acid: it curdled if the milk was not the right temperature or if it was added too quickly. When first starting in the food room, the nurses had to acquire the technique of putting the teats on with forceps, a very clumsy and slow procedure. If a nurse was found measuring the powdered milk 'heaped' and not smoothed by a knife, Sister Rogers made her throw it all down the sink and start again, a lesson never forgotten.

Dr Vernon Collins was concerned that baby formulas were too complicated and wrote the book *Infant Feeding*, which became a 'bible' to medical staff and nurses alike. The nurses were expected to know the principles that were adapted into the Maternal and Child Health book, *Child Care*. In the late 1950s, Mothercraft nurses did some of this work in the food room and tended to needs in the Baby Wards.

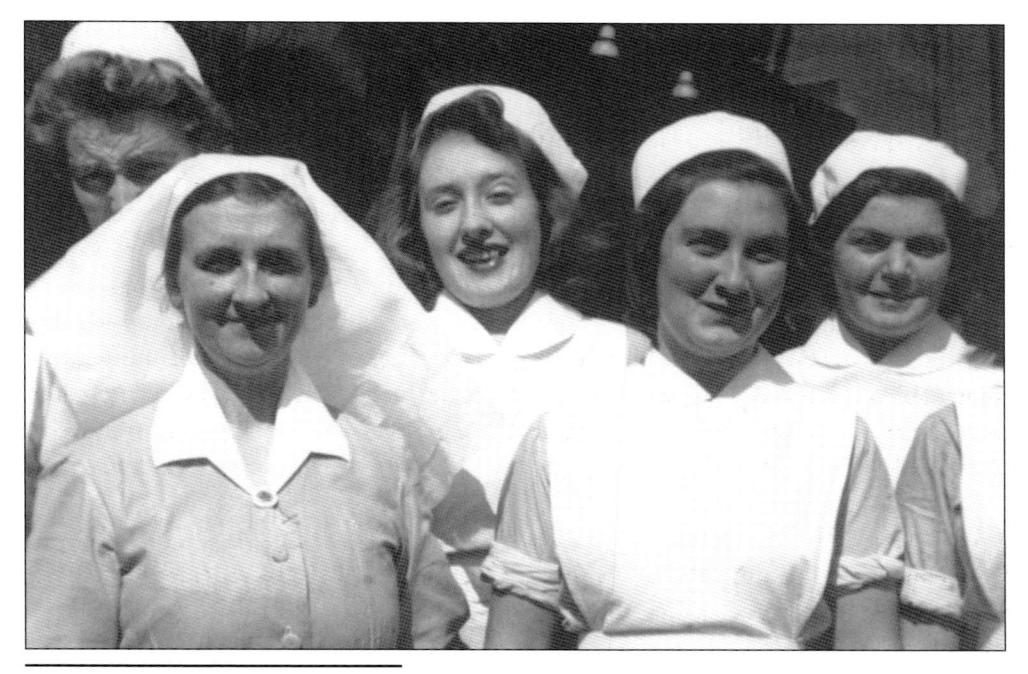

Food room staff, 1942.
Back L–R: Cecily Smith, Elizabeth Jenkins, Barbara Morris.
Front L–R: Sister Rogers, Pauline Brearley.
RCHA/Morris Family Collection.

Visitors

Visiting days were very difficult in the Medical Wards (the children were usually in and out more quickly in a Surgical Ward). The children screamed in all the wards after three o'clock when visitors left, but for longer-term children the parting was traumatic.

Until the 1950s, children were not allowed visitors until they had been in the Hospital for between four and six weeks. After this time, only the parents or guardians (no siblings, friend or other relatives such as grandparents). Visiting was each alternate Sunday between the hours of 2 pm and 3.30 pm. Parents of dangerously ill children were allowed as often as the doctor considered necessary. The Resident Doctor was available for an interview at 1.20 pm except on public holidays or Sundays. However, the child's name had to be lodged at the Enquiry Office between 1 pm and 1.20 pm on Saturdays. No allowance was made for parents living in the country or in distant suburbs.

Visitors to Baby Wards and Infectious Diseases Wards were required to have special permission from the Medical Director or his deputy. The rules, also extended to Sherbrooke and Frankston, were considered to be in the best interests of the patients in the Hospital. No visitor was allowed in the ward without a ticket from the Manager bearing the day's date, and visitors had to comply with the Hospital regulations for a ticket to be issued. The Sister-in-Charge directed the visitors in the ward.

Lollies, cakes and biscuits were banned. The lockers were cleared immediately after a visitor left. Eggs and nuts and other nourishing foods were acceptable and handed to the Ward Sister but it is doubtful if the child ever saw the food the mothers so lovingly prepared. Former members of staff remember: 'Sunday afternoons were a nightmare, hysterical children screaming, vomiting jelly or anything the mother had spirited in. The children did not know where they were, or where their mother was. Many became silent, a sign often misinterpreted.' Sister Castellan said of the children in Ward 7: 'I could not believe how good the children were usually. They just sat in their bed or cot.' Nurses knew they were witnessing severe deprivation, depression, detachment and terror and sometimes overheard mothers telling of their distress.

One mother reported 'her three-year-old rejected her'. She was heartbroken when the little girl died a week later. She had not seen her for days.[39] The nurses thought that 'when open visiting came in, it was terrific'. Nevertheless, some of the attitudes of Senior Staff in the wards were extraordinary. Elizabeth Coombes remembered an incident: 'We had a little two-and-a-half-year-old girl in [the ward] who had a prolapsed rectum and mother came in and breast-fed her. The whole of the staff didn't like this at all, and I couldn't understand why it mattered.' She thought it was good that the mother was holding that child and came every day. She was the happiest child in the ward. But the objections really masked another anxiety on the part of the staff: 'It was because she had teeth and was two-and-a-half. The staff felt she shouldn't be breast fed.'

Fortunately, some antiquated beliefs changed and access became more liberal. Dr Collins was well aware that the lack of personal attention and separation from their families in early childhood was devastating for young children and their parents. In the old Hospital there were no parent waiting rooms and no quiet place for the Sister to inform them of the progress of their child. In the event of death, the bad news was delivered in the corridor of the Hospital, more often by telegram. Soon after his appointment as Medical Director in 1949, Dr Collins implemented an interview process with the parents after the death of their child, supporting them in their quest for answers.

Casualty

The major emergencies in Casualty in the 1950s were meningococcal septicaemia and meningitis, obstructed breathing (broncho-laryngeal tracheitis), poisonings and burns. Children's Hospital nurses developed acute observation skills and were at that time very aware of the meningococcal septicaemia with its tell-tale petechial spots and a possible fatal outcome; sometimes a child with a sore throat and flea bites was admitted for an overnight stay. To detect the signs, the tell-tale purpuric spots, the nurses lifted the child's singlet. Elizabeth Coombes experienced this responsibility:

> …no marks at all and you were worried but had no proof and kept them there in Casualty for hours on end and sometimes you sent them home and they came back dead. [With antibiotics] meningitis virtually disappeared. Mary said it was because the new Children's Hospital was built and Camp Pell disappeared.

If an intrathecal antibiotic was given in time, the child could usually be saved. The nurse was essential in assisting the doctor while carrying out this procedure on a very distressed child.

But it was in the treatment of poisoning that Sister Coombes became expert. There were no lists of antidotes or records when she came to Casualty in the late 1940s and she began a register. 'I went to the pharmacy and acquired a big pharmacy book with an alphabetical listing of drugs and gradually built up a profile of the most common substances and products implicated in child poisoning. Any known antidotes were recorded but the most commonly used treatment was an emetic such as ipecac, and a stomach washout.' Before modern publicity campaigns, the most common poisons presenting to 'Cas' were corrosives, washing liquids and drain chemicals from backyards and furniture polish and iron tablets in the house. In the 1960s a major culprit was antidepressants. Sister Coombes' work was the beginning of the Poisons Register as we know it today. When she was interviewed in the 1980s, her memories were vivid:

> The trauma was terrible. Once we did eight [stomach washouts, involving a tube forced down the child's throat causing untold trauma] in two-and-a-half hours. The mothers were sitting around chatting and I ticked them off saying, 'you don't know what your child has been through' and they all burst into tears. [40]

Phil Thomas (née Richey) remembers when she was invited back on the staff at the end of her training and worked in Casualty where many migrant families came for assistance. A child from a road accident presented not with a great deal of injury, but accompanied by all his concerned noisy Italian relatives, none of whom spoke English, and bedlam reigned. Phil had a brilliant idea and rang Chef in the kitchen to ask for someone who spoke Italian. Joe arrived and talked to the parents in an animated way for some time but unfortunately it was discovered he did not speak English either, so the whole exercise was futile. Another time a non-English speaking mother with a toddler with a bloody finger wandered around looking rather lost in

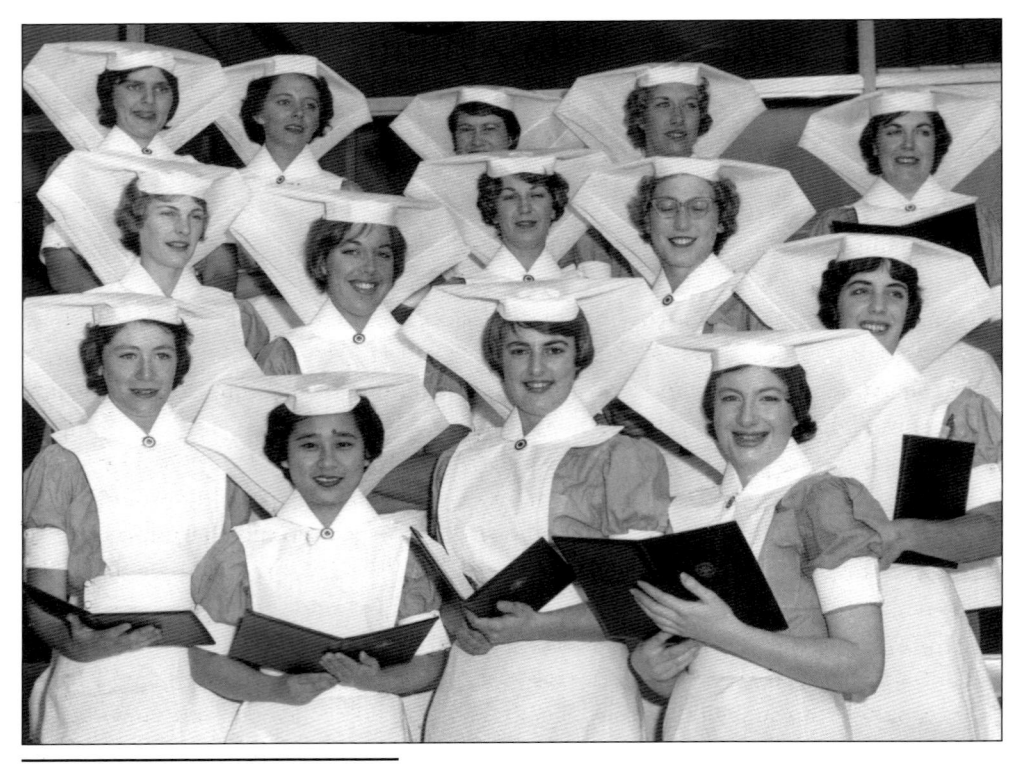

Graduation, 1959.
Back: Patricia Grieve, Marie Sheehan, Jennifer Holland, Barbara Ditterich, Rosanne Davey. *Middle Row:* Janet Colley, Gillian Salter, Helen McElhinney, Margaret Long, Elizabeth Allan. *Front Row:* Jennifer Hall, Oi Yuet Ng, Dawn Jenkins, Elizabeth James.

the Out-patients Hall. They were directed to Casualty where the nurse began a tetanus test. Phil said 'when I checked on what was happening I discovered that they had been to an Out-patients Clinic and then to Haematology for a blood test. Very embarrassing!'

Weekends in Casualty were hectic. With all the seats full, people waited quite some time to see a doctor. The Sisters could usually fix the problem with a simple remedy such as a wad of gauze for a bleeding tooth socket or, in the absence of a medical student, a suture for a simple wound. Children came back again and again. One of Phil's favourites was a three-year-old Italian child, Gian Carlo, whose lovely young mother taught him to greet her with 'havarya' the equivalent of 'how are you'.[41]

A New Era

Nurse education at the RCH and the Royal Melbourne Hospital
In her Annual Report of 1951–52, Lucy Sechiari said:

> The importance of having enough nurses well trained in Paediatrics cannot be too strongly emphasised. In addition, it is therefore essential that girls of the right social and educational background should be encouraged to train in a hospital which caters especially for this training.

Most nurses do not remember anything about the social part except that there was a pecking order between hospitals and according to which school you had attended. All have vivid memories of the PTS (Preliminary Training Scheme); some good, some lukewarm.

Marjorie Allnatt taught in 'extension B' of the Nurses' Home, two bright sunny rooms, one for lectures, the other for practice procedures, and set high standards in nurse education. Known for her meticulous detail in everything the nurses had to learn, she always insisted on the child's comfort first and the importance of the explanation of a procedure about to take place.

Some felt that they 'were taught lots of stuff that was useless when confronted with the reality'. The theory taught was basic: anatomy and physiology and 'a lot of time was spent on such procedures as carbolising a bed'. This occurred every time a child was discharged or died. In practice, there was no time to place newspapers on the floor, to wash, dust and sweep, change the mattress, scrub and dry the mackintosh. 'You gave the bed a good slop over with Zephiran solution and that was it.'[42]

In the wards the nurses soon found a pecking order. Staff Nurses wore yellow and Ward Sisters wore blue; doctors wore long white coats, students wore short coats. Social workers and physiotherapists were confused with doctors in long white coats. Honoraries wore a suit. Administration staff wore long sleeves, and Matron wore white. Probationers did not realise until later that it was all very military and there was great relief when another school came into the wards so that they were not the most junior. They learnt very quickly that some Ward Sisters were kind, others terrifying 'and even abusive bullies'.[43]

Above all, there were three cardinal rules drummed in that nurses broke at their peril: never leave a cot-side down, never leave a baby on a bench and never leave a child unattended in the bath.

Gwen Coventry (1948–52) thought that 'the PTS was very good at teaching the basics of general nursing given by Children's Hospital tutors'. Lectures were sparse, mostly given by doctors in the nurses' own time, some good, others not so good: 'We learned from the senior [nurse], an apprentice style training.' The greatest fear was that on senior night duty, a young nurse's ignorance or inexperience might lead to a child's death. Similarly, she feared not knowing how to relate to grieving parents when a child died. In the late 1940s and 1950s nurses were taught to use initiative, to be innovative. Years later when Gwen was involved in helping set up the first hospital in Western Nepal and training the nurses in that area, an American doctor and a Canadian doctor at different times commented on the quality of Australian nurses. They felt that they were able to handle emergencies and take initiative. Gwen thought of the many nights on Surgical Ward duty, when the Surgical Doctor was in theatre while the Surgical Nurse had to make decisions and deal with emergencies such as suckers (electric suctions apparatus) and underwater drainage not working.[44]

Some of the lecturers were remembered with affection, others abhorred. Mr Raymond Hennessy was a favourite; not only was he kind and gentle, but he gave high marks to everyone in ENT (ear, nose and throat). He claimed to 'fan' the exam papers and let them slip down the stairs. The first one to be retrieved was awarded 100 per cent. No one received less than 90 per cent.[45] Always cheerful, he whistled in theatre and addressed his nurse as 'dearie'. The big jar on his office desk was a curiosity; it contained his trophies: toys, safety pins, beads, coins and even a Mickey Mouse brooch extracted from the noses, ears, throats and bronchi of unfortunate children.

The 'study block' system of training was introduced in August 1949 before the first and after the final exams. The PTS extended from one month to two in 1951 and remained basic, with visits to the wards for demonstrations only. A very welcome diversion and an extension to public health education were the excursions: the Ideal Dairy, Kew; a food factory in Richmond; the Werribee Sewage Farm; and Janefield, a Home for children with intellectual disabilities at Lower Plenty.

Nurses were fiercely loyal to their Nursing School and conscious that the entry standards were specifically raised higher than the Royal Melbourne because of a common perception that children's nursing was not in the mainstream of general training.

The six months at the Royal Melbourne Hospital (RMH) were a contrast. Children's nurses received no lectures or supervisory visits from their Tutor. Commonly feeling aggrieved and neglected, many were used as extras in their first week, relegated to backroom jobs such as laying out the dead. The majority were male victims of heart attack and stroke, sometimes several of them a week. Industrial and road accidents—all were dreaded on the early shift from 6.30 am, the most likely time for these events to occur.

Night duty came early in the six months at the RMH. Life in the comfortable Charles Conibere Nurses' Home abruptly ended with the transfer to 'Biltmore', a rat-infested, creaky, five-storied, rabbit warren of an old place in Albert Park backing on to the Gordon Boys' Home. It was possible to work and sleep nights at a stretch in the winter without ever seeing daylight. But if anything, night duty brought out inner strengths of endurance, particularly when nurses worked the ward alone caring for adults who required pain relief for cancer. As 'extras', RCH nurses also worked

A New Era

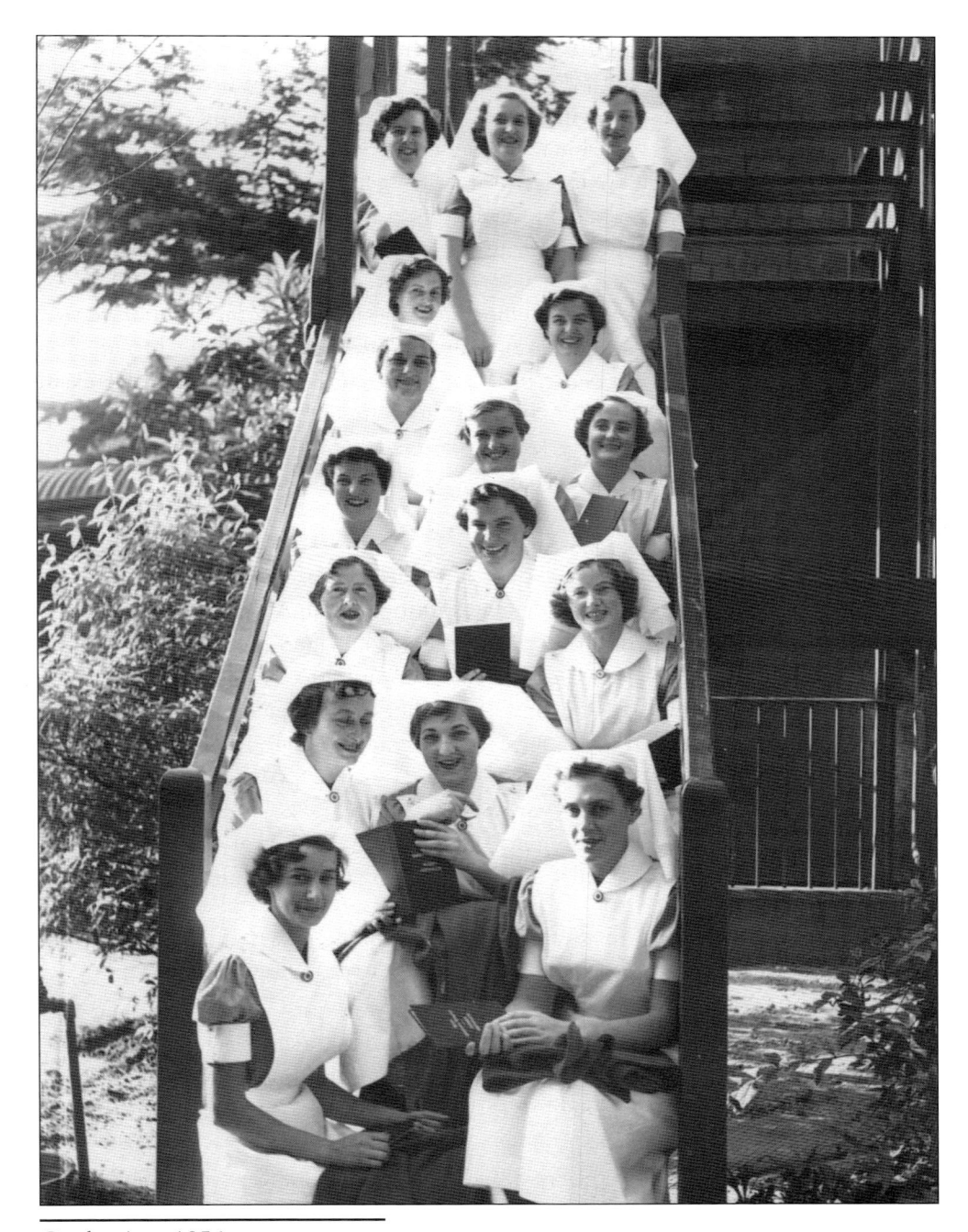

Graduation, 1956.
Back L–R: Gwenda Payne, (unknown), (unknown), Cathie Wall, (unknown), Janet Robertson, Myrna Cobbin, Meryl Hogan, Faith Street, Berenice Bon, Judith Wilson, Janet Campbell, Verna Wright, Josie Frizon, Sheila Jess, (unknown).
Gooderham Family Collection

the rounds, set up breakfast trolleys and generally became a 'dogs body.' Of course, there was lots of fun being invited to the Resident and student parties.

Many RMH nurses were not impressed with their three months' rotation at the Children's, some claiming they were 'just minding children.' In 1956, the picture changed. Nancy Jacobs (1956–60) recalled:

> I found the nurses from the RMH and St Vincent's were happy to be at the RCH. Sometimes at the Melbourne there was some friction, but I found the Ward Sisters valued the nurses from the 'Kids' as good team members. I believe the training we received was excellent, as our patients could not always communicate. We had to anticipate their needs, therefore developing our powers of observation.[46]

On the strengths of the training at the Children's, Peg Bellair (née Mitchell) remembers:

> We were taught to OBSERVE [and] not to rely on pathology. The training fitted girls very well for adult training: Children's nurses, above all, had to be caring and observant. The atmosphere was happy, because sick children did not worry over the future. The best thing, which came out of the training, was the allegiance we had for the Hospital. We were proud to be trainees of the Children's Hospital.[47]

Living in

Everyone knew each staff member around them. Jane Altmann recalled that the Children's was small during her training days: 'We knew everyone involved in the running of the Hospital. This built up lasting friendships that many of my non-nursing friends cannot understand.'[48]

The dining room staff guarded their domain with watchful eyes and 'told Sister' (Flower) if a nurse was not cleaning up her plate. Bella, a lovely, kind lady, was the self-appointed boss of the kitchen and dining room who tried hard to make Jane put on weight. Scones with honey and a fresh cup of tea were highlights for those on early morning shift. Bella watched the nurses carefully, and fed Jane up at meal times with scones, jam and cream, with Aktavite for morning tea. Jane said: 'If only she could see me now. I still enjoy a slice of raisin bread with mashed banana on it late at night, à la canteen under the stairs in the Nurses' Home.'[49]

Nurses led a narrow life: there were no newsletters, newspapers or bulletin board. The sitting room was barely used; bedrooms were preferred for a good gossip. One of the things the girls liked most about their time at the RCH was life in the Nurses' Home. A reason many chose nursing was to get away from the restrictive

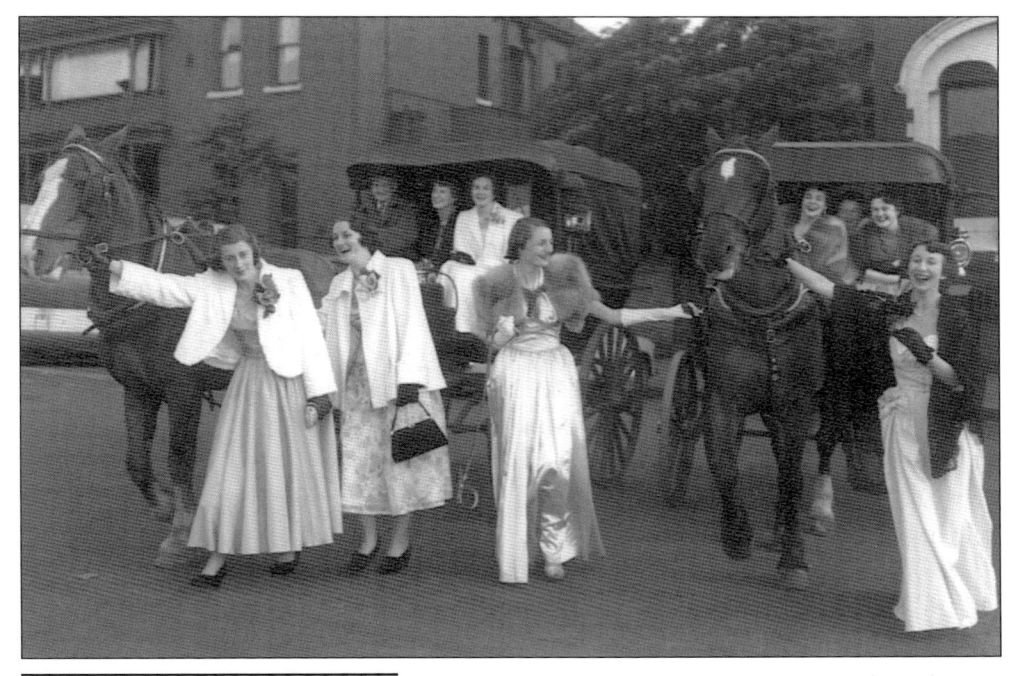

Graduation Party, 1952. Leaving Pelham Street.
RCHA/Black Family Collection.

environment at home. They could do as they wanted (within the rules), with no one to quiz or query them. There was always company when you wanted it or needed it. This was especially the case after a difficult episode on duty. Whether it was the death of a child, a bawling-out by the Sister, a doctor or other things that were too hard for an eighteen-to-twenty-year-old to deal with, most said that the company of others kept them sane and from becoming too hardened by what they had to deal with. No one thought of counselling in those days.

In the 1950s, seniors lived at the Terrace during day duty, where there was a more relaxed atmosphere. No one locked a door. Jean Cusson remembers a Hans Heysen painting hanging over the mantelpiece in the two-bed room. 'I saw it many years later in the office of the Director of Nursing, Elaine Orr.'

Some sneaked out after 9 pm after coming off duty. Patricia Pex recalls how 'once we took a skeleton out of the PTS and propped it in the front seat of my VW and we all piled up, five or six of us, and drove around getting weird looks. We used to change into ski pyjamas and pile into the car with a bottle of sherry and go to the Drive-in for the late show.'[50]

Night staff lived at the Murdoch home, 'Heathfield', in Toorak, which became the residence for the PTS students, six to a room. They were bussed to and from the Hospital for the duration of the eight weeks. All enjoyed the luxurious baths, the ballroom and the lovely meals provided by the housekeeper, Mrs Hope. The only problem was that it could be tedious waiting outside in Pelham Street for the bus to go to 'Heathfield' after night duty. 'One morning while waiting outside in the bus, one of the nurses, who later became a DON [Director of Nursing] at a famous interstate hospital, decided to take us around the block.'[51] No one was any the wiser when the real driver returned.

In 1953, the Children's Hospital became 'Royal' by Charter in anticipation of the visit of Queen Elizabeth. Living in close proximity to the Exhibition Building, many were able to have a good look at the reception and were invited to watch the Queen arrive—an unforgettable experience. A select few were invited to Government House to form a Guard of Honour as she left at the end of the tour.

Lucy Sechiari De Neeve (as she had become by that time) was greatly admired and found to be sympathetic. Small nuisances such as burnt saucepans and broken thermometers were very tedious when nurses were 'sent to Matron'. However, she also had a great sense of humour. When two night duty nurses decided to 'fix' a certain doctor on the prowl, they crept out the front office and lifted a moveable but heavy '2-hour parallel parking' sign used by the ambulance men in Pelham Street. Dragging it up into the doctors' quarters, they placed it outside the offending doctor's door. The next morning at breakfast, Lucy asked for those responsible to own up. Both nurses did, and were reprimanded. As they were leaving, Lucy called out to ask how they got the 'the damn thing' up the stairs.

Forward planning

Big issues occupied the Lady Superintendent. In the 1940s, the main Hospital had three branches with a total of 280 nurses, thirty-eight of those at Frankston. By 1950, the number had diminished to 271 (trained and in training). The Nurses' Home, then nearly fifty years old, had accommodation for only fifty nurses, hence the need for off-site accommodation.

Technical advances and developments in clinical paediatrics were making an impact on children's diseases, hospital procedures and length of time patients spent in bed. Although nurses had to know more and carry out increasingly complex tasks, the actual practice had changed little. They were still working within the same hierarchies, obeying the same rules and working the same shifts established in the nineteenth century.

The significant expansion, rebuilding and refurbishment of hospitals throughout the State, including the new Children's Hospital, created a planning crisis. The competitive labour market of the 1940s and 1950s forced all hospitals to be more creative in finding ways of attracting women and, after 1952, men, to nursing. More than 3,000 £50 nursing bursaries were awarded in Victoria in the 1950s to encourage nurses to stay at school and eventually enter a nursing career.

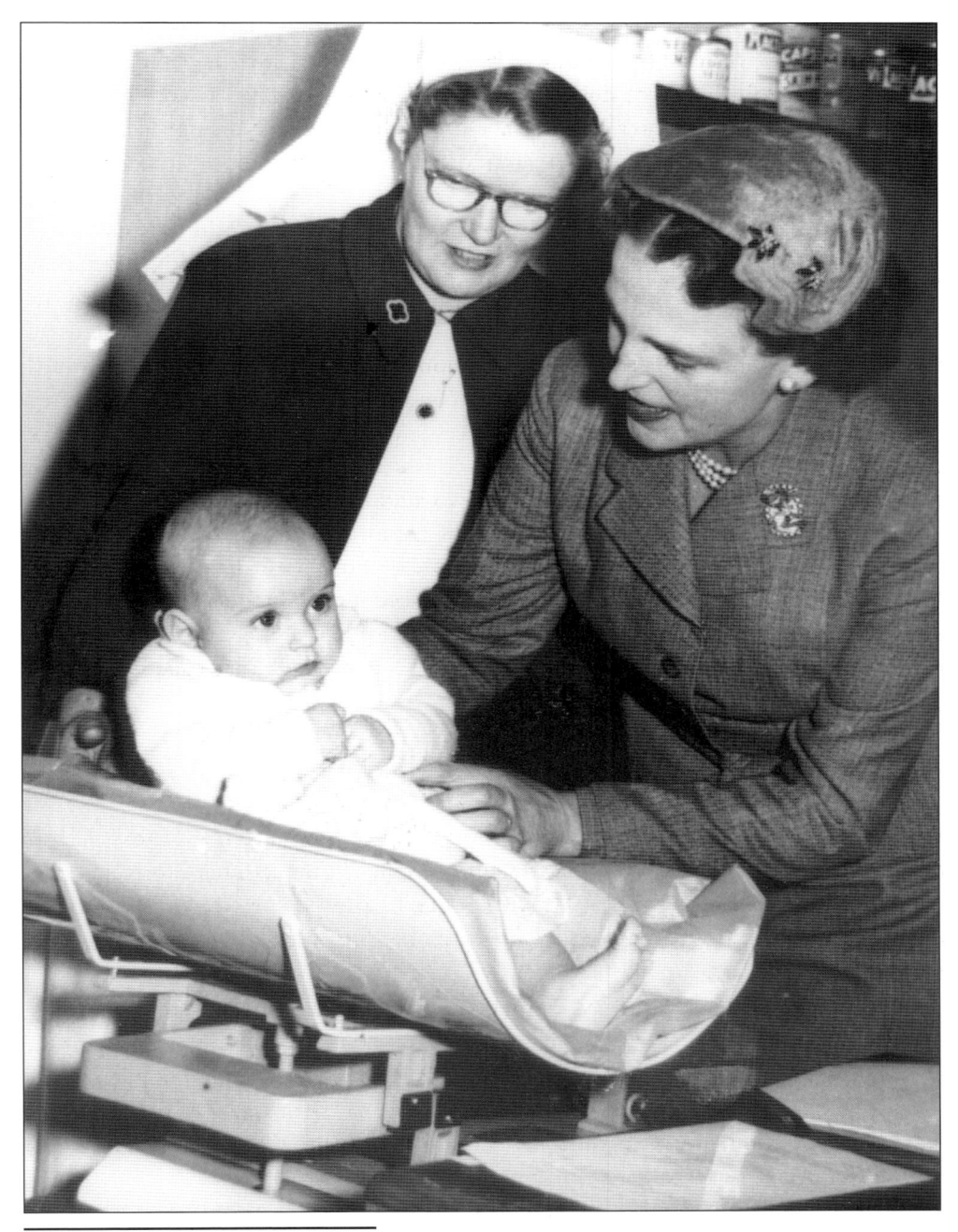

Sister Elizabeth Chalmers (née Sadlier), BEM (RCH 1946–49), with Violet, Lady Brooks (wife of Sir Dallas Brooks) and baby Lillian Sanders at the Infant Welfare Centre, Lilydale, in 1958. Sister Sadlier was awarded the BEM in 1981 for many years of devoted service to Maternal and Child Health in the communities of the Shires of Upper Yarra and Lilydale where she became a legend.

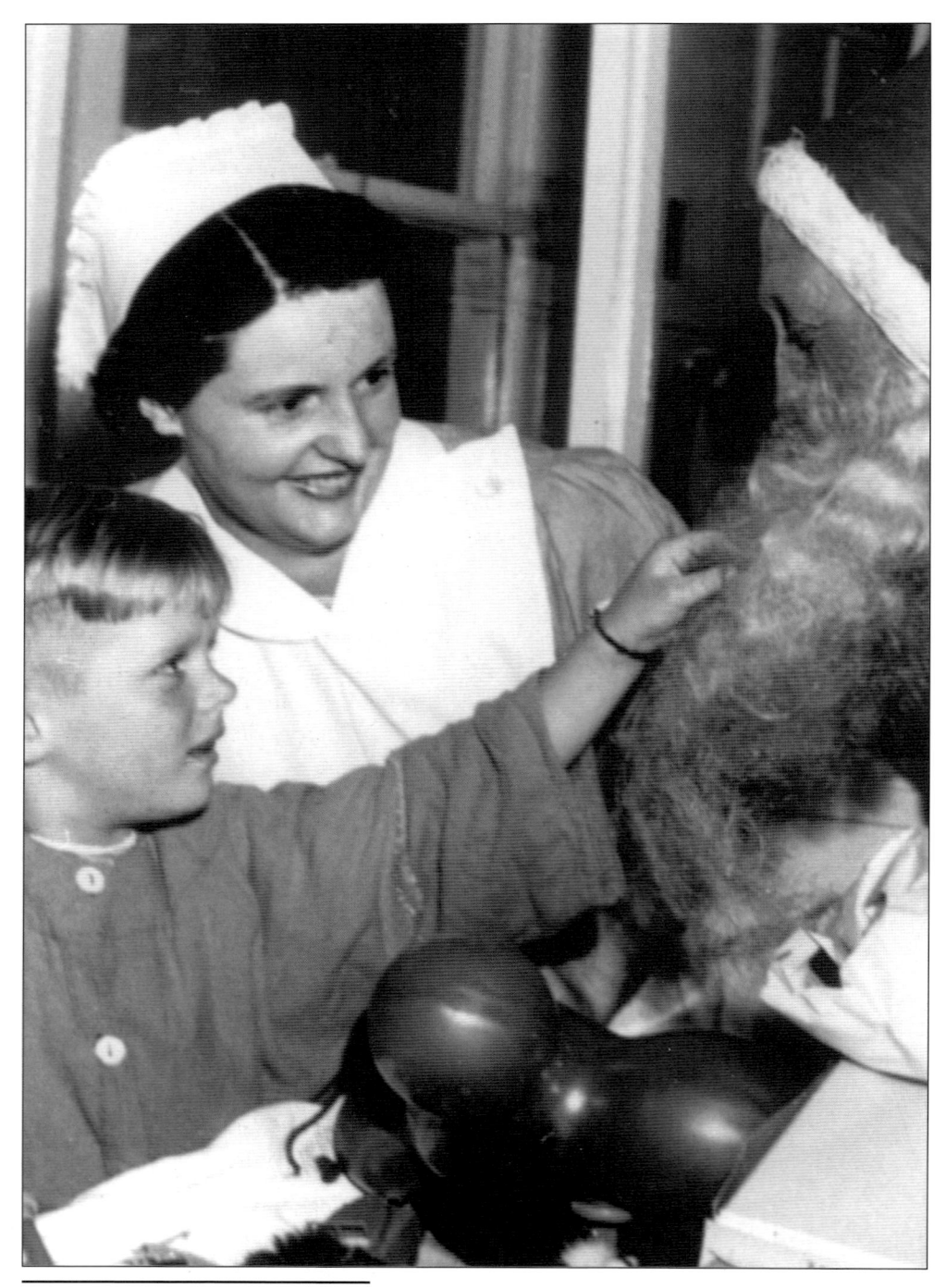

Nurse Margaret Playfair (RCH 1947–50) and her young patient. Christmas, 1949. The Jeffreys Wood gold medallist for 1951, Miss Playfair became the Director of Nursing at the Queen Victoria Hospital.

To solve the crisis, the Hospitals and Charities Commission decided to classify nurses into two divisions: those who undertook highly skilled nursing treatments (State Registered Nurses) and those who did routine care which did not require a high degree of professional knowledge and skills (Nursing Aides). The second category applied to girls who may not have attained the required educational level.[52]

In 1945–46, the Medical Superintendent of the Royal Melbourne Hospital, Dr John Lindell, and Miss Gwen Burbidge SRN, advocated revision of the whole system of nurse training: a central school, an extension of the PTS, the introduction of the 'block' system of study, and transfer of certain elements of the training to the postgraduate sphere. In 1949, the Hospital and Charities Commission worked on a new approach and in 1950 this culminated in the formation of the Northern School of Nursing, Bendigo, and the Melbourne School of Nursing. In Melbourne, the participating hospitals were the Royal Melbourne, the Women's, Fairfield, Queen Victoria and the Children's.[53]

The idea of training away from traditional hospital bases had opponents: the Medical Honoraries of the Royal Melbourne Hospital (with a two-year waiting list for nursing) saw it as the closing of a successful training school, and the RMH Matron Helene Grey, a very influential member of the Melbourne nursing scene, disapproved too. There was also historical antagonism between the Alfred and the Melbourne Hospitals, who vied for teaching honours. The reason for the opposition to the new School was that the individual Hospital Matrons could not select, supervise or discipline the trainees, and therefore lost control. Trainees had no sense of belonging and so were perceived to lack loyalty. These factors, together with the School's inability to attract sufficient recruits, resulted in its closure in 1960.

The Children's had never really lost momentum in popularity; in 1955, Lucy De Neeve reported more than 250 applicants on the waiting list and the numbers were steady.[54] The problem was the high wastage. Many with low educational levels were encouraged to become nursing aides.

'We came a long way'

Under the leadership of Lucy De Neeve, the Children's Hospital largely maintained the integrity of its own Training School throughout these years of change. Lucy became influential on the Board of the Royal Victorian College of Nursing. In 1952, she alerted the Committee of Management that paediatric nursing would become a postgraduate course, a world wide trend. She proved to be thirty years ahead of her time.

The nursing curriculum was governed by the requirements of the Victorian Nurses' Registration Board but individual hospitals relied on creative and innovative tutors to incorporate the unique philosophy of the individual hospital and the training of its nurses. Lucy De Neeve gave Tutor Sister Kathleen Wilson freedom to develop her ideas. By the mid-1950s, the undergraduate curriculum was almost unrecognisable to nurses of previous generations.

On 7 October 1958, at the age of seventeen years and seven months, Nancy Gray entered the Nursing School with her Leaving Certificate. Her results in maths and chemistry gave her an excellent start in the three months' Preliminary Training School. She had also completed a Cookery Course at Emily McPherson College while working at the Hampton Branch.

Nancy successfully completed theoretical and practical instruction in April 1962 after forty-two months. The course contents included anatomy and physiology, bacteriology, immunology and pathology, chemistry and urinalysis, health education (principles of teaching), psychology and mental hygiene, pharmacology and therapeutics and the maintenance of a healthful environment. Surgical included general and infants, gynaecology nursing, operating theatre, ear, nose and throat in general surgical, genito-urinary and first-aid.

Many class hours were devoted to nursing arts and twelve hours to the history of nursing, for which the nurses presented a special project. Nancy spent twenty-one days in the block system, 184 days in affiliation courses and 927 days in clinical services. One aspect that did not change was the six months at the RMH.

Further education and post-basic courses

The College of Nursing became national in 1949 and paved the way for senior staff to be groomed for more senior positions in administration, ward management and nursing education. Lucy De Neeve wasted no time and negotiated with the Committee of Management for time release for her most senior and promising staff. In 1949–50 she reported that Miss Gertrude Newing, who was in charge of Ward 15, had been granted a one-year scholarship for study for Ward Sisters. She was the first of a long line of Children's Hospital nurses who made their mark throughout Australia.

In 1957, Sister Kate Wilson began a post-basic course in paediatrics for outside applicants. This was successful but, for some reason in 1959, ceased. It was said that there was a financial issue. These students, some from overseas, completed six months as full-time students in class and became supernumeraries for six months on the wards on full pay.

The new Hospital at Parkville was imminent and Mrs De Neeve fought to be included in the planning and to increase the knowledge of the staff in anticipation of the move. She was quite dispirited by the lack of support for paediatric post-basic nursing education, study leave and sabbatical periods for her senior staff. Many doctors, sponsored by various foundations and clubs, travelled overseas for study, meetings and congresses; each year the number grew steadily. Only two nurses were given the same consideration, Dorothy Saunders and Elizabeth Jackson, both sponsored by Committee members. Most took leave without pay.

In 1962, on the eve of the move to the new Hospital, Lucy De Neeve resigned in favour of Joan Gendle, a Children's Hospital trainee. She remains, in the memory of all who met and worked with her, as an innovative woman well ahead of her time.

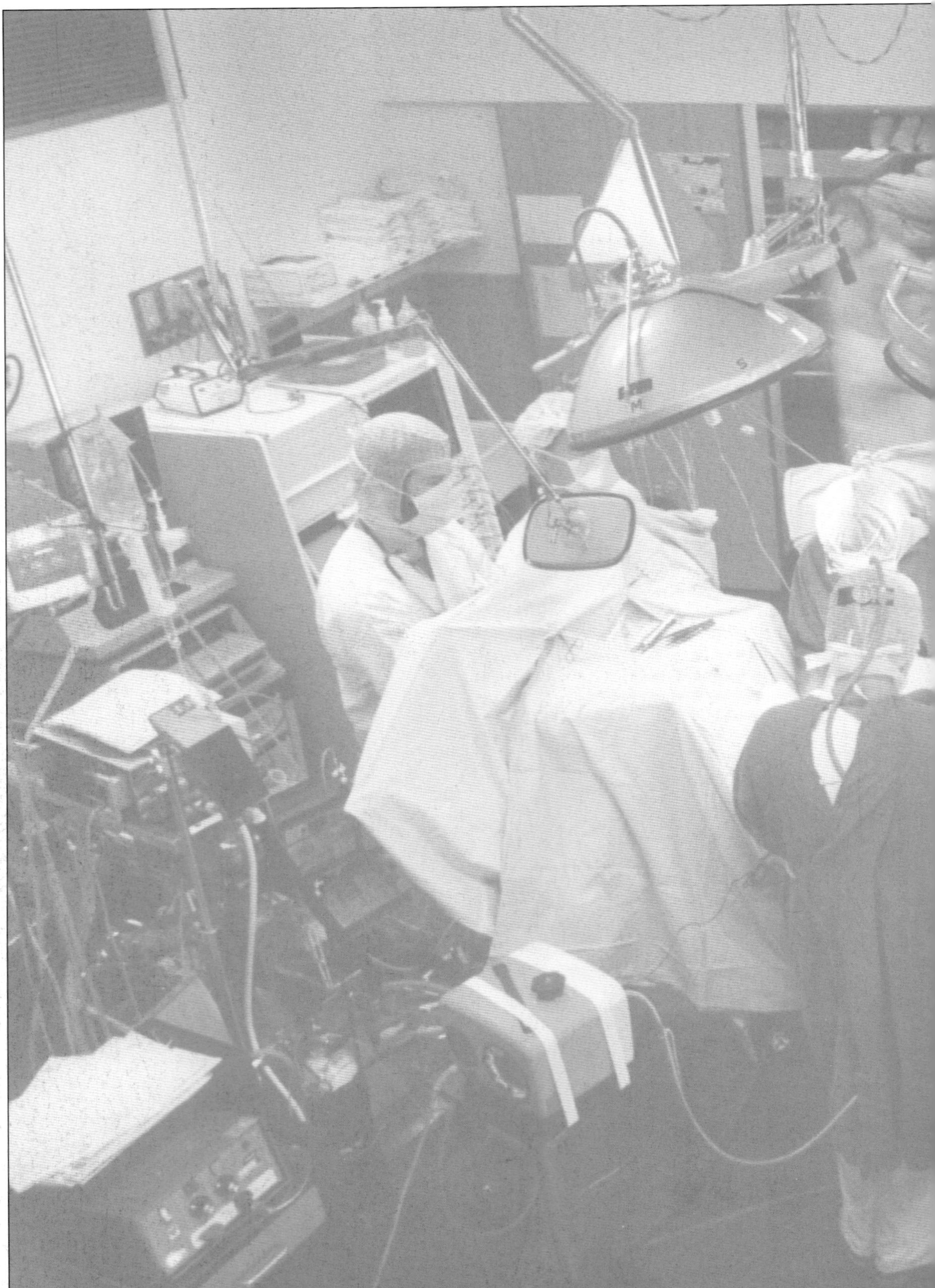

Part 5

1963–1987

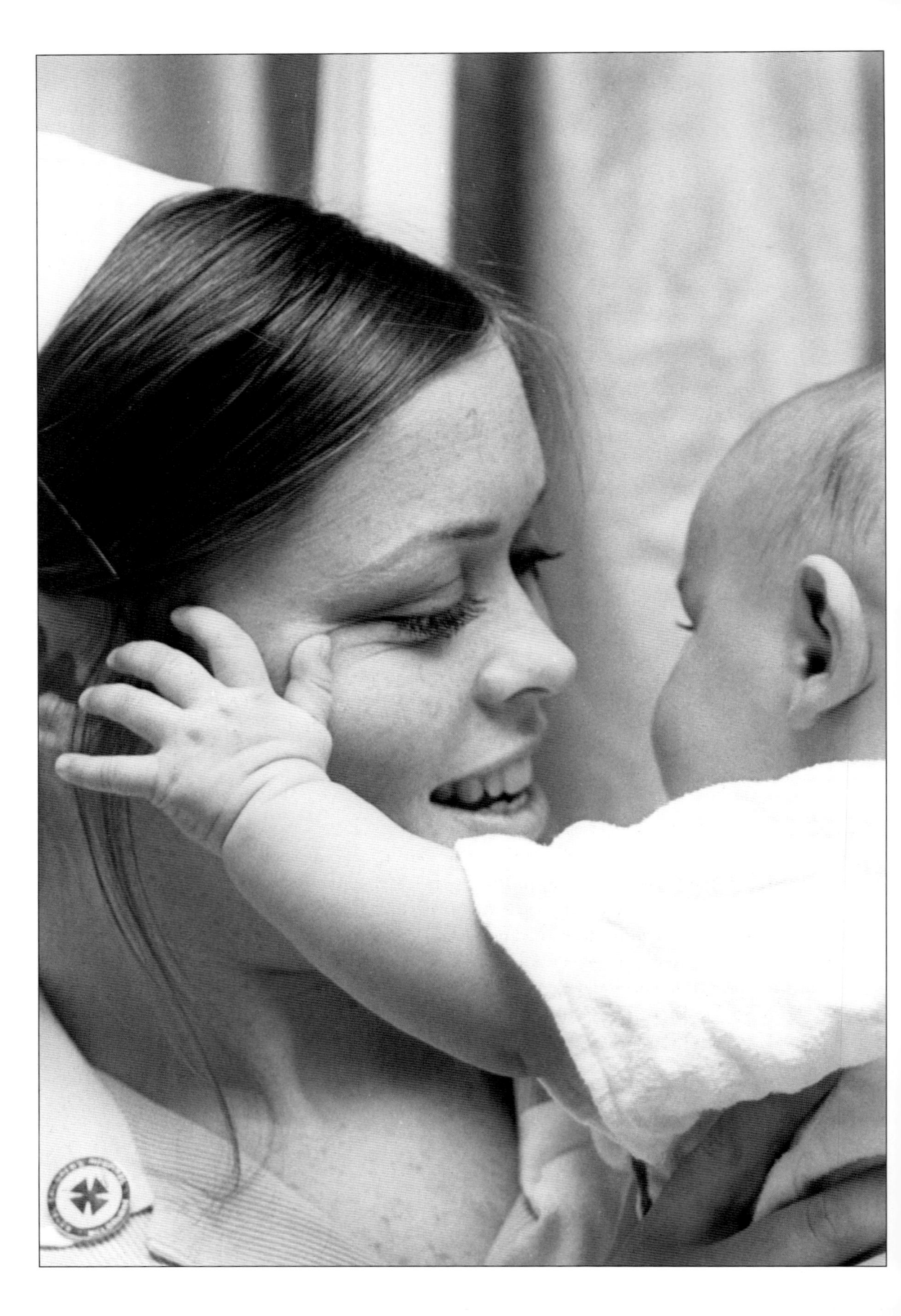

CHAPTER 11

A New Hospital

1963–1987

*I*n 1963, more than 400 nurses transferred to the new Hospital in Flemington Road, Parkville. The Director of Nursing, Miss Joan Gendle, the first Children's Hospital-trained nurse to obtain this prestigious position, was challenged by the complexities in a rapidly changing social world, the growth of medical specialisation and the implications for the modernisation and direction of the Nursing School.

A new Hospital—20 January 1963

Nance Gooderham was a Staff Nurse at the time of the transfer to Parkville. She assisted with the Sunday morning convoy of ambulances, moving sixty-one children on stretchers with their medications, belongings, records and equipment.

Leaving the Carlton site was an emotional experience. Many respected Senior Nurses chose to retire or move on. Lucy De Neeve had resigned after fifteen years, initially as Lady Superintendent and two years as the Director of Nursing.[1] The brilliant Sophie Brodie, looking for a new challenge, resigned from her position as Matron at Frankston Orthopaedic Hospital to become principal of the Nursing Aide School at Mayfield in Hawthorn. Her good friend, Kate Wilson, was Chief Tutor but resigned to care for her mother. Nance said, 'we felt somewhat leaderless'.[2]

Nurse and her baby patient, 1960s.

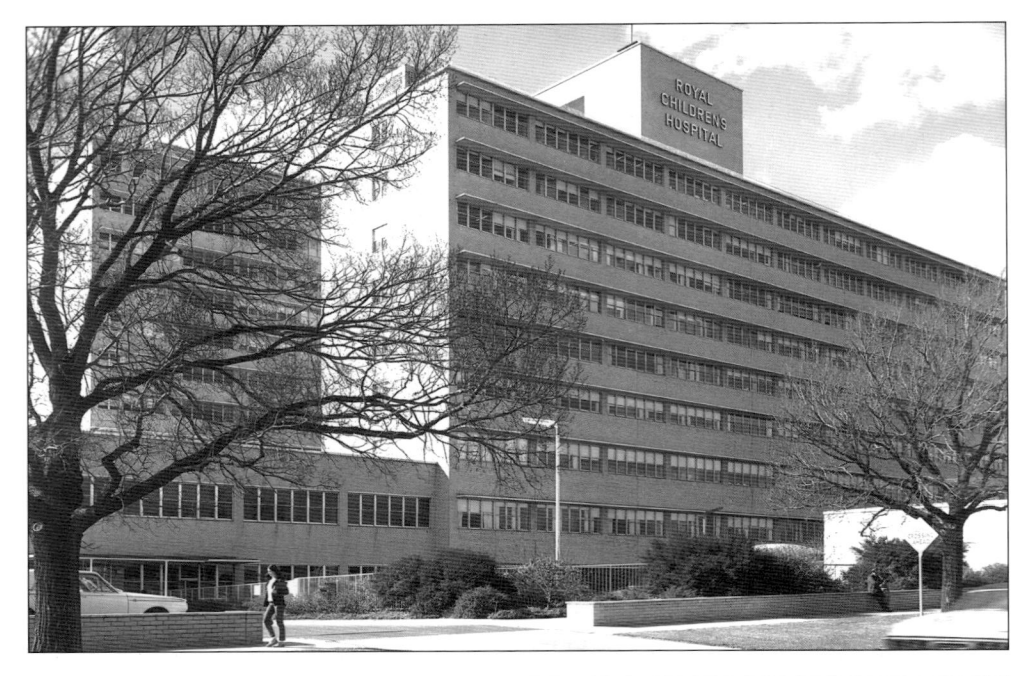

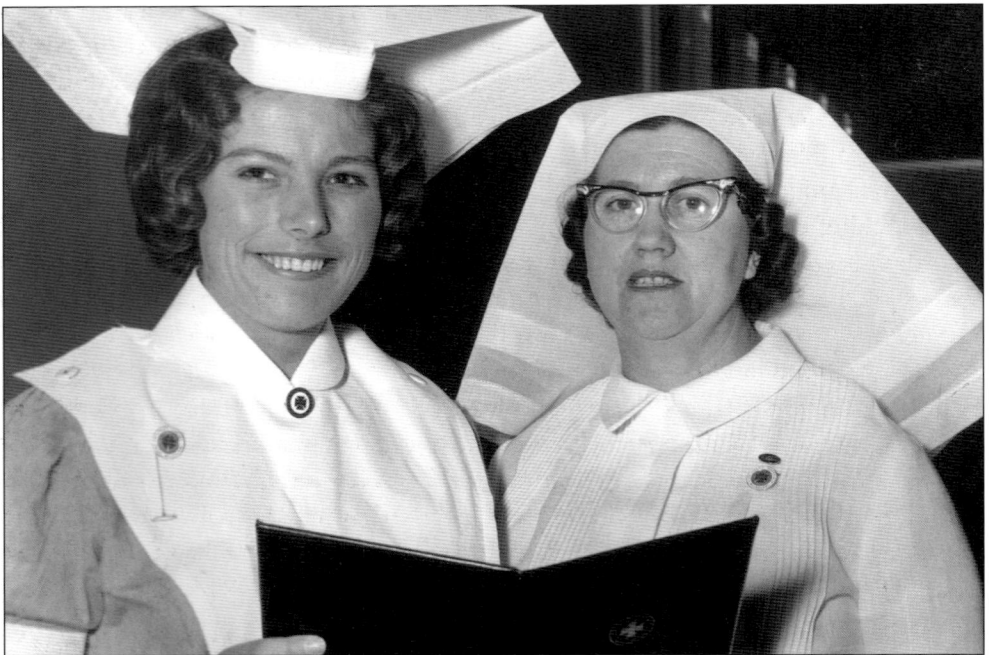

Top: New Hospital Parkville, 1963.
From the Collection of the National Archives of Australia A1200, L81210
Bottom: Director of Nursing, Joan Gendle and Libby Rodda on her graduation.
The Sun News Pictorial, 1964.

This was a double blow for Joan Gendle, a contemporary and friend of these women; as it turned out, she would need all the support she could muster in her formidable new role as Director of Nursing in the new Hospital, where she faced great changes for which the staff was ill-equipped.

The move to Parkville was premature because of Queen Elizabeth's visit. An acute shortage of equipment in the first few months resulted in departmental chaos for the better part of a year. For example, air-conditioning was not at first applied because it was untested and the risk of the spread of infection unknown. Four years were to lapse before it became operational.

A monument to the vision of successive Committees and to the architects Stephenson and Turner, the Hospital was more than twenty years in the planning but somewhat lagging in design by the 1960s, a time of immense developments in specialist medicine. Built in an 'H' shape, the Children's Hospital was one of the largest in the world, with a bed capacity for 490 children. The wards and operating theatres had a wide outlook to the northwest over the ancient river red gums in Royal Park, while the administration, laboratories and other departments faced Flemington Road. Car parks surrounded the Nurses' Home.

The wards left a lot to be desired. During the building phase, Lucy De Neeve and her senior staff had not been extensively consulted by the architects. Once a week, however, Lucy De Neeve called the Sisters over to look at a mock-up of the facilities and the general design. Sister Elizabeth Coombes and other senior staff discovered many design faults, one of which was that the washbasins and toilets were adult height. Their protests brought a response that 'children could stand on steps', until it was pointed out that some children would be on crutches.[3] Subsequently, all the plumbing had to be re-done. The original plans had the utility rooms opening into the Sisters' offices, turning them into a walk-through to the wards. Dr Vernon Collins said bed pans should not be a problem (carried through Sister's office) because they were going to be stored in the children's lockers, an idea he had picked up in Boston Children's Hospital.

Miss Elizabeth Jaffray decided to go the United States to see for herself. In 1959–60, she went with a friend on an exchange programme to Boston Children's Hospital. It was true! Bedpans and urinals were flushed, cleaned, and placed back in the lockers, and each locker cleaned and sterilised when the patient went home. 'There were special staff to do that and if that person was not available, this was not done. The American nurses certainly did not do the cleaning.'[4] This idea, of course, was not adopted at the Royal Children's Hospital.

Within one or two years of the opening of the Parkville Hospital, the rough wall surfaces and benches were condemned as unsuitable for cleaning and curtains were replaced with washable blinds. Very ill patients seldom used the toilets. The flushing attachments for bedpan rinsing over the toilet produced fine sprays condemned by the pathologist as a likely spread of infection.

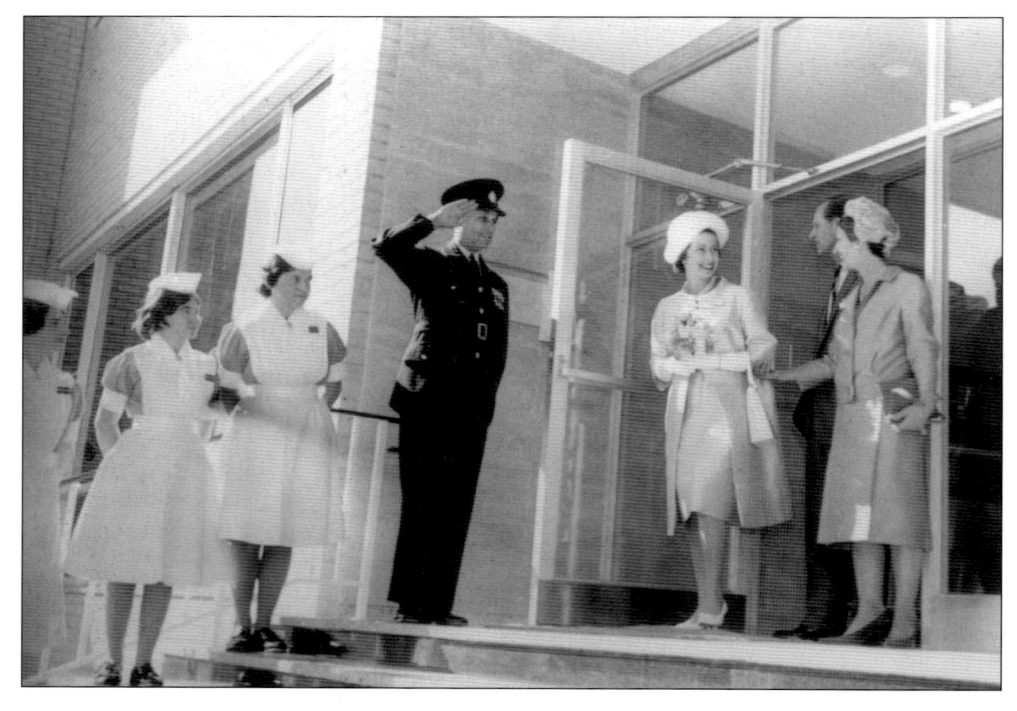

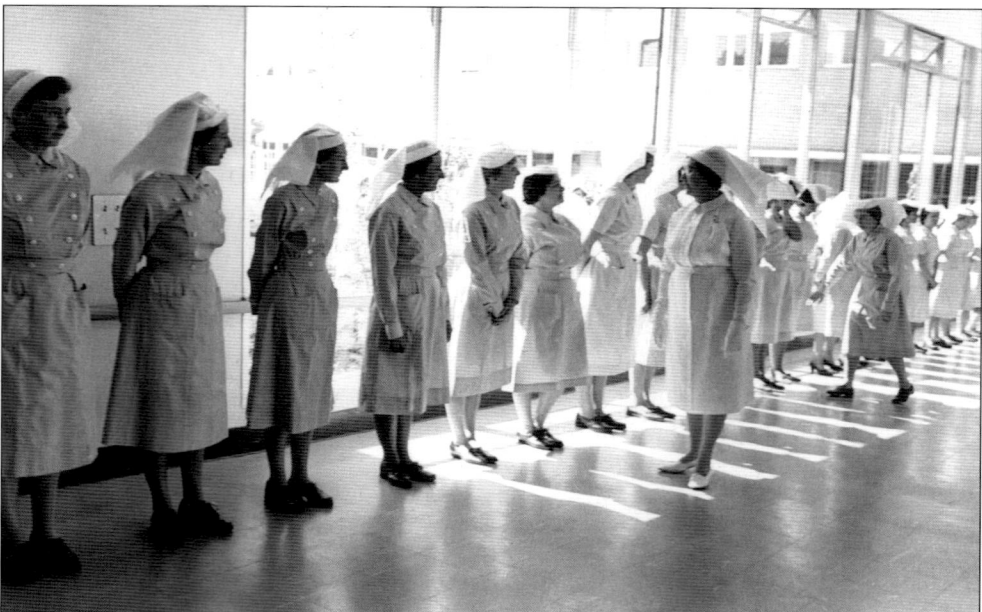

Top: Opening of the Parkville Hospital, 25 February 1963.
Queen Elizabeth and Lady Murdoch (Dame Elisabeth).
Bottom: Matron Joan Gendle inspecting the guard of honour.
Sisters Cogan, Fearon, Thompson, Pollock, Harden, Chrisfield, Jaffray and Jackson.

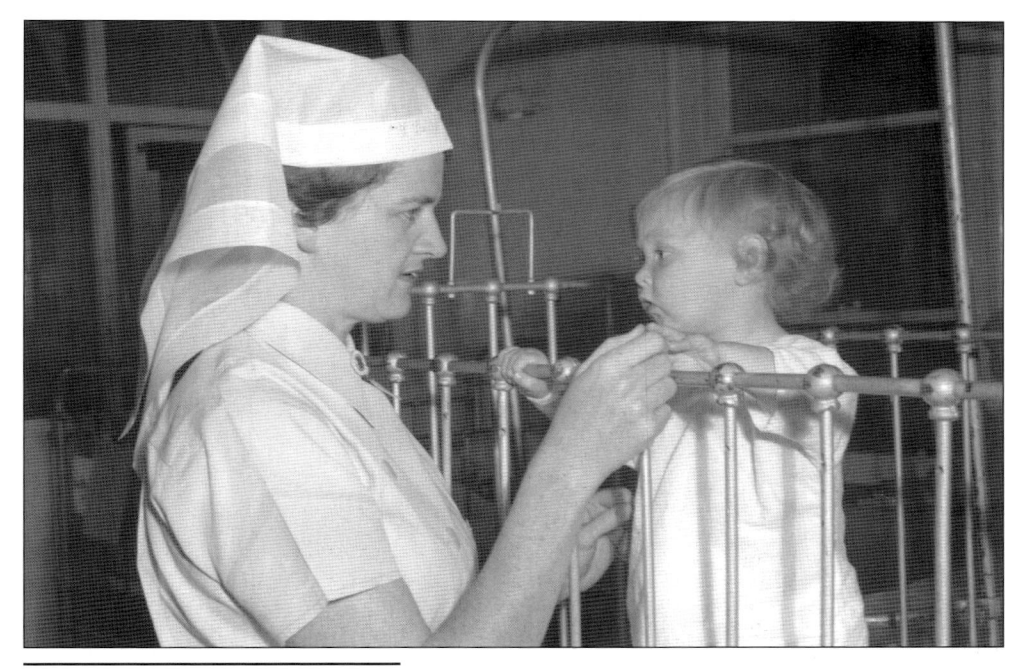

Sister Elizabeth Jaffray, Dip. Nursing Admin, CNA. FINA, NSW and ACT. RCH Distinguished Service Award, 1995. Shown here with a patient, c. 1959.

There were other obvious practical and 'comfort' problems: very ill children could not see outside into the garden because the windows were too high; there were no safe balconies or suitable play areas. Lucy De Neeve's recommendation for a low-rise Children's Hospital in a garden—a *Kindergarten*, where children could be wheeled from the wards into the fresh air and sunshine—fell on deaf ears.

Dr Collins suggested the inclusion of playrooms, and although playrooms were attached to each ward, they were not equipped or staffed and instead were used as storerooms. For nearly forty years, since 1926, the Annie Stirling Kindergarten had become a tradition, providing morning sessions for children who could be taken to the Hospital playroom. In the afternoons, a kindergarten teacher visited the bedridden patients with toys. However, in 1959 the Kindergarten closed when Occupational Therapy merged into traditional kindergarten 'territory' and the therapists did not wish to be known as 'play ladies'.

There was so much concern about the practical problems for nurses working in the wards that Sister Val Duke, a floor supervisor, was prompted to write an article in the *Nursing Journal* titled: 'The Perfect Ward'. She pointed to hundreds of factors that should be considered in hospital planning, particularly for children. For example, the number and type of patients, the quantity and quality of staff, the rostering, and the amount of research and teaching to be carried out in the wards. Central storage areas, central services, and the frequency of delivery of store supplies, bench heights, bathrooms and toilets, were essential issues. She recommended that linen and refuse be dispatched by chutes and special lifts to cancel the need for through traffic.

Her final message was directed to the holders of the purse strings in the building of ward units:

> To consider the band of nursing personnel, who alone, of the vast number of Hospital employees, provide a twenty-four-hour, seven-day week, bedside service to the patient in the ward. Surely, this warrants a hearing and a heeding on any planning committee, which sets out to design the perfect ward.[5]

Despite the irritations of the settling-in period, the nurses were enormously proud to be part of an organisation so respected in the community. Chris Fautley was touched by 'the pure innocence of the children and their helplessness and dependence on the nursing staff, the bonding that occurred with patients at all levels, nursing and medical. The reward of the speed of the recovery and resilience, or inability of recovery of young patients was treated equally.' The fact was that children had names and were not merely bed numbers was another source of satisfaction.[6]

The concept of visiting changed in the 1950s and 1960s. The presence of parents was encouraged during doctor's rounds, providing more interaction and interview time with the medical staff. Long-term patients reacted in different ways. While some became 'institutionalised', others never adjusted to the regulations of visiting hours, the ward routine and the coming and going of their mothers. The wards became more family oriented but, for some children, the distress of separation remained a sad memory. Overnight accommodation for parents was not possible except for those children in crisis.

The Director of Nursing, Joan Gendle, had an immense task ahead of her, not only the administration of the wards and the comfort of the children, but also that of the nurses. She chose the analogy of the family in her first Report to Management: 'Like all new householders, we have taken time to settle in—now we are reviewing the situation and sorting out adjustment problems. [T]o uproot 400 young women and place them in a new setting without some repercussions would be impossible.'[7]

> JOAN M. GENDLE, FCNA, was the first and only Royal Children's Hospital-trained nurse to become Director of Nursing at the Children's Hospital, 1963–69. She trained at the RCH from 1934 to 1938, coming first in the State Final Examination.[8]

Although there was no actual change in basic nursing care, the daily life and routine of each staff member was affected. Due to the move, they had to learn to use many new types of gadgets and equipment. The layout of the Hospital and the higher staff ratio to patients meant that many staff changes and movements were necessary. Many left because of an undefined and unacknowledged feeling of insecurity brought about by the physical changes and the introduction of new ideas.[9]

While some were disoriented, others loved the novelty. All agreed they were over-awed by the size of the place. 'We used to have a separate sitting room at Carlton to talk and get to know everybody. You passed on the paths, but here you went to your floor and that was it.' Despite memories of the overcrowded and run-down aspect of Carlton, staff felt dislocated and lonely, missing the well-known, intimate environment which was like the corner shop.[10] In the old days, the Committee ladies had a phenomenal input. Dame Patricia Mackinnon and Mrs Erick Grimwade visited the Carlton wards at least once a week, listening keenly to the requests and needs of the Ward Sisters. In the vast new location, the House Committee became less important in the scheme of things, although Dame Elisabeth Murdoch was always very helpful in offering suggestions to improve the ward environment.[11]

Other suggestions for interior design were not always helpful; curtains were unsuitable in Children's wards where nurses needed perfect access and continuous observation. Nevertheless, some well-meaning folk who brightened the environment with plastic flowers found they 'did the rounds', turning up again and again in different locations, even in Casualty.

The 1960s were dramatic years in paediatrics, with many firsts in cardiac surgery. A wider variety of congenital abnormalities was being treated since the days of the first patent ductus operations. In the early 1960s, Mr George Westlake performed the second Mustard operation in Australia and the first to be successful on a child in which the function of the transposed great vessels was reversed to correct the circulation problem.[12] The child, Brendan Waddington, had turned blue after birth at St Vincent's Private Maternity Hospital and was rushed to the Children's to the care of Dr Alex Venables.

Working in the wards

The work changed dramatically with the evolution of specialist medicine. Gone was the mundane, ordinary medicine from the old Children's; there were fewer children requiring long-term nursing with pneumonia or rheumatic fever and cardiac complications. It was a different atmosphere. The modern generation never knew the frightful odour of pus while packing a suppurating tibia with gauze, or gagged at the suffocating body odour of rheumatic fever patients. Not only nurses, but also medical students, never saw a child choking with diphtheria.

Nurses encountered many situations they had not expected and, as in all large hospitals, Intensive Care was a whole new area. Emergencies were commonplace as one nurse found: 'I was working in ICU where a child suddenly haemorrhaged—never seen anything like this before—vomiting blood. People came from everywhere. I don't know what I did but remembered feeling part of the "saving team".'[13]

There was no counselling and no debriefing. Entering a busy public hospital at the age of seventeen to do nursing, some girls tended to become over-involved and attached; the death of a patient was naturally the most upsetting event: the sight of a father in Casualty on his knees begging the nurses and doctors to save his daughter when nothing could be done for her. Other stressful scenes were witnessed too: the heartbreak of children who had been abused by their parents; traumatic accidents such as the boy who came in on a trolley with his sawn-off foot underneath wrapped in newspaper; watching a child with cystic fibrosis die.

The most terrible was in Casualty: two little girls admitted, thrown through the windscreen of the family car driven by a drunken father. They arrived in the cubicle, and the Nurse had to tend to the poor traumatised little faces, 'I will never forget touching the nose of one of them—it simply moved sideways entirely, almost completely severed. I was distraught. The drunken father was distraught. The RMO was furious. He tore strips off the drunken father for drunk driving.'[14]

Most challenging of all was the Burns Unit, which began in 1955 under the leadership of Mr A. Murray Clarke, in Ward 9 East. In the late 1960s, the treatment of burns was becoming more humane. Nurses looked up to Sister Win Menadue to help them cope when children were admitted from Casualty smelling of smoke and burning flesh.

Within a few weeks of specialist care, their pink skin showed through and children started smiling again. The strictest infection control was practised and nurses wore gowns, masks, caps and boots. Following the Lara bush fires, the work was heartbreaking; nurses felt bound to console the parents in some small way. At least they felt able to be of some little help. This was to be repeated in the Ash Wednesday fires in 1983. Many nurses were traumatised 'seeing the burns children in the bath having dressings changed'.[15] Fortunately, safe anaesthetics could be administered if necessary.

The team widened to include Drs Julian Keogh and John Solomon and, in 1971, Sister Wendy Swift. The treatment of burns became quite complex and the management involved many facets: the treatment of shock, acute surgery, medical care, infection control, nutritional needs, psychological and psychiatric support for the child and family and particularly for parental distress and feelings of guilt. In addition, there were well-recognised problems of child abuse: in 1981, John Solomon suggested that about 6 per cent of all admissions to the Burns Unit were the results of deliberately inflicted burns.[16] Many children had cigarette burns on their buttocks and legs. In 1968, silver sulphadiazine began to be used 'with great enthusiasm and success' in the control of infection.[17]

The nurses who worked with surgeon Julian Keogh in the operating theatre found him very gentle. As he carefully explained the process of skin grafting, the nurses could only look on with wonder.

Neil McGeachin worked as a nurse in the Burns Unit and in the Surgical Wards. He believes that one of the most dramatic changes for the better was the development of efficient post-operative pain control. Although small improvements occurred in the 1970s, it was not until 1984 that opiate drug infusions were introduced in the General Wards by Dr Jim Tiballs (intensivist) and Mr Alex Auldist (surgeon). This allowed, for the first time, continuous analgesia for children. Drs Ian McKenzie and Philip Ragg with Kate Brereton, the Pain Unit Nurse, initiated the development of an acute pain service, which has been of the greatest benefit following surgery.

The atmosphere at the Children's was such a contrast from the Melbourne Hospital. Marge Thomson remembered the awful days in the late 1950s when she was put off adult nursing 'a bit'. Her first day there she was literally thrown in head first to look after an adult in a big box respirator. A Melbourne nurse handing over said, 'it's all yours' and walked out. The patient's neck was raw because nothing soft had been put around it and the big rubber collar had rubbed all night. The poor patient had been trying to get a drink but the nursing staff had not released the valve for pressure. Each time a mouthful would come out and run down her neck. 'You were left with fifteen to twenty patients at night—impossible.'[18]

Marge was ready to walk out of nursing at the Melbourne but her friend Wendy Bond was there at the same time. 'We said "wouldn't it be easy to throw yourself out of this window?" That was the stage we got to.' Her cases were packed two days before her six months were up, the taxi booked, and she went home.

Nurses felt that at the Children's patients were treated with more respect. 'For example, if you were doing dressings you would at least warn the child, so that when you were doing it he or she was much more comfortable. That seemed to be unheard of at the Melbourne where two blunt needles were used to give injections for the whole ward.'

Marge returned to the Children's after she did her midwifery training at the Women's, which she said 'was like a factory where the treatment of women was shocking: "Mrs Brown" could come in one night and be shot out the door the next, to go to Aftercare at Henry Pride, or home on the train. The babies were parked in the nursery overnight while "rooming-in" was limited to two hours a day by the mother's bed.'

Marge had no time to apply her acute observation powers to mother–baby interaction or temperament. She puzzled why babies turned up at the Children's with feeding problems and failure to thrive. No one had time for anything. Eventually, she discussed this with Dr Frank Bishop, the Children's Hospital psychiatrist 'to work it out'.

One night at the Women's, Marge had a great surprise; she saw an old granny with her hat on come to the window of the nursery.

Marge signalled 'which baby?' and, holding up to the window the one indicated by 'granny', remarked that he was settling down and looking fine. But, despite Marge's entreaties that visiting hours were over, the 'granny' ambled around into the nursery, replying: 'It's alright dear, I wish I was grandma. I'm Dr Kate Campbell.' How was Marge to know she was talking to one of the most famous neonatal specialists who, for the sake of a sick baby, would come at all hours?

She continued her career as a Staff Nurse and Tutor for four years. She felt a little hesitant. With some advice and wisdom from the Senior Tutor, Sister Kate Wilson, 'that the experience of talking to people was vital in the apprenticeship system where the one above taught the one below', she became more enthusiastic.

One of Marge's mentors was Nancy Hardy, Ward Sister in Ward 9, Surgical, at the old Hospital. Nancy was of significant help in teaching her about running a ward and used to say 'As far as parents are concerned, if you are in doubt as to what to say, reverse the position and put yourself in their shoes. Ask yourself "what is it they want to know?"'

Eventually she became Sister-in-Charge and Supervisor on the entire seventh floor East and West: Dr Mostyn Powell, Cardiology, and Dr Alex Venables, General Medical. The other end was Neurosurgery and Cardiac Surgery. But there were still many difficulties: 'I was down one end not knowing what was going on at the other end—the ward was too long and so I could not control it. It was almost impossible to know which end to work.' The ward units averaged twenty-seven children each.

MARGE THOMSON, trained at RCH 1952–55, was a meticulous nurse and tutor. She is chiefly remembered for her outstanding work in Neuroscience Ward 6. She introduced the idea of continuity of care for families of cancer children from the time of surgery through the time of treatment, whether it was radiotherapy, chemotherapy or rehabilitation. She specialised in the care of children with brain and spinal tumours.[19]

Everything appeared to happen so quickly after the move to Parkville that Charge Nurses' jobs were never really defined. 'Ward planning soon fell apart and people were sent in all directions. Friendships and communication broke down.' Joan Gendle and others noted that Medical staff began to build up little kingdoms, and everything became 'mine and I', instead of 'us and ours'.[20]

Staff thought Joan Gendle was a wonderful person but she had such tremendous challenges. For example, 'everyone was fighting for their own niche. Two great

A New Hospital

divisions grew: administration and management versus nursing and medicine. New specialist departments grew overnight. There were always meetings.' On the Medical side, the Medical Director, Dr Perry, left after he became ill. After that, there was instability for quite a long time.[21]

From the Nursing point of view, Joan Gendle was juggling many balls, the education of staff required fitting the curriculum into the available hours. For the doctors there were never enough nurses, no matter how many were provided. Very soon it was realised that merely increasing the numbers of staff was not the only answer; quality was uppermost.

The administrative problems escalated as the constant shortage of nurses was incompatible with the uneven demands, the peaks and lows. Each January, the operating theatres were closed or short-listed while surgeons were on leave. The Intensive Care Unit was in the developmental stage and required additional trained nurses. In 1968, a proposal to build a three-storey building in the northwest corner to house a Psychiatric Unit and long-term Medical and Surgical cases would increase the number of beds to 520. Further extensions provided care for disabled children, some of whom had been abandoned by relatives.

In the 1960s, Neurosurgery patients were nursed in the wards; intensive care was not available for head injury patients. Intra-cranial pressure was not monitored, and children with cerebral tumours received methotrexate intrathecally. Some came back to the ward to die. The quality of life was not good for hydrocephalics. Children returned to Hospital frequently; arterial ventricular shunts were often blocked. It was

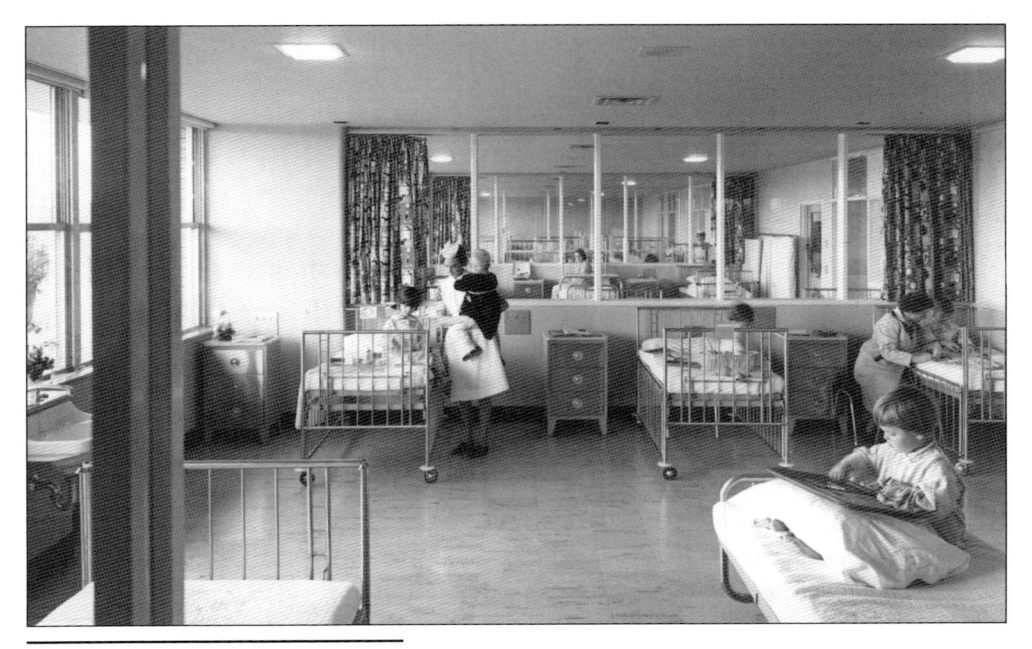

Ward 4 West, 1960s.

a busy, heavy area all the time. The spina bifida babies and children were all in the same ward, which was not desirable. All spina bifida children were treated, some of whom would be classified as untreatable today.

Dr Keys Smith, who used to come up from Frankston weekly to get patients sorted and settled, set up the Spina Bifida Unit. The biggest change was that parents had somebody who understood their children's condition, and to them, Dr Keys Smith knew all the answers and he was able to refer them to the appropriate department. They had a clinic that was theirs and they met other parents and talked to them, whereas before they were scattered around. The nurses did not see the follow-up patients; they saw only those with blocked shunts. If the child presented with a temperature, it was automatically presumed the shunt was blocked and the child was put in the nearest Surgical Ward.

Nursing rosters became particularly difficult in the operating theatres for the February–March 'catch-up' case list. Ward Sisters began to relay their dissatisfaction directly to management rather than work towards a solution and were frequently absent on leave for training and other purposes.

Joan Gendle had no time to visit each ward individually. To add to the confusion, there were many other people in the health team; it became rather crowded with occupational therapists, social workers, play leaders and physiotherapists, to name just a few. Nurses had traditionally covered many of these tasks and, while they welcomed the expanding services for children, not all these therapies were useful.[22] The extra attention the children received during the week ceased at the weekends and nurses once more reverted to filling the gaps.

The numbers of nurses grew steadily: in 1965 there were 282 in training. By 1972, there were 707 nurses, eighty-three nursing aides, sixty-two assistants and eighteen orderlies.

The Gatehouse Street Nurses' Home

As in any Hospital before nurses lived out, the Nurses' Home formed a hub of their sleeping and waking activities.

The seven-storey Nurses' Home at Gatehouse Street opened almost five years before the main Hospital. In the interim, buses transported nurses to Carlton; very inconvenient for those on 'crazy' broken shifts. For many, this often involved climbing aboard on dark winter mornings wearing only the uniform dress, completing the dressing process *en route*. 'Fortunately it was still dark for those on early starts, a skill that stood us in good stead for many years—dressing and grooming in a moving vehicle.' Transport was within thirty minutes of each end of shift, adding up to a lot of travelling with little time for leisure. 'If you were late for the bus, walking was the only option, otherwise—an expensive taxi. Lots of time was spent at Genevieve's café bar and restaurant in Faraday Street if walking to and fro.'[23]

A New Hospital

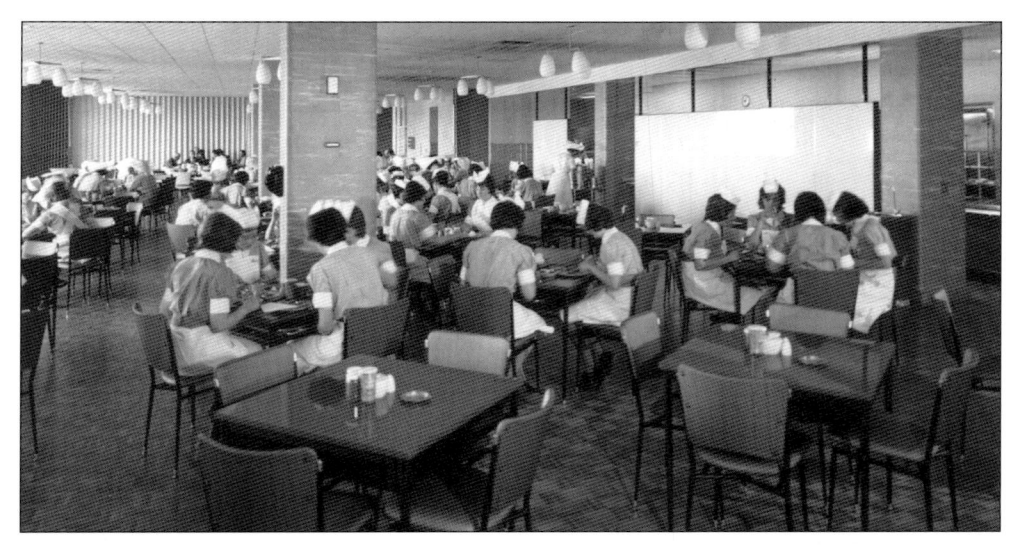

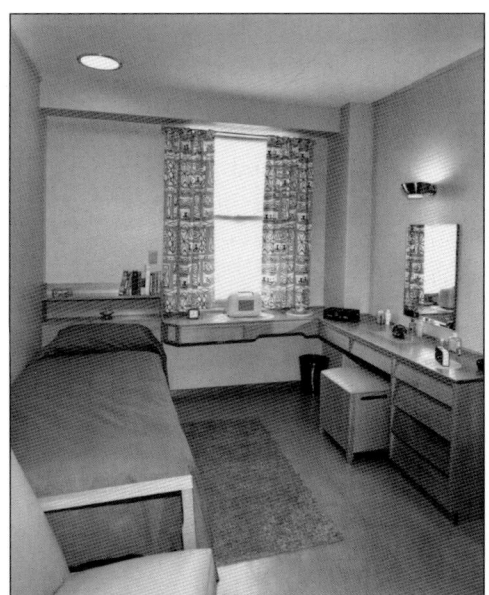

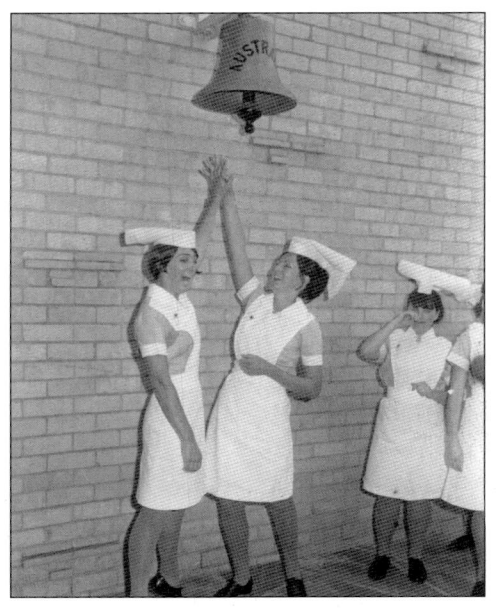

Top: Nurses' dining room/cafeteria, Parkville. *Photo by Wolfgang Sievers.*
Bottom left: A nurse's bedroom, Parkville. *Photo by Laurie Richards.*
Bottom right: Graduation 1969: 'Ringing the Ship's Bell'. *L–R:* Helen Arnold, Marg Smith and Sue Neilson. The bell was salvaged from RMS *Australia* wrecked off the coast in 1904 and presented by the Honorary Secretary Mrs F. White. It was first used to announce mealtimes at the Carlton Hospital site and it became a tradition until 1988 for nurses to ring it when celebrating success in their exams. The bell was preserved as a fixture in the grounds of the Parkville Royal Children's Hospital by the League of Former Trainees in 1990.

In 1960, the Nurses' Home was still quite new and, for many, the first experience of having a room of one's own, living and sharing bathrooms with other than one's own family. However, it was like an extended family, which overcame selfishness and shyness and created long-lasting friendships. Everyone remembers how 'copious amounts of white bread and jam were consumed as we sat in sitting rooms which overlooked the main entrance of the Home. The comings and goings provided us with 50 per cent of the conversation. When a curfew presented some problems, the hessian bags on the tennis court doubled as a bed on warm nights.'[24]

Hundreds remember the fun times of the 1960s; the borrowed clothes for special dates, checking out each other's boyfriends from the sitting rooms, living on toast and coffee when away from the Hospital dining room, a great deal of smoking indoors (if one was a smoker). Playing jokes. They loved or hated the RMH for their six months' adult training, relaxed a little at Mt Eliza, and could spend time with the children who were there long-term. Girls covered for each other when the late pass book needed to be signed, confided in each other, and matured together from school girls to women, capable of responsibility.

When locked out, access was easy at 6.30 am—staff nurses were kind and sneaked people in. But the rules seemed out of date for the 1960s: lights out while in PTS (Preliminary Training School), no transistors, late passes and signing false names in the book to avoid reprimands. Some slept at Ormond College if no late pass was obtained.

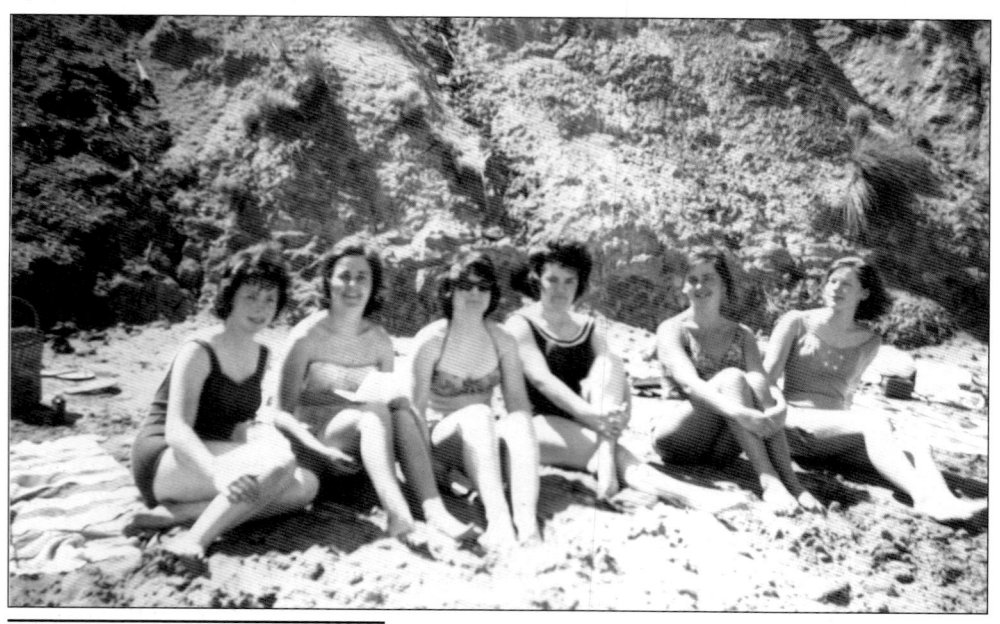

Having fun off duty at Frankston beach, 1964.
Menzies Family Collection.

Other students, those above twenty years old, found the quizzing by one of the administration staff intrusive: where have you been, who were you with, what did you do? Being addressed by surnames was considered old-fashioned and hierarchical, much like a boarding school.

In 1967, Anne Bryan's parents arrived to drop her off on the first day. Her father was not allowed beyond the reception area and was therefore unable to visualise where his daughter was going to spend the next few years of her life. Groups were moved *en masse* from floor to floor: the most junior to the first floor, night duty to the seventh floor where it was 'supposed to be quieter!' Anne spent a lot of time studying in her room. The intercom, room to room, called nurses for work and private calls; this worked better than today's sophisticated pagers.[25]

The first Supervisor at the Gatehouse Street Nurses' Home, Mayne Bodycomb, trained at the Children's in 1926. Several of the nurses were postgraduates from other countries. Despite the generation gap, Mrs Bodycomb, who seemed more like their grandmother, was looked upon very kindly. As far as the young nurses were concerned, she was an elderly lady who sat at the front desk in the reception area, quite easily duped but certainly very sympathetic. Mrs Bodycomb modelled the style of Mrs De Neeve who was deeply admired for her way with the nurses.[26]

The piano was moved from the old to the new Nurses' Home and permission was given to hold a dance but later drew a warning 'that more care must be taken to prevent cigarette burns on the floor'.[27] A similar warning was issued at social functions at the Nurses' Home at Frankston, where staff was told 'that damage was to be prevented from stiletto heels'. By September 1963, there was a desperate need for a recreation room for the nurses—there were approximately 230 nurses in the building at any one time with one TV room and a piano: an unlikely mix.

This nursing hierarchy continued into the 1960s, providing security for some and instigating rebelliousness in others. Student nurses, staff nurses, Ward Sisters, nurse assistants, Mothercraft nurses and nursing aides were ranked by the style, colour and cut of the uniforms, their caps, veils and badges of office. Nurses were predominantly female; most were single. Rules and regulations dominated their lives. Doctors, medical students and allied health professionals were known by name and status; the length of their white coats signified rank. It was not until 1969 that the first remarkable change occurred: the symbolic Sisters' veil was discarded.

When nurses became engaged to be married in the 1950s, they were expected to be interviewed by Mrs De Neeve who invariably asked to see the ring. She would say 'oh, it is just like mine'. This was a joke, because her ring was a big pearl. Most girls had a very small diamond. In Miss Gendle's time, most did not tell. In 1968, the Committee agreed that Miss Gendle should have full discretion in deciding when to agree to the marriage of trainees.[28] However, in practice that was rare. Some married secretly. It was not uncommon to become engaged, marry, finish training and, in more than one case, become pregnant without discovery.[29]

In the 1960s, subservient rules and broken shifts perpetuated the nurses' role as servants of the Hospital and as a cheap source of labour. There was a strict order about where to sit (unwritten rule) in the dining room: the most junior near the door of the 'Ella Latham'; no slacks allowed; uniform to be worn at all times, except weekends, in the dining room. The 2 am curfew was a treat; all other hospital curfews were at midnight and at St Vincent's, where nurses were now going for adult training, it was 10 pm. The tenth floor Doctor's Residence at the Children's was out of bounds but everyone knew about Friday nights!

Uniform inspections were mandatory. An administrative staff member had a personal rule: there was to be no hair on the collar, and short uniforms were viewed as an outrage. Anne Hardham recalls that in 1970 'each morning we knelt for inspection as the hems were measured with a ruler from the floor. Once inspection was finished, we got away and hitched up our dresses under our belt. In the days of mini skirts, long dresses were so daggy. A girl was badly caught—she had nothing to hide—she cut off her hem.'[30]

The Nurses' Home rapidly became crowded and, in March 1963, Joan Gendle found there was a serious shortage of accommodation for trained staff. In the years when all the effort went into the establishment of the new Hospital, the quality of some of the bed-sitting rooms at Park Court had deteriorated. Within a few months there was so much concern over lack of nurses' accommodation that the Committee decided to make use of the nursing mothers' bedrooms on the seventh floor for nurses' accommodation.[31]

Nurse education in the 1960s

In 1964, an inquiry into technical education, the Martin Committee,[32] opened the way towards federal funding of basic nursing education. This was the beginning of a political alliance with the Royal Australian Nursing Federation (RANF). The Committee included Pat Slater, Director of the College of Nursing 1965–76, a former Children's Hospital trainee, and Mary Pattern, Secretary of the RANF. It was to have a profound influence in bringing the two organisations together, leading to many reports, inquiries and recommendations.[33] Ultimately, Pat Slater and the Committee led nursing education in Victoria into the tertiary sector.

The nursing curriculum became subject to major revision. The need to produce more thorough knowledge for the nursing trainee and, at the same time, improve the quality of patient care provided extensive access into the basic sciences and, to a lesser extent, into some of the more specialised fields of medicine and surgical nursing. In theory, the plan provided a sound theoretical knowledge base almost equivalent to university standards, with no more than two or three days a week for actual nursing. The reality was harder to implement.

By 1968 there were 300 nurses in training, and the lectures were being

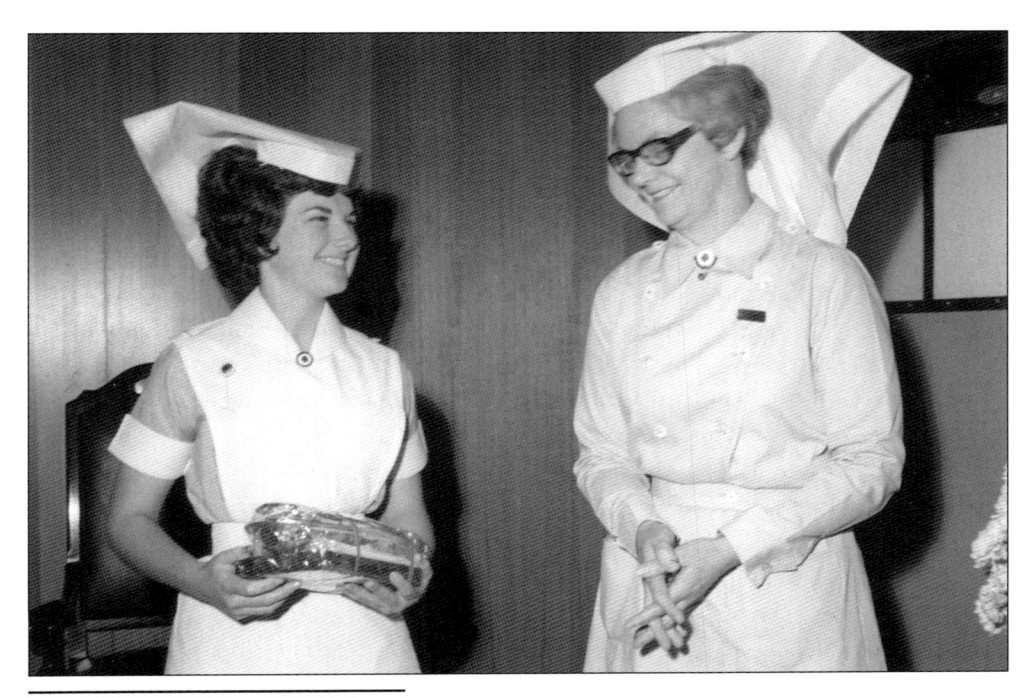

Nell Chrisfield, Tutor, with Ruth Bram.

conducted in the Hospital lecture room instead of the Nurses' Home. One half-day study a week was granted during Hospital time as well as an educational allowance for lectures taken off-duty. Before first-year exams, study blocks were re-introduced. With nurse trainees spending only two or three days a week in the wards, the Medical Director became concerned about the reduction of the Hospital's role as a trainer—in other words, the loss of control. Nurses would be away at other hospitals for fifteen months of their course. This meant a massive increase in the numbers of nurses needing to be employed.

To compound the serious shortage of tutorial staff, none of the six Nurse Tutors in the School had trained in a children's hospital.[34] This was thought by some to be a disadvantage as their teacher's knowledge of paediatrics appeared limited, although individuals were admired: 'they were young, caring and good teachers'. One of those was Nell Chrisfield, an Alfred Hospital trainee (1940–43) and Senior Nurse Educator at the Children's, favoured by the nurses for her kindness, her teaching and understanding. Unfortunately, she died in September 1966, but such was her reputation that the Nell Chrisfield Memorial Prize was founded to honour her name.

Throughout the 1960s and early 1970s there were sharply contrasting ideas about the course content: most of the curriculum was based on adult nursing. Girls went to the Children's because of their love of children.

Juniors straight out of PTS nearly always went with babies, a great learning experience, feeding and bathing six babies at 10 am. This practice continued well into the 1970s.

Newcomers sometimes found the buildings confusing. Kathy Purcell found the layout of the wards on the north side of the building very different to that in Ward 2 West; became disoriented. With a tiny baby to bath, she asked the Charge Sister where to wash the baby—she saw no bath—and Sister stated crossly: 'in the sink'. A seemingly impossible feat, she attempted to bath the baby in the huge bath used for older children. Sister stopped her saying, 'in the sink, in the sink'. Kathy then filled up the small basin by the door used by staff to wash their hands, but she was stopped again. The Sister pounced on her and pulled her all the way down to section 3 and 4 where the large sinks were. 'If only she had shown me!'[35]

Many have recorded how very tired they were when going off duty at 3 pm only to be stopped by a certain Ward Sister who would say: 'There is a chart that has no 10 am temperature recorded. When you bring it to me and show that it has been done, then you can go', and, 'There is a child that has not had its regulation fluid [whatever it was—for example, 600 ml], and when that child has been given the right amount of fluid then you can all go.' Although there were older nurses, very strict and staid, none of them equalled that particular Sister's harshness.

Others remember a notorious 'blue' sister, an Army Major type who gave nurses a hard time; she called them from their sleep in the Home after night duty, to 'get fully dressed in uniform, come over to the ward, and fill in the charts!' So terrified were they of her and the likely repercussions that one or two nurses were observed running around filling in the TPR and BP charts before going off duty. As a measure of the impossible, with so few staff, sleeping babies assessed as being more able to miss an early feed were allowed to sleep in favour of those most frail.

After PTS there was one lecture a week, 'fairly useless, about adult nursing, because we nursed children!' There was some paediatric nursing course content but the main point was that 'when sitting finals, the questions were about myocardial infarction, coronary disease and all that sort of thing, it was all adult'. The educational backgrounds of nurses during the 1960s improved enormously. Most had at least Leaving Certificate and many had HSC with a science subject, more commonly, biology. Dr Kester Brown lectured in anatomy and physiology between 1968 and 1972, and claimed he had educated every nurse in the Hospital. He noticed that the students had a serious lack of science subjects, chemistry and physics.[36]

Admired and respected for their youth and freshness, gentleness and kindness to children and their skills in observation and nursing ability, Children's Hospital nurses nevertheless had a high dropout rate.[37]

Educated, independent and militant, products of the liberal, open classroom *laissez faire* school teaching methods of the late 1950s and 1960s, these young women found the subordination and harshness of a few Ward Sisters unacceptable.[38]

Being in PTS there were no frills on their caps; the general feeling among the student nurses was of utter inferiority, reduced to their school day systems with long unfashionable uniforms. But going into the wards, being subordinate was even more traumatic. 'The Staff Nurse in yellow expected doors to open for her and to be invited for morning tea.'[39] As a measure of the unpopularity of the old types of Ward Sisters, who brought their unchanging attitudes with them, the attrition rate was very high. Of the July 1963 group, for example, the first to start training at the new Hospital, only eight out of twenty-eight student nurses sat their finals.

St Vincent's Hospital

For more than twenty years, RCH nurses obtained basic adult nursing experience exclusively at the Royal Melbourne Hospital. In 1966, the nursing workforce had expanded and the Victorian Nursing Council approved RCH nurses to receive adult training at St Vincent's Hospital. Until 1960, when St Vincent's opened their own Children's Wing, there was a reciprocal arrangement with the Children's.

Initially RCH nurses went in twos. Many people at St Vincent's said they enjoyed having Children's Hospital nurses over there because they had been taught to observe, not just to learn from books. As children cannot always articulate their ailments, Children's nurses had extra skills in observation.

The experience of night duty at St Vincent's for a Children's Hospital 'acting senior' was traumatic when a patient died nearly every night. They were generally required to lay out the body and, occasionally, and alone if there was no help available, to wheel the body to the morgue to be placed in the fridge. Some nurses have said that to this day they do not really like visiting St Vincent's. Nevertheless, many enjoyed their days at 'St Vs'.

War service—Bien Hoa, Vietnam

The social and political changes accompanying the women's movement and the Vietnam War had a significant effect on young people during these years. Several Children's Hospital nurses answered advertisements from the Federal Government to volunteer in civilian medical teams to work in war zones. Among them was Jo Van Valen.

Jo was twelve years old when her parents settled on a farm near Yarram in South Gippsland after migrating from Dordrecht, south of Rotterdam in Holland. She trained at the Children's and Royal Melbourne Hospitals from 1960 to 1963 and followed this with six months' experience at Yarram and St Andrew's Hospital in East Melbourne. Her midwifery training at Royal Hobart Hospital was distinguished by her graduating with top marks in August 1965, and followed by experience as a midwife in New Zealand. But her love for theatre work, first kindled in her student

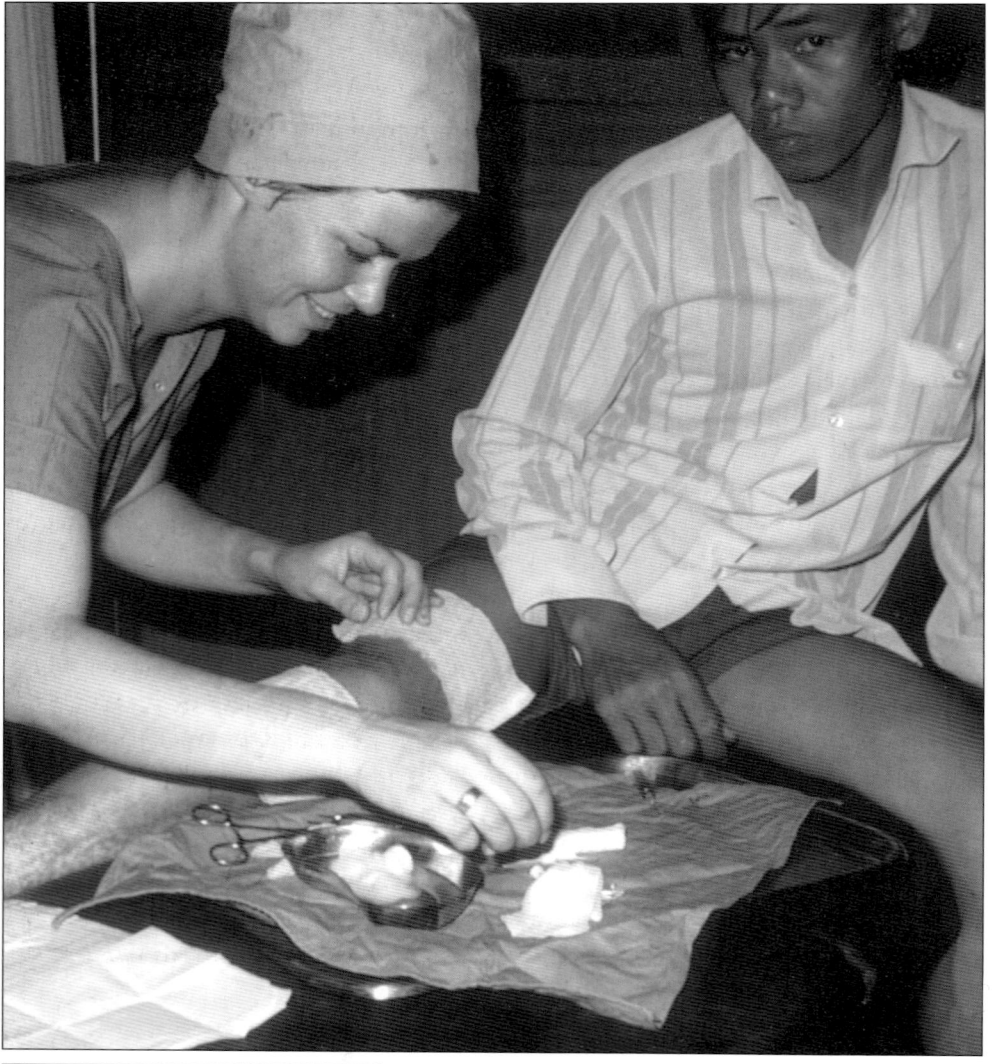

Bien Hoa, Vietnam: Jo Van Valen and patient.

days, brought her back to Melbourne and the RCH, something that was to last until the end of her nursing career.

Throughout the 1960s, Jo worked with surgeons in all surgical disciplines, but predominantly with Mr Durham Smith and in her two specialties, Cardiac and Neurosurgery, with Mr George Westlake and Mr Reginald Hooper. It was early days in cardiac surgery and, whilst exciting, there were many conditions that were still inoperable. Open heart surgery was often complicated and required very long hours for patients and staff.

In late 1968, Jo saw an advertisement for work in Vietnam. The government needed volunteers. She had long nurtured compassion for others in unfortunate circumstances, especially in war, and had watched TV and reports of the plight of the Vietnamese while longing to serve and help. With the encouragement of all including Director of Nursing Joan Gendle, she applied and joined an Alfred Hospital medical team in January 1969 for six months' service. She said: 'it changed my life and direction'.

A few weeks after arriving in Bien Hoa, the team's lives were endangered when the small town was invaded by the Viet Cong. Work conditions were primitive, with dirt floors; supplies were readily available from the American Air Base doctors: blood, serum, oxygen and other requisites. Australian surgeons did magnificent surgery—not only war injuries but cleft palates and lips as well. There were road casualties too, 'everyone drove like maniacs'. As horrific experiences unfolded—held up by gunmen, surrounded by small mortar bombs, street casualties and whole families appearing at the door to become a casualty clearing station—Jo not only learned to live with fear but also developed a personal strategy.

The team, seventeen in all, consisted of doctors, surgeons, anaesthetists, nurses who had to be prepared for anything, and three to four builders. One morning a week, they flew to a French outpost in Viet Cong country, to a leprosarium where surgeons operated on patients with Hansen's disease. It was spotlessly clean, with beautiful tiles. The French nuns and priests were very thankful. Jo visited orphanages and her mother sent children's clothes from Australia. She became very friendly with a translator in Vietnam whose husband had been killed. They still correspond today.

Jo's work at the Children's Hospital was good preparation for Vietnam. However, returning home was a shock. After resting in Hong Kong she arrived all alone at Essendon airport. She became very disillusioned by the life style and riches in Melbourne, by 'the luxurious amount of supplies in hospitals' and left RCH at the end of 1970.[40]

Civilian life

Jo commenced Infant Welfare training at Queen Elizabeth Hospital for Babies in Carlton in 1971, after which she managed a crèche in Collingwood for a year. While there she was pleased to be involved with Dr Kester Brown, the RCH anaesthetist in a safety trial of anti-depressant packaging—tablets in bottles which were a prominent cause of poisoning in children presenting at the RCH Intensive Care Unit. This research eventually resulted in legislation to change pharmaceutical products to foil packs.

Her love of theatre work enabled her to work at London's Great Ormond Street Hospital for Children and she became operating theatre manager of three floors for seven years but retired due to ill health in 1979. In her view, RCH Melbourne was a wonderful place to work in, and the basis of all she achieved: integral to her career and to the growth of her personal humanity.

Like most of the nurses who served in Vietnam, Jo had not thought about the long-term health consequences from exposure to chemicals. There were more immediate dangers, although she said: 'We were in an area that was defoliated—all the trees had been razed and at the back of where we lived there was a big pond and some of our cooks used to go down and pick herbs from the ponds. You had to wonder what we were eating and all of the chemicals that had been used to raze the trees were in the soil.'[41]

Jo developed health problems; in 1978, closing the door on her beloved theatres, she turned to another significant interest, first inspired by her work at RCH in the 1960s: care and support for her staff and colleagues. She returned to Melbourne, became a hospital chaplain and devoted the remainder of her working life to patients and staff.

Nursing in the community

The Children's Hospital has always experienced competition with community work, an area where Children's Hospital nurses are in high demand. As Melbourne grew there was considerable demand for Maternal and Child Health Services, School Health and Child Welfare Programmes. In 1975, eighteen Early Childhood Development Programmes (ECDP) were established in the city and in regional Victoria. Royal Children's Hospital nurses were ideally suited for these roles and many found work in such centres preferable to travelling to a city hospital.

Employment was plentiful in the 1960s; further education was possible through Commonwealth scholarships and allowances. For those who did complete the training, travel became an option as wages improved.

In 1961, an experienced Ward Sister in a large hospital could expect to earn £19/2/6 a week with free board, uniforms and lodging, while a first-year nurse earned £7/9/0 for a female and £9/18/6 for a male.[42] In 1965, there was a substantial internal pay rise for trained nursing staff in response to staff shortages at the Children's Hospital and, in September, there was an award pay rise for nurses according to duties undertaken and classified accordingly.[43] However, these wages were not competitive with other professions.

As the RCH drew towards its centenary in 1970, it was noted that many of its former nurses had an impressive community record in their contribution to the health and welfare of Victorian women and children. Many became Maternal and Child Health 'institutions' throughout the State. Una Allen relieved in country and city on the Victorian Baby Health Centres' Association (VBHCA) Travelling Caravan and became an Inspector of Infant Welfare Centres from 1951 to 1975. Lesla Sutton

A New Hospital

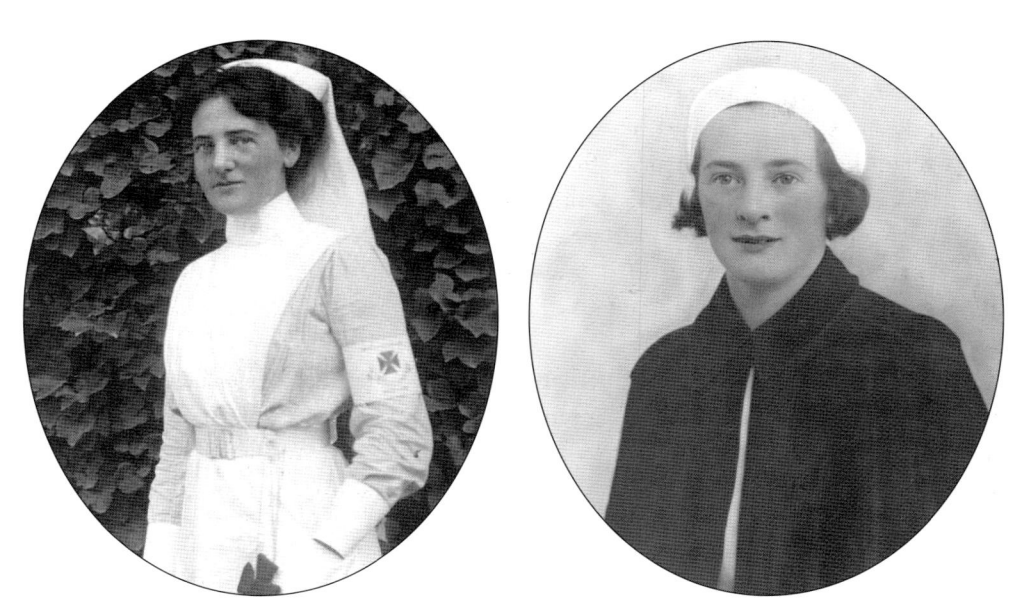

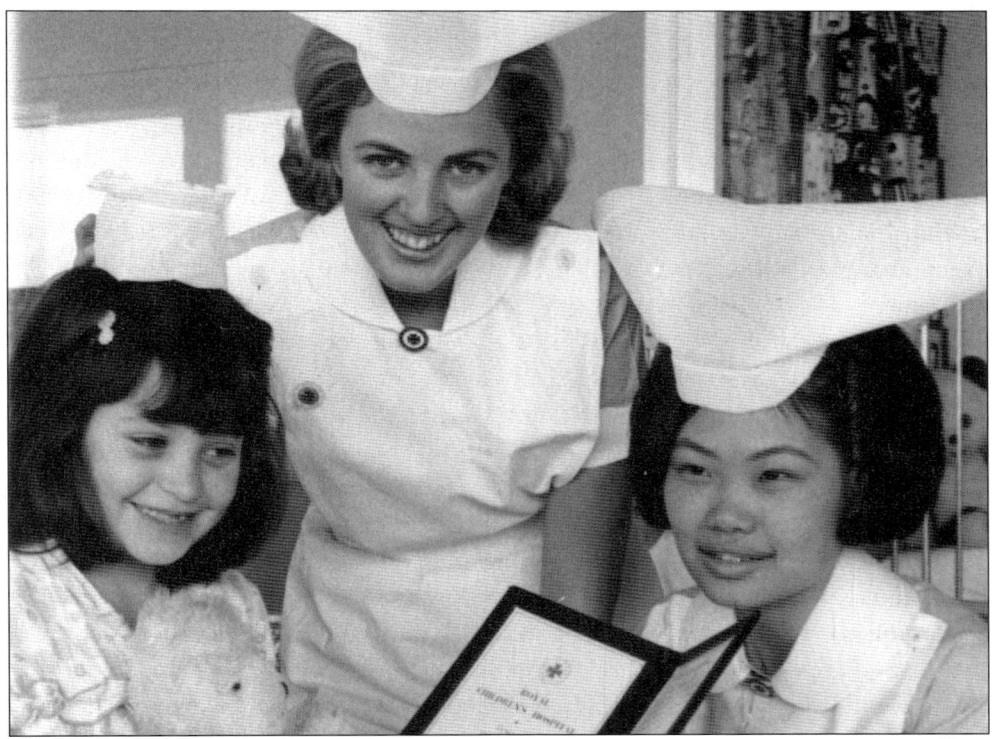

Top left: Irene McCausland, 1911. Grandmother.
Top right: Kate Menzies (née Carew), 1936. Daughter.
Bottom: Janet Leckie (née Menzies), centre, 1967. Grand-daughter.
Menzies Family Collection.

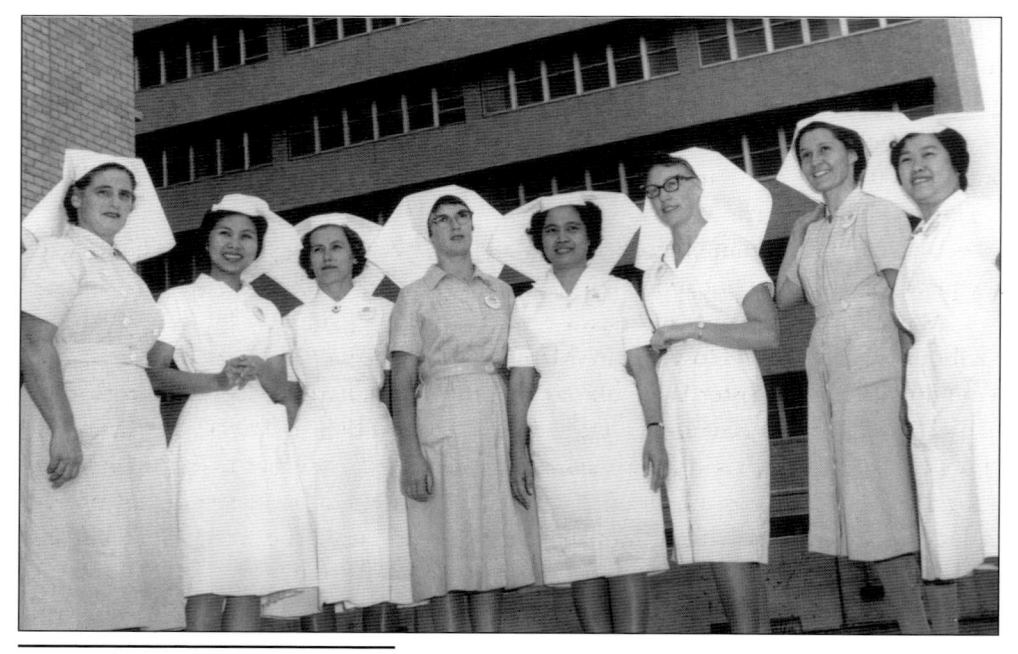

Sister Val Duke (L) and members of the Post-Basic Course group, 1969.

(RCH 1935–38) directed a very large Children's Centre in Hawthorn until the 1970s. Muriel Lewis (RCH 1933–38) cared for the women and children of Pakenham and attended the Bush Nursing Hospital from the 1940s to the 1950s. Thekla Kirschner (RCH 1932–36) founded the first Baby Health Centre at Chadstone in the 1950s and worked there for nineteen years.

Following several years in the Maternal and Child Health service at the City of Knox, Audrey Grant won a Centaur Scholarship and gained her Masters Degree in Special Education at Monash to become a lecturer in the School of Nursing in the Department of Nursing at La Trobe University.

Elizabeth Sadlier, known as 'Sad', became very much a part of the local community from the 1950s to the 1970s in Yarra Glen, Lilydale and Healesville. In 1981, she received the award of the BEM for her long outstanding service in Maternal and Child Health. Others celebrated include Joan Waters, Mary Buxton and Gwen Mackintosh (née Easton). Beryl Shannon worked at the Royal Women's Hospital in 1947 and remained a charge midwife until she retired in 1972.

Adele Brain commenced Family Support Services for City of Melbourne and received an OAM in 2002 for her work for services in the community. Marjorie Tomlinson (RCH 1942–43) received many awards, including the OAM for services on the Mornington Peninsula.

Future directions

As the Hospital approached the centenary year of 1970, additions and alterations were being planned for further building in all of its precincts.

The closure of the Frankston Convalescent Hospital was imminent and provision was made to transfer convalescent and asthmatic children to a villa in Chapman Street, North Melbourne.

But the most immediate plan was the first-class Intensive Care Unit, with adequate space for patient monitoring and a work area for the busy staff.

Many overseas and interstate-trained nurses gained experience at the Melbourne Children's Hospital. In March 1967, the post-basic paediatric courses recommenced with Sister Val Duke as the Tutor-in-Charge. Medical Director Dr Lionel E. G. (LEG) Sloan predicted that, as with other fields of medicine, the knowledge in paediatrics was advancing at a rate where it was becoming increasingly difficult for medical and nursing staff to adjust. But despite the development of new technical devices, 'individual humane bedside care must be the prime consideration'.[44]

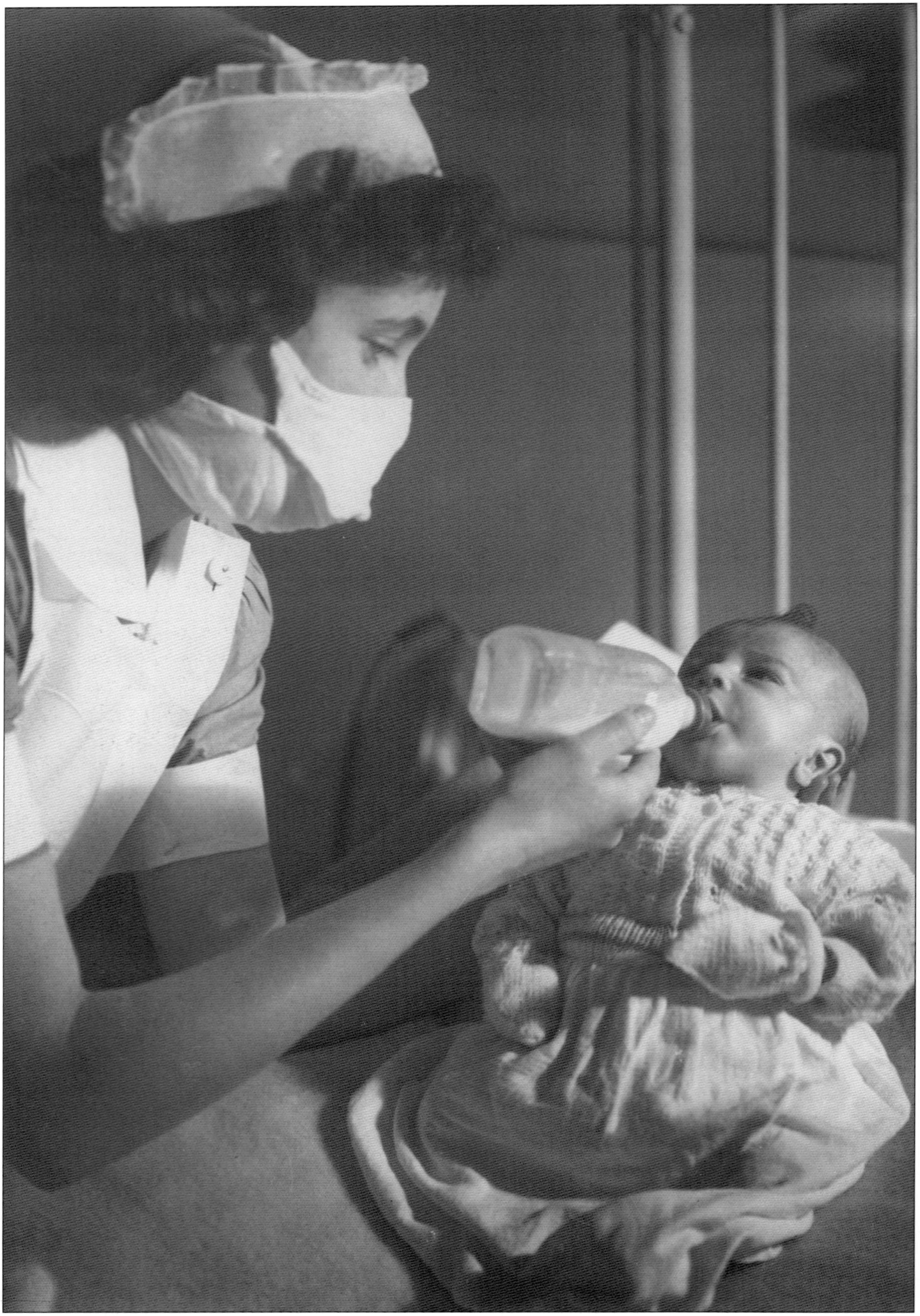

CHAPTER 12

Intensive Care and Theatre Nursing

1963–1987

*A*very important development in patient care since 1963 at the Royal Children's Hospital has been intensive care. An Intensive Care Unit (ICU) is a component of modern hospitals where patients are admitted to receive special and sometimes complicated treatment, which is unavailable elsewhere in the Hospital. This can be a routine admission following cardiac surgery or as a result of an emergency, for example a serious accident, a near-drowning incident or the ingestion of a poisonous substance causing respiratory failure.[1] The prolonged use of nasotracheal intubation to maintain the airway and ventilation is the cornerstone of modern intensive care.

None of the advances of the 1960s could have been accomplished without the development of this unit in the Department of Anaesthesia, and the assistance, knowledge and expertise of the nurses caring for the patients. They not only learned new techniques with modern technology, but also to handle crisis situations in ventilated children and to respond to their psychological needs and those of their families. These were revolutionary years in paediatric nursing at the Royal Children's Hospital.

Nurse Joan Hatswell with the youngest baby to receive a tracheotomy, c. 1949.
Collection, Claire Taylor.

Historical background

Tracheostomy and endotracheal intubation have long been known to medicine. In 1848, a Parisian physician passed a catheter via the nose and condemned tracheotomy (nowadays universally called tracheostomy)[2] as unsuitable.

In 1879, the New York physician, Joseph O'Dwyer devised a tube which sat in the larynx and did not come out of the mouth. Dr A. Jeffreys Wood of Melbourne Children's Hospital observed this technique to prevent suffocation and found it could easily be learnt.[3] The method became less popular in the twentieth century when Chevalier Jackson of Pittsburgh designed brass tubes which passed though the larynx and were intended to make tracheostomy safer for children.[4]

With the introduction of anti-toxin in Melbourne in 1895, laryngeal diphtheria, one of the most common causes of obstruction, became less common.

Background to nursing in the ICU

To understand the historical development of and background to the ICU/RR (Recovery Room) nursing at the Children's, it is useful to consider the recollections kindly provided by the first ICU nurses and others.[5]

At the old Carlton Hospital, children returned from the theatre following major cardiac surgery to be 'specialled' by a senior nurse in the ward. A screen was wheeled around the 'operation' bed the nurse had prepared with warm blankets, mackintoshes,

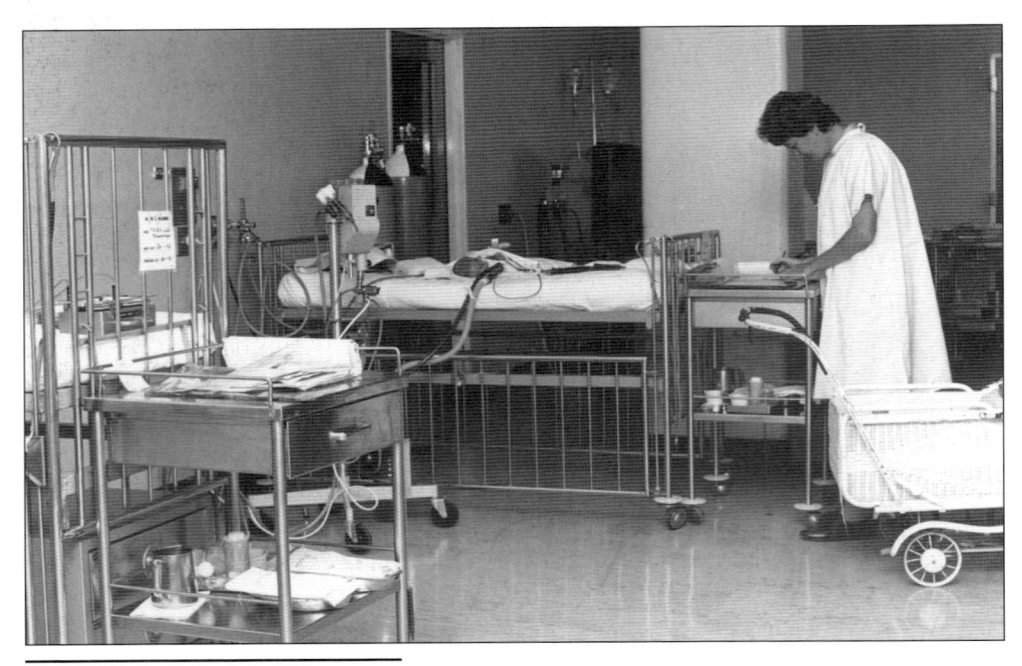

Elizabeth Jaffray. Early days in the Intensive Care Unit (ICU).

draw sheet, a kidney dish, towels and tongue forceps. She recorded the pulse, blood pressure, colour and general condition of the patient and kept the airway clear of vomit. If oxygen was needed, a heavy black oxygen cylinder was wheeled to the bedside. In those pioneering days of complex cardiac and other surgery, the patient sometimes died. Ward activities continued as usual, those around oblivious to the drama being enacted in their midst.

When Miss Elizabeth Jaffray[6] returned to the Carlton Hospital in 1960 from a one-year exchange in the United States, she was appointed as the Charge Sister of Surgical Ward 9 at Carlton, which was located on the floor below the operating theatre. Of the four sections to this ward, one was devoted to the children who had undergone cardiac surgery, another to children with neurosurgical conditions. It followed later, given the familiarity of the Ward 9 nursing staff with the post-operative care required by surgical patients over a range of specialties, that some of the nurses and the equipment would be transferred to the ICU at the new Hospital. Miss Jaffray, from her position in Ward 9, was appointed to be the Nursing Supervisor of the proposed ICU/RR.

Children with laryngotracheal bronchitis (croup), some with tracheostomy in place, were nursed in steam tents in Ward 16. Diphtheria, although rare, occasionally presented at Casualty but, if the condition was not urgent and breathing adequate, was usually transferred to Fairfield Hospital.[7]

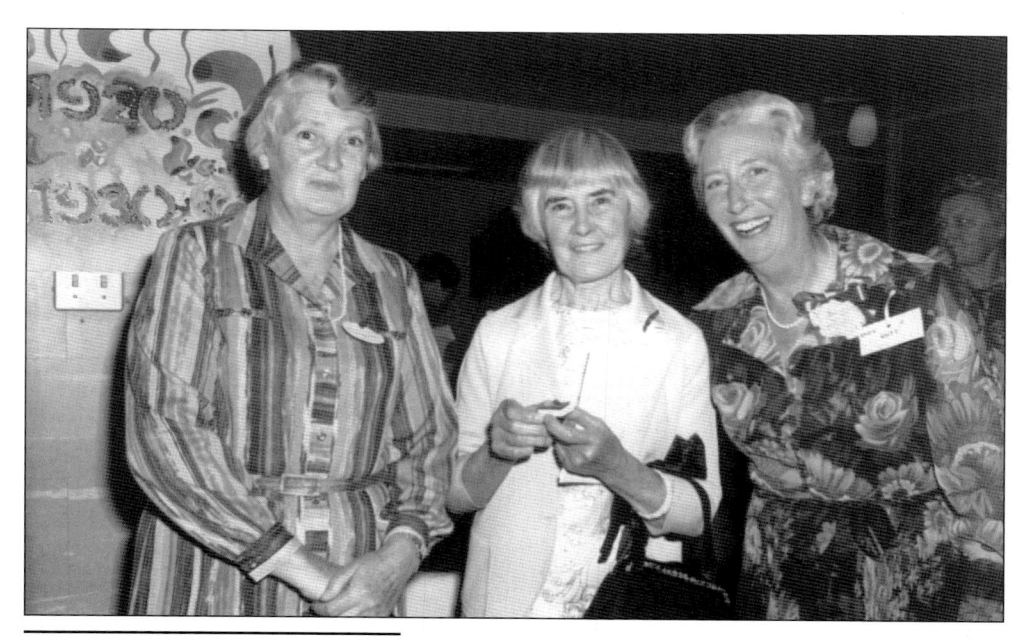

Re-union: Former RCH Theatre Sisters Noreen McKay, Dorothy Saunders and Judith, Lady Court. Centenary dinner 1970.
Dr Kester Brown Collection.

Tracheostomy was far from ideal and problems could occur. The patient could develop respiratory obstruction to the extent that the tube had to be replaced. This was a retained tracheostomy. Surgeons were careful not to remove any cartilage at operation; but the cartilage was often softened from the initial operative damage and sometimes collapsed when the tracheostomy tube was removed. There were still about thirty tracheostomies performed every year at the Children's in the 1950s, mainly for croup. During this decade two Registrars, Doctors Nate Myers and Ian Aberdeen, developed a tracheostomy tube at the Great Ormond Street Hospital in London that reduced the number of retained tracheostomies in their unit to one per cent.

In 1960, two years before the move to Parkville, the Sister-in-Charge of the theatre suite, Dorothy Saunders, observed world trends in hospital and theatre management on a study tour but did not see one intensive care unit. This was a new

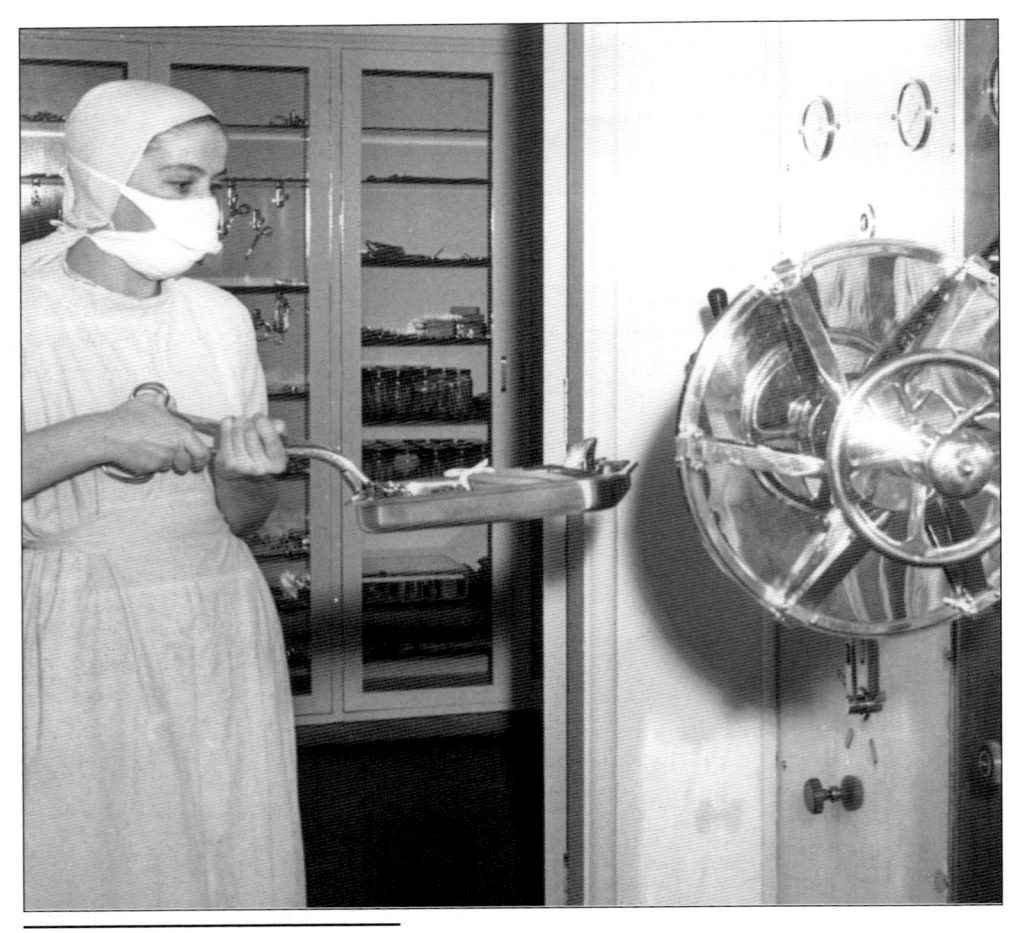

Old-style theatre autoclave, 1953.

McInnes Family Collection.

concept internationally, and in the time lag to the move to Parkville in 1963, dramatic developments in medicine and surgery occurred. Unfortunately, an ICU had not been included in the original planning and construction of what was becoming the RCH, Parkville.

Almost on the eve of the move to the new Hospital, Miss Jaffray spent ten days as an observer at the Sydney Children's Hospital. One thing impressed upon her by the Charge Sister of that hospital was that there must be 'no curtains' in an ICU for children. Visibility of patients was paramount at all times. As it happened, on her return, the move to the RCH Parkville now having taken place, she walked into the empty ICU to find workmen installing curtain rails. She said, 'some high-level representation was required, but the rails came down'.[8]

As moving day to Parkville approached, an ICU was considered close to the operating theatres that could accommodate patients after major thoracic, cardiac and neurosurgery. It was believed that those children presenting in Casualty (now Emergency) with severe head injuries, could appropriately be admitted to a unit that was adjacent to the operating theatres. Therefore, one half of the Recovery Room would be allocated to the future ICU, which at the time was visualised as being a Surgical ICU.

Setting up the ICU

During the outfit and set-up of the ICU in the few days following the move to Parkville, all but emergency surgery was suspended. The new unit proved to be small and makeshift: there were just six beds—often squeezed into eight for surgical cases. ICU and RR shared staff. The unit was in the charge of the Department of Anaesthesia under the direction of Dr Margaret McClelland, assisted by Dr John Stocks.

Such cramped space was far from ideal but at least it allowed the Sister to see what was going on, to keep an eye on the patients. However, this was offset by safety considerations, poor infection control and working conditions. Before overhead heaters were introduced, babies were nursed crosswise on cots, fully dressed, on an electric blanket to maintain an ideal temperature. Piped oxygen was available but had to be mixed with air which was not piped in.

The work of intubation began in Melbourne in late 1963, when the anaesthetist, Dr Ian McDonald, used endotracheal tubes in the post-operative management of two patients. One, a neonate with intrathoracic extension of a cystic hygroma, was returned to the ward with an endotracheal tube in place, but subsequently died.

By 1965, fifty children were successfully treated for over twenty-four hours. The range of patients at Melbourne Children's grew in the 1960s: cardiac, thoracic surgery in children with head injuries, breathing difficulties, epiglottitis and, in 1967, the first baby with tracheo-oesophageal fistula.

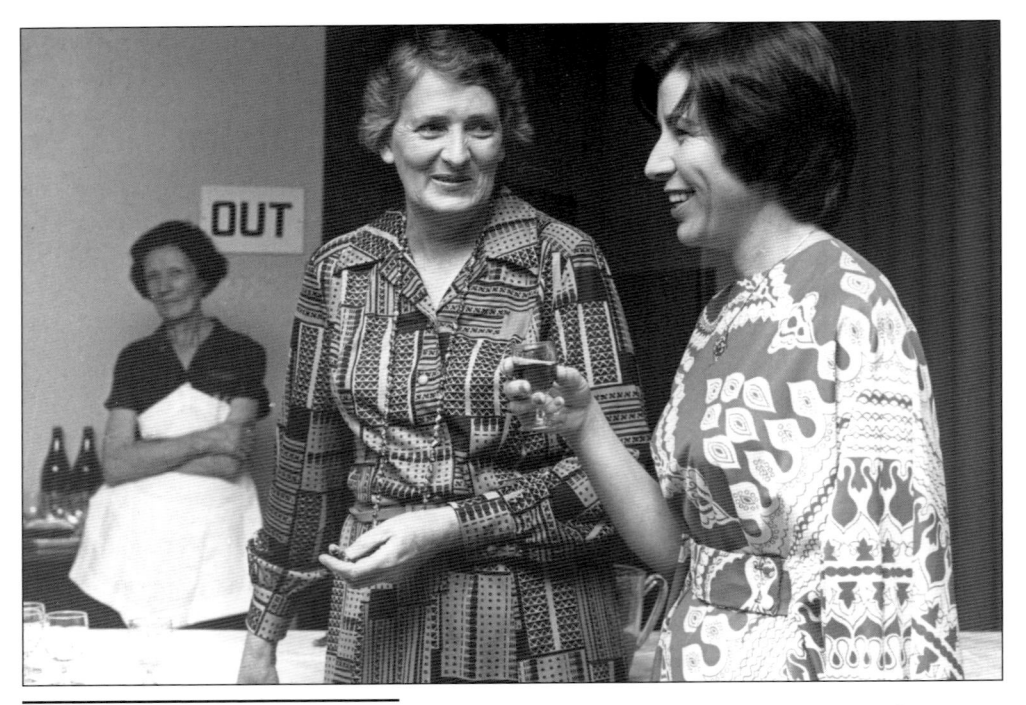

Doris Flett, PhD (Neuroscience, ANU), Melbourne School of Nursing and Associated Schools of Nursing 1956–59. Supervisory Sister, RCH ICU 1974–82. Shown here on the right with Noreen McKay (theatre) reminiscing, 1970.
Dr Kester Brown Collection.

Work in the ICU

In February 1964, Doris Flett, an experienced emergency theatre nurse, was asked to work as Charge Sister in ICU. She had trained at the Royal Melbourne Hospital and Associated Schools of Nursing (Melbourne School of Nursing) from 1956 to 1959, completing three months' training in each of two other participating hospitals, Fairfield and the Royal Children's. After staffing at the Royal Melbourne in the operating suite and in the wards with several years in Casualty theatres, she was appointed Charge Sister of the Professorial Unit Ward for two years at that Hospital. She returned to the Children's following midwifery training and was immediately asked to work as the Charge Sister in ICU. She succeeded Miss Jaffray as Supervisory Sister of that unit in 1974.

On Doris Flett's first day, the RR was in full operation and there were several patients in ICU.

Sister Jaffray, of course, was on duty, as were two staff nurses—in their yellow uniforms and white veils. One of these was Nan Oliver, who later became a Senior Sister in the unit.

A cardiac patient was received from theatre after bypass surgery, to be nursed in a Melco Oxygen Tent. A large machine stood at the foot of the bed and circulated air and oxygen through a large plastic tent that was tucked into the sides and top of the mattress. The patient, conscious and of good colour, was attached to the Electrodyne ECG machine. Venous pressure was also recorded and blood balance charts kept, in addition to the usual fluid balance charts. The patient was over five years old, because at that time the available equipment did not allow younger patients with cardiac anomalies to be brought to bypass surgery.[9]

Doris was unfamiliar with the commodious, humming Melco machine and the child seemed lost in the tent to her eyes and ears; she felt rather uneasy about this, telling her flatmate that evening that she could not see the patient for the machinery. She discovered that her feeling was not unusual for first-timers entering the unit.

The introduction of nasotracheal intubation

Within a few days, and from the far desk where she was discussing something with Miss Jaffray, Doris saw Dr John Stocks (then Assistant Director of Anaesthesia) bring an isolette in from the theatre, quietly park and stand alongside it. When she went across she saw a post-operative baby with a plastic nasotracheal tube in place and, without being quite aware at the time, began to understand the technique of long-term endotracheal intubation and its potential as an artificial airway, that is—if it could be managed successfully. 'And this', she said, 'turned out to be the crucial issue'.

Up to that time and beyond, patients with a severe airways problem such as potentially life-threatening laryngotracheal bronchitis or epiglottitis were subjected to tracheostomy. At the Children's, a group of doctors experienced with that operation in children and its subsequent management maintained a 24-hour on-call roster and the children were operated on if necessary in ICU. Because the unit was so small, the babies were returned to be nursed in Ward 9 East where Sister Eileen Morton was second-in-charge to Sister Lois Murray. The responsibility for these children was considerable, as they were nursed in oxygen tents with a humidifier. Antibiotics were given, extra care taken to keep the tracheotomy tube clean and the tapes in place. Eileen recalled the parents were very frightened and needed reassurance. It was usual that these small babies were graded out of oxygen and on to normal feedings within a day or two.[10]

The ICU really got under way when nasotracheal intubation was introduced to maintain the airway to assist these breathing problems. One of the things that made this possible was the use of plastic tubing that softened to body temperature and moulded in place to the shape of the patient's own warm airway—the more rigid anaesthetic tubes were quite unsuitable. Much of the specialised stock came from overseas and the nurses quickly learned to keep extras on hand in case of a shipping strike.

The patients remained under the care of the referring consultant/specialist with Dr John Stocks to determine the best way of dealing with the management of intubated patients.

Among the worrying details were: how to strap an endotracheal tube securely to the face of the baby or child and even what type of strapping it was best to use. At one point, it seemed possible that the whole procedure would have to be abandoned with neonates altogether, because the strapping excoriated their skin. In one case, the nurses were relieved and pleased when it was found that the skin could be protected by first painting it with compound tincture of benzoin (Friars' balsam). It was a small but important win.[11]

A story of a child told by Doris Flett indicates why this was so important. A neonate had oesophageal atresia and tracheo-oesophageal fistula, a split larynx and hemi-vertebrae when first admitted to ICU in 1967. The initial operation was successful but the repair of the oesophagus had to be delayed until the baby had grown a little. During this period she was nursed in a sitting position, with a nasotracheal tube *in situ*, the position and the tube being necessary to protect her airway from the excessive pharyngeal secretions that frothed and bubbled out of her nose and mouth. Constant suctioning of the tube, nasopharynx and pharynx was required. The strapping holding the endotracheal tube in place was constantly moist, the tube would loosen and had to be re-strapped, causing a constant problem for her delicate skin. Keeping her environment happy and secure was difficult in these circumstances, and could be a very exhausting experience for her bedside nurse.

Heather Telfer knew this baby well. The surgeons looking after her were from Ward 5 West where Heather was the nursing supervisor and she often visited ICU. After nasotracheal intubation for seven months, the baby had her oesophagus repaired and subsequently, the ETT (endotracheal tube) removed. She was transferred to Ward 5 West instead of the Neonatal Ward only because Heather knew her.

The respiratory care of individual patients, oxygen and humidity, were determined by Dr Stocks while the nurses then learned the basic concepts and techniques. Most important was the prevention of blockage of the tube. Another potential hazard was that a sub-glottic stenosis could be caused if the tube fitted too tightly into the patient's airway. The trick was to select a tube slightly smaller in diameter than the patient needed (judging from their age and/or size). The doctor intubating would listen for an air leak when ventilating a patient by hand bag. The trained nurse in charge of the shift would also carry out this check after new intubations and, from time to time, there would be an insistence that 'the tube was too tight and should be changed'.[12]

It was not long before Dr Stocks was driven by necessity to intubate and ventilate as well. Initially, some small pieces of equipment were not always readily available and many a time staff hunted around for bits and pieces among anaesthetic equipment. In 1964, an adult Bird respirator was in use. The Bennett PR2 ventilators with modified breathing circuits were introduced in 1966. The use of the muscle relaxant, curare, allowed more effective, mechanical ventilation.

In former days when the patient went back to the ward, as has been noted, the outcome was poor. It was thought by many medical people that intubation could not be used with children because it would be too difficult to obtain the right sort of tubes and children would tear them out at the first opportunity. As the staff became more adept at management, cases gradually began to be referred from other parts of the Hospital. The unit became crowded very quickly.

In 1965, Drs Ian MacDonald and John Stocks praised the work of Elizabeth Jaffray and her staff in the ICU whose attentive care made the procedure possible.[13]

Doris Flett noted that it was not just the putting in of the tube; that was only the beginning: the nurses had to look after the care of the child and the tube. They had to manage it.[14] Thereafter, about 400 children were admitted a year.

Patients in older age groups were intubated for many reasons, neurosurgical and cardiac, meningitis and, in 1964, a toddler and an older child required intubation after swallowing a poisonous substance. A boy was in need of urgent attention because he had an upper respiratory tract obstruction, the lower half of his face and his neck were grossly swollen with angioneurotic oedema and it was thought that he had been bitten by an insect.

Some children were nursed with an endotracheal tube *in situ* for varying lengths of time. Apart from caring for the patients as their needs arose and as their medical and surgical condition demanded, the ICU staff was occupied in working alongside Dr Stocks to determine the best way of dealing with the management of prolonged intubation.

Nurses became attached to the children who stayed a long time. Doris Flett 'specialled' a child who was admitted at six weeks old. Born with haemangioma of the larynx, she was, to her, the dearest little baby who found it difficult to breathe. The family lived outside the metropolitan area but her mother visited often with the baby's siblings who played quietly in the room as the staff endeavoured to make the ward as homelike and normal as possible. Her first birthday was celebrated in the Doctor's office with a party—a big milestone.

The ICU had excellent ward assistants, or 'Pinkies'. These women worked until quite late in the evening, and took great care to avoid cross-infection by ensuring the clean operation of the unit and the ventilators.

By 1967 there was serious overcrowding in the ICU, and medical staff reported an urgent need for improvement and development of the Neonatal Service. A deep concern was expressed about the serious actual dangers of cross-infection. Intensive Care became an autonomous unit in 1974 and a sixteen-bed unit opened, utilising the areas of Ward 2 East, the Plastics Theatre and a portion of the Central Sterilising Department (CSD).

Changes since 1969

In the very early days blood for transfusions came in bottles and the amount given was measured by a tape on the side of the bottle. When bags came into being, the blood bag was hung on a spring and the weight of the blood infused was recorded. Previously IV drips were recorded as macro drops per minute, then progress was made to micro and next to infusion pumps.

There was very little disposable equipment—in the 1950s and early 1960s, needles and syringes were autoclaved, as were rubber endotracheal tubes, rubber urinary catheters and rubber chest drains. Arterial lines, when initially left in place for monitoring purposes, had to be syringed every fifteen minutes.

Louise Blewett returned to the RCH in 1969 to work in Surgery. However, she was immediately posted in the Paediatric Intensive Care Unit (PICU). She held the position of Charge Sister from 1974 until 1984.[15]

Louise and Lucy Cuddihy described those early days: the long-term ventilation of neonates required that they devise a system to keep the infants warm yet have them accessible. 'We nursed them across a cot lying in a nest, the lowest layer being an electric blanket, their body enclosed in a Perspex headbox (bodybox) and an overhead "Terry" light shining on to the Perspex for added warmth.'

In the very early days of the unit there were no technicians. One of the procedures to be mastered initially in ICU was to take to bits and re-assemble a 'Bird' ventilator. There was some improvisation; theatre technicians became the nurses' help mates while bio-med engineering helped design and modify equipment. Theatre technicians originally under the nursing administration eventually moved into the Department of Anaesthesia with Dr Kester Brown.

Changing patterns of illness

The annual numbers of children admitted to the ICU grew rapidly from 1980 to reach 1,605 in 1992, after which they began to decline.[16] The lowering of the incidence of meningitis, the control of epiglottitis with introduction of the Hib vaccine, the fewer numbers of children injured in car accidents and the opening of the Neonatal Intensive Care Unit contributed to diminishing numbers in the 1990s. Nevertheless this has been offset with a different pattern of patients treated, for example, transplants and other major surgery. There have been hundreds of children who otherwise would not have survived.

The nursing trainees generally felt that the ICU staff held key roles in the Hospital. They relied on them totally for guidance and as mentors, as they seemed to be crucial to the whole drama of medical breakthrough.

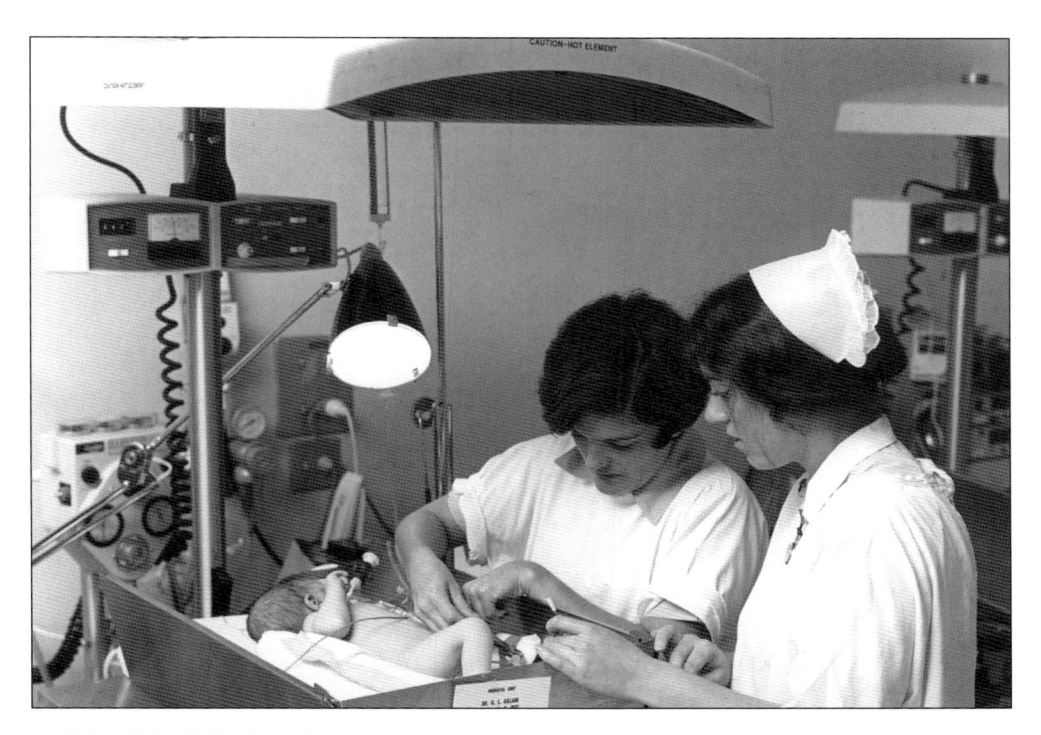

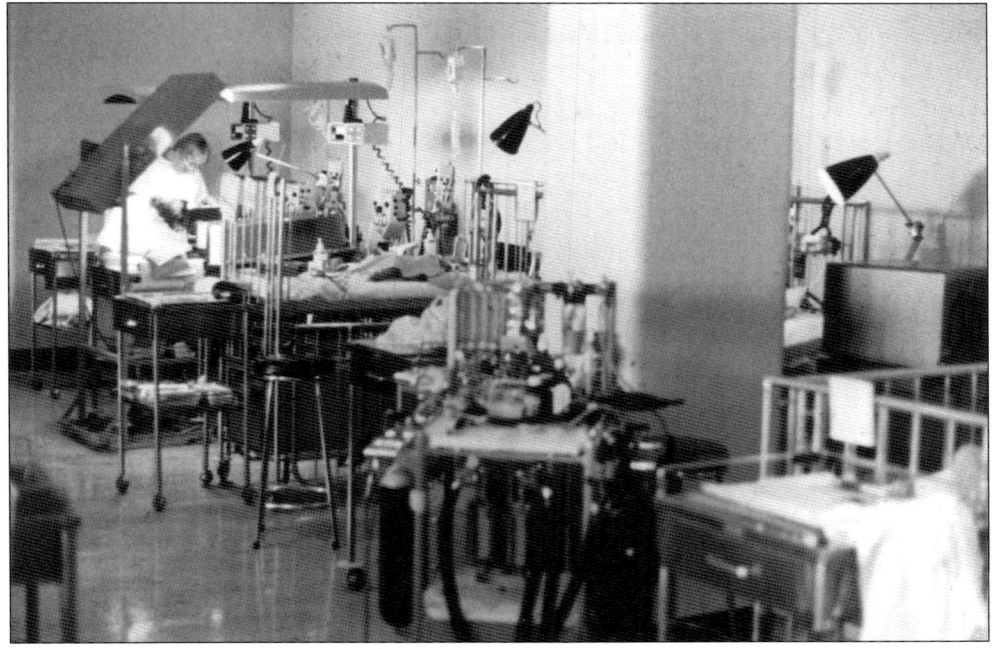

Top: Ohio overhead heater in the Recovery Room. Third-year nurse receiving instructions from Louise Blewett.
Bottom: Theatre Recovery Room, c. 1975.

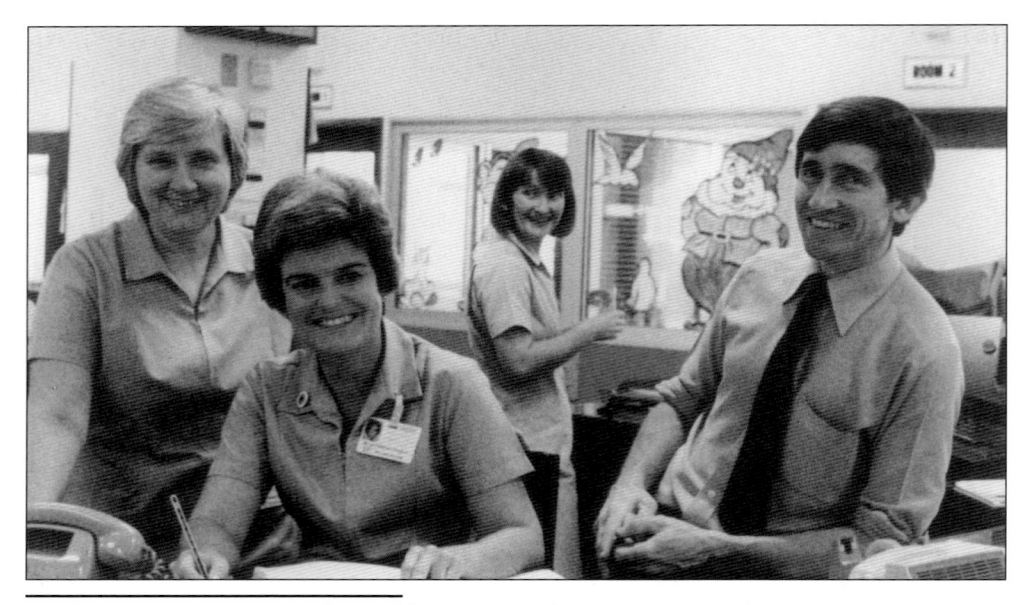

Intensive Care Unit: Heather Telfer, Louise Blewett, Lucy Cuddihy and Dr Jim Tibbals, 1970s. Heather Telfer—(RCH 1948–52) B. Ed. (La Trobe), Dip. Nursing Education, CNA, Chairman's Medal 1987—was in the clinical teaching area of Intensive Care for about eleven years. Louise Blewett—(RCH 1963–66) Charge Sister PICU 1973–84, Chairman's Medal 2003—spent many years there too.

Clinical nurse teaching

A great deal of effort was needed to train the staff as the number in the unit grew quickly: 457 children in 1964 but 836 in 1972. Initially, the Staff Nurses were rostered to the unit for six weeks and worked in either ICU or RR, according to need. First and second-year nurses were rostered to ICU for three or four weeks.

In 1975, Doris Flett and Heather Telfer combined their knowledge of the management and education needed to function effectively in this setting and developed the first paediatric intensive care nursing course to be conducted in Australia. In the beginning the focus was very much on the intensive nursing skills and a group of experienced nurses experimented with the course content.

In the 1970s there had been growing concern amongst nursing staff that the introduction of the general nursing curriculum in 1976, followed by the phasing out of that programme in 1987, would lead to a decline in paediatric nursing knowledge and skills. The provision of post-registration programmes, paediatric nursing and paediatric intensive care nursing in the 1970s was very new. They were seen as progressive and advancing the standards of nursing practice and education. The apprenticeship arrangements existing then were purely practical in nature but still thought to be best learnt on the job. The arrangement that existed for the basic programme eventually shaped post-registration education and the way nurses worked.

A graduate nurse year and orientation to paediatrics course was commenced in 1986 and became a twelve-month programme in 1989 with an intake of forty to fifty students per year. In 1987, the paediatric nursing course was changed from six months to twelve months so that the curriculum could be broadened to take account of the growing emphasis on the normal needs of the child and family and changes in the cultural backgrounds of the patients. Clinical Nurse Educators were appointed to most clinical areas of the Hospital under the leadership of Heather Telfer, who played a major role in the transition from the student workforce to a registered nurse workforce.

Paediatric and adult accident and emergency course

A paediatric and adult accident and emergency nursing course was eventually established in July 1986, with both the Austin and the Alfred Hospitals collaborating with the RCH during the five years it was conducted. The course recognised that children presented to many Accident and Emergency Departments around the State but that few of these employed nurses who had the necessary paediatric skills. It was successful, but funding difficulties ended it in January 1992.

Working with parents and children in ICU

Very often a parent would ask to bring in another member of the family. The parents could sit in a small waiting room between visits if they wished, an essential facility obtained by dint of Miss Jaffray's having the end of the passage blocked off. In this room, staff members spoke with the parents of newly admitted children, recently operated-on children, critcally ill children and with the parents of a child who had died. The parents accepted this facility without a comment. Their distress was such that the focus was on their child.

Parents were often outside ICU when so much was going on inside. In the end, the clinical staff was instrumental in finding a place where parents could sit. They saw the parents in the extreme stages of fear, chronic anxiety, isolation and loneliness. The nurses had to work out how they could alleviate or lessen these fears.

Assisting nurses in their interaction with parents was done very much on role modelling. The trained nurses took students with them at the point of direct contact, talking to people, making sure at any point of the child's treatment that parents were involved within reasonable limits. During a crisis, obviously there was no physical room for them to be included.

When any child enters an institution such as a hospital there are many considerations and children can be very frightened. Before older children go to theatre, the

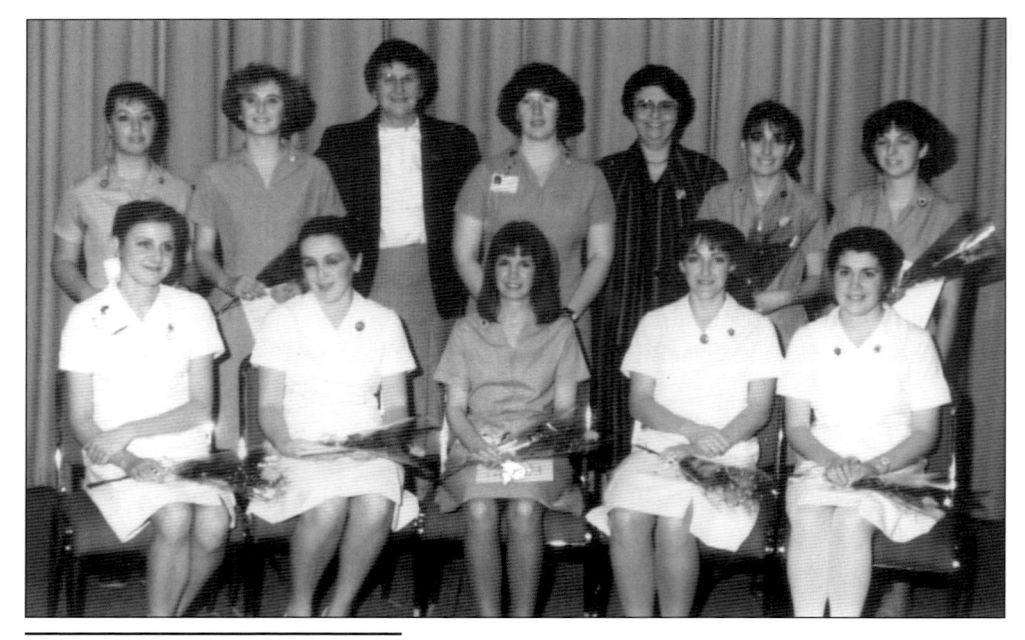

Graduation of the first combined hospitals, Accident and Emergency Course at the Austin Hospital. *Back:* third from the left: Miss Rae Anstee (RCH 1957–61), Assistant Director of Nursing (RCH 1970–77), Director of Nursing at the Austin Hospital (1977–95). Miss Mary Patten third from the right, Director of Nursing at the RCH (1982–95).

procedure can be explained to them just enough to gain confidence in the presence of the parent, to allay most of the anxiety. Nurses must fine tune their knowledge of the stages of development in babies and young children and anticipate the result of separation from the mother. The parent also needs to know what is happening, to have fears allayed when the child becomes anaesthetised, when there are complex procedures, and to be alerted to the expected outcome. The anaesthetist is very involved at this stage.

The four nurses committed to these values, Elizabeth Jaffray, Heather Telfer, Doris Flett and Louise Blewett, had practical concern for the children and parents, and commitment to bedside teaching and formal education for nurses. The unit grew with this very caring group of people and gained a huge reputation. However, to other staff within the Hospital, it was something of an elite group.

The new Intensive Care Unit opened in 1978 with sixteen beds and was later extended to twenty-four. Today, a PETS (Paediatric Emergency Transport Service) retrieval service established in 1978 brings seriously ill children to the Hospital accompanied by an ICU doctor and nurses.

Neonatology

Neonatal nursing began in Ward 14, a General Ward for babies at the old Carlton Children's Hospital. In the 1950s, it was likely a baby with haemolytic disease of the newborn, erythroblastosis, would arrive severely jaundiced and die a few hours later. The father would quietly come in the night to see his perfect, beautiful newborn child laid out with a ruffled gauze shroud in the wire bassinet, a tiny flower placed in the hands by the nurse. At night, this was a cheerless little premature babies' room overlooking Drummond Street, so far away yet so near to the Women's Hospital where a mother lay grieving for the baby she would never see.

The first exchange transfusion was carried out by Dr Elizabeth Turner in that little room in 1954 under the watchful eyes of Sister Kate Hardham. The outlook for these babies was much improved by the 1970s.

Originally at Parkville, half of Ward 4 West was devoted to neonates, with responsibility rotated among the medical units and a junior consultant running the ward. In 1971, part of the tenth floor was refurbished to become the Neonatal Ward to care for thirty-nine babies, though sometimes up to fifty, where Doris Milliken became the Supervisory Sister. Blessed with a phenomenal memory for patients and their conditions, Sister Milliken maintained contact with her patients for years after. She was even invited to one patient's wedding.

Unfortunately, Ward 10 West was planned before future needs were recognised. By 1976, 550 neonates were admitted compared to 150 at the Queen Victoria, eighty at the Royal Women's Hospital, and forty at the Mercy Women's Hospital. The ward rapidly became a conglomeration of equipment; staff members were practically tripping over each other and there was a danger not only of overcrowding but of cross-infection. The ward had effectively become another ICU.

The Neonatal Emergency Transport Services (NETS) provides continuing treatment during transport from outlying obstetrical hospitals. The RCH Unit is one of four tertiary units in the State of Victoria. The department treats babies from Tasmania, southern New South Wales, and country and regional Victoria.

In 1982, 600 babies were treated from Victoria and Tasmania with congenital malformations, birth asphyxia, low birth weight, convulsions and jaundice. About 13–15 per cent died, causing stress among the staff. A separate unit south of the ICU was established for neonates in the late 1980s. Sister Geraldine McDonnell was the supervisory nurse where about 750 babies were admitted per year. Dr Neil Campbell believed the unit had

---

Doris Milliken, 1993.

to be near the operation theatres and, in 1990, his wish was granted. Geraldine McDonnell became Supervisory Sister in the Neonatal ICU on the second floor. This unit pioneered work in the use of high-frequency oscillatory ventilation in Australia. The technique allows optimal lung volumes by applying continuous distending pressure while a rapid oscillatory wave facilitates the elimination of carbon dioxide. The method, introduced in the 1990s, followed the training of staff—including nurses—in animal laboratories.

With modern advances in treatment, the nurses and doctors are forced to face ethical dilemmas almost on a daily basis. Sometimes babies born with severe disabilities who otherwise may have died, were kept alive. There is always wide consultation. The issue came to a head in 1989 with the 'Baby M case' and the threat of charges of manslaughter when the life of a severely disabled child was not artificially maintained. The protocols of the Hospital and the Department of Neonatology were upheld by the Coroner's Court.[17]

Operating theatres

Anne Bryan began nursing in 1967 when Dorothy Saunders was still in charge of theatres. When Anne finished her training and married in 1971, married women were not welcome back on the staff and she spent some time working in Croydon Child Care. That was not very satisfying but some time in the mid-1970s, she was invited back to nursing. There had to be many compromises, particularly for those staff with children who needed consideration.

> DOROTHY SAUNDERS Trained RCH 1928–32, Midwifery Cert. 1933, Theatre Supervisor 1934–72, one of the longest serving nurses at the Royal Children's Hospital—thirty-eight years.
>
> When Parkville Hospital opened in 1963, Dorothy took charge of six operating theatres and fifty staff. To many, she was a reserved, private person appearing to have few interests outside theatre work. In fact, she had a great interest in music, which she introduced into the operating theatres.[18]

Following the birth of her daughter, Anne was able to negotiate with theatre management to work at weekends. Shirley Dunne was Nurse-in-Charge. Cliff Buchanan, who was assistant to Elaine Orr, the Director of Nursing, gave Anne her first job in theatre and she has stayed ever since.

There have been many changes in nurse training and protocols in theatre. One of the most significant developments mentioned by nurses with many years experience has been in pain prevention and control. Other notable developments include greater accessibility for parents, who are able to see their children into the theatre and be there when they wake up, and the additional care and attention given to the needs of non-English speaking parents and children.

In the 1960s, junior nurses spent minimal time in theatre because there were so many trainees. As a requirement to fulfil the curriculum, nurses needed to spend at least some time scouting and scrubbing for small cases that were well supervised by the senior staff. But there is doubt about how much they actually learnt.

On weekends, the juniors scrubbed the surgeons' shoes (they wore white runners), washed down the walls and trolleys in theatre and generally did the housework. Folding of towels and other linen was a big part of the day.[19] In the late 1970s and as a student, Judith Smith remembers being in the Central Sterilising Supply Department (CSSD) packing endless white paper bags with cotton balls and gauze—five to a pack—as well as doing tray packs.[20]

At Carlton, nurses carried from the wards heavy bins packed with towels, dressings and other necessary theatre linen. They took them to the theatre autoclave room, placing them in the autoclave along with the trays of instruments. Cheatles forceps were used to lift towels, gowns and sheets. Autoclaving (flashing) is considered unwise today. The trays are pre-set and sterilised in the CSSD department, no longer on open shelves where surgeons chose their instruments. Australian standards (AS4197) rule the theatre nurses' lives.

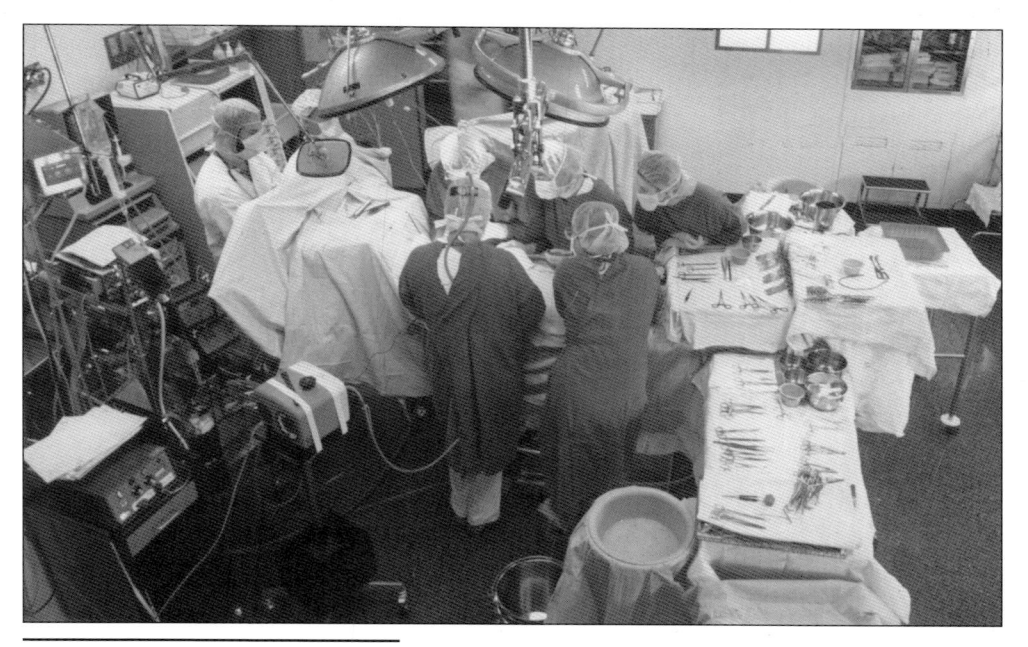

Cardiac theatre, c. 1987–89. Taken from the viewing room above. Surgeon Roger Mee and May Chan, the Theatre Nurse, in attendance.

In the 1960s, juniors were permitted to scrub for tonsillectomies and herniotomies and, if they were very proficient, towards the end of the time allocated, they might assist with an appendicectomy. Nowadays an appendicectomy is one of the first 'scrubs' done by the graduate nurses. Non-nursing duties came into being and theatre assistants took over most of the cleaning duties, attracting a 'nauseous linen' allowance payment. Anne said: 'We [the nurses] never thought of that, I guess!'

Formerly, children were collected from the ward by a theatre assistant, on a trolley big enough for an adult. Well pre-medicated, they arrived in the corridor of the theatre area where Noreen McKay kept a watchful eye. Parents were not present. The Recovery Room was a small area, half of which was Intensive Care in the early 1970s. Nursing staff rotated in both Theatre and Recovery. Six theatres faced onto a large set-up area with open shelves and instruments.

Nowadays, children come to the pre-operation 'hold', a purpose-built area equipped with TV, video, games and toys. The parents, and sometimes brothers and sisters, nearly always accompany the child. Parents go with the child into the anaesthetic room and may even hold their child on their knee. The use of Angel Cream, a local anaesthetic cream on a small patch on the back of the hand, facilitates a vein some time before operation and, when the induction occurs, the child is free of anxiety and pain. The child is told that their mother will be there when they wake up. Meanwhile, the parents are escorted to the waiting area. As soon as their child is awake, they are called to the Recovery Room. There are also volunteers to assist if parents are not available.

The nurses believe the unit is recognised for its expertise in major surgery and transplants. Minimal surgery, involving laser and keyhole surgery, requires different technology for which the nurses have now successfully adapted with help from clinical educators/supervisors.

Over the years, several nurses have given much of their life to theatre work: Hilda Jergamanis and Elaine Salter (both retired in 1994), Shirley Dunne, Noreen Mackay and Jo Van Valen. Nurses have much more say now that there is a career structure. Claire Collins noticed many changes since she started in 1972 arriving from an adult hospital in Adelaide. While the culture then was generally quite relaxed, with people addressing each other by their first names, nurses were still subservient in theatre, standing with their hands behind their backs. Siok Chew was in the theatres during the Barry Catchlove era, the 1980s and 1990s, and found him most supportive of intensive care and cardiac surgery. She believes 'he was an agent of change who forced the Hospital to modernise'.[21]

Since the 1950s the theatres have attracted male nurses too: Kevin Curtis, who became the cardiac heart–lung machine nurse technician assisting Dr Kester Brown, and John Tonzing and Paul Kelly. In 1977, John became the Sister-in-Charge of the Ear, Nose and Throat Theatre, challenging, for the first time, the notion of the title of 'Sister', the last vestige in the hierarchical system of nursing.

Day Surgery

There are now six general theatres, two cardiac theatres, one radiology theatre, and two procedure rooms in a purpose-built Day Centre. Day Surgery was introduced in 1977, in Ward 4 East, by Sister Elizabeth Fearon who was described as an inspiration for her calm, reassuring and gentle manner. She was also very firm in the management of the unit, ensuring that anaesthetists visited every child some time prior to the actual surgery. A film was developed in conjunction with Dr Kester Brown to explain to parent and child every step of the event. There is special attention as well to the developmental age of children and their needs.

This facility provided an easy transition for children having day procedures. Kim Lee took the position when Elizabeth retired and today Paula Howard runs the Day Surgery Unit.

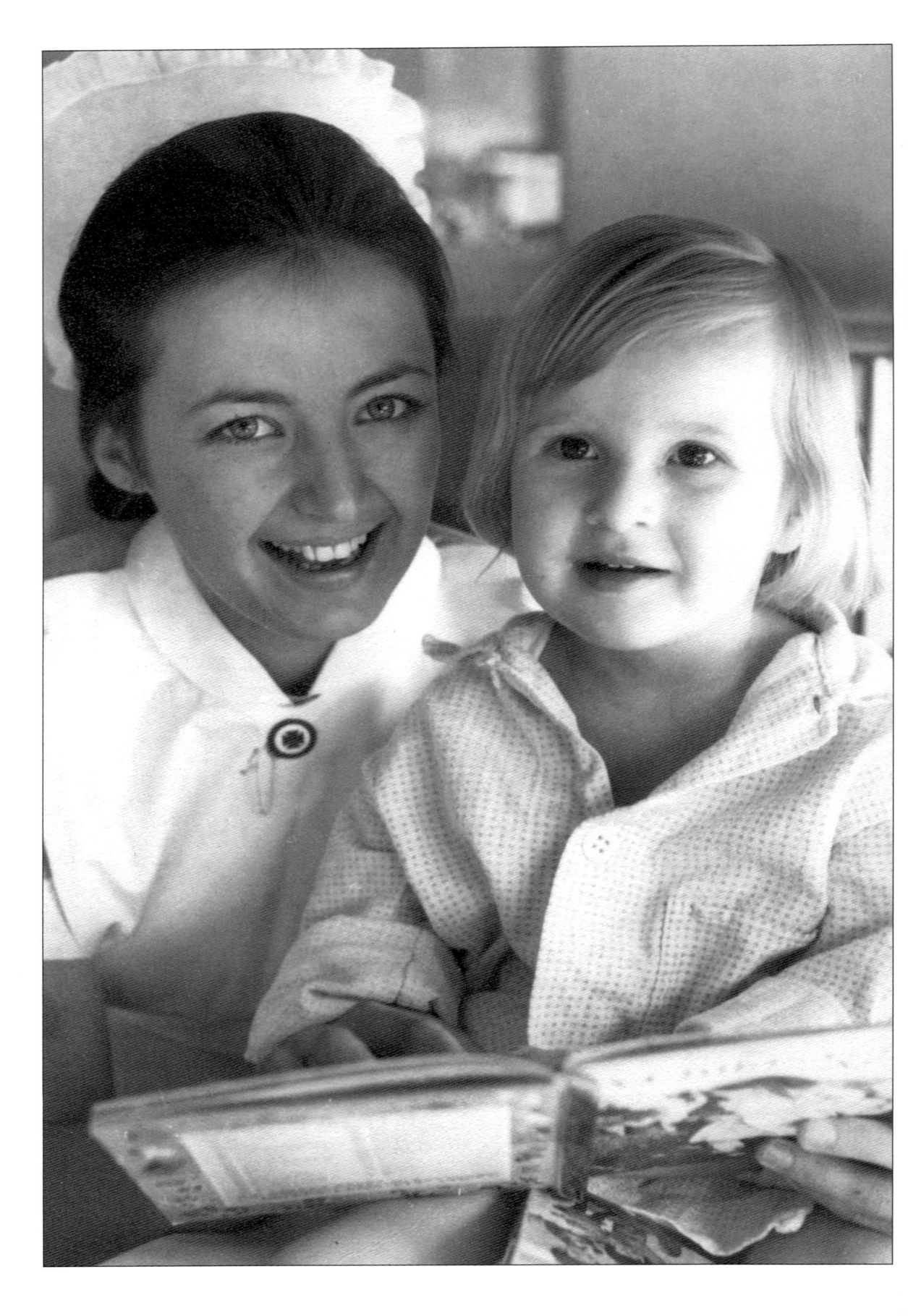

CHAPTER 13

Transition to Tertiary Education
1970–1987

The 1970s to the 1980s were years of reform in nursing. Despite a general shortage of nurses throughout Victoria, eligibility for entry to the Royal Children's Hospital Nursing School became more complex under the Director of Nursing, Elaine Orr. Academic excellence was encouraged, vocational and psychological aptitude tests became mandatory.

Anne Hardham (née Coventry) was representative of the transition between the old hierarchical apprenticeship system and the tertiary educated, modern nurse. From the top grade of her school, a junior nursing scholarship, a nursing bursary and dux for two years, Anne had Matriculation scores necessary to enter the Preliminary Training School (PTS) on 27 January 1970. She had always set her sights on nursing and loved the Nightingale legend. Her role model was her mother, Jennie Coventry (née Armstrong), who trained at the Children's Hospital in Carlton from 1944 to 1947, and successfully combined a career in nursing with family life. Anne's experiences were to be, in many respects, very different to those of her mother.

Anne commenced training at the Royal Children's Hospital four weeks after leaving school at the age of seventeen and was required to undertake a series of tests:

Robyn McLaren on her graduation day with her patient, 1969.
Robyn graduated top of the State in her finals and was awarded the A. Jeffreys Wood Gold Medal (1969) and the Nell Chrisfield Prize for 1970.
Herald Sun, 1969.

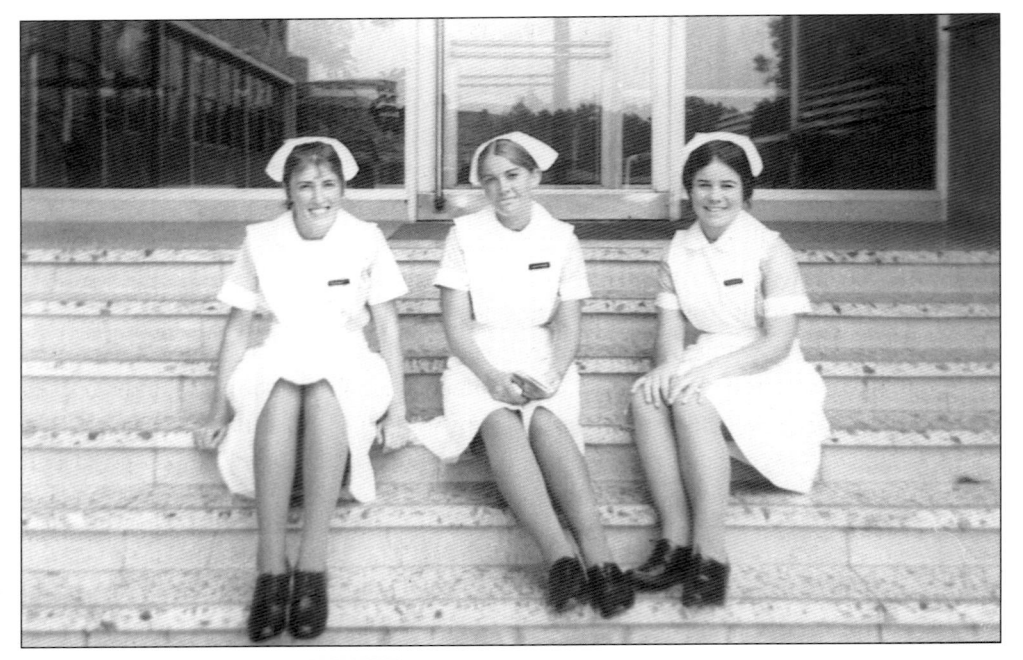

First day, Preliminary Training School. On the steps of the Nurses' Home, 1970.
L–R: Helene Bond, Anne Fischer and Anne Hardham (née Coventry).
Anne Hardham graduated top of the State in her final examination in 1973 and top of the State in midwifery in 1976.
Hardham Family Collection.

an IQ in logic, mathematical problem solving and psychological competency. Matriculation was simply not enough.[1] Miss Orr constructed the tests and personally conducted all the interviews. She believed that medical advances required nurses to have a higher general standard of education to be better equipped to take their rightful place in the hospital team of the future; and that repetitive and domestic duties had to be eliminated so that the nurses could be educated to give maximum patient care. She said: 'When medical staff is assessed, the Committee of Management look at qualifications and experience, so why shouldn't they do the same for nurses? Look at the spread of nurses' experience.'[2] She pointed out that the two top jobs, DON (Director of Nursing) and Deputy, as well as the teaching jobs, had usually gone to outside people. There had been some excellent nurse teachers but, again, they had been totally paediatric orientated: 'While this hospital is a general training school of nursing, you have got to have a far wider spread of experience to rise to the top jobs in the field of nursing.'

Miss Orr was appalled at the high wastage of nursing students. Theories for explanations abounded: higher education and higher expectations appeared to lead to greater wastage. She believed 'a real problem of recruitment of students was the concept of sick children strengthened by the Good Friday Appeal that attracted the gentle, overprotected, non-academic, immature, and the "doubtful" about adult nursing, especially men'. The reality of a paediatrics teaching hospital sent many students into shock. In Miss Orr's view, parents were often to blame: the RCH had an image as socially elite, and nursing children was regarded as 'sweet'.

The problem of reciprocity of registration with other countries had never been resolved. Career-oriented paediatric nurses were required to receive at least one additional year of adult nursing before travelling overseas and many transferred over to general training during their paediatric training. From almost every PTS, at least one trainee transferred to the Alfred Hospital. Miss Orr's theories extended to changes in family structure: students came from smaller families and were unused, or never exposed, to sickness, death and dying. Traditionally, the sick and injured and aged relatives were cared for in the family; now that many more women were in the workforce, they were cared for in institutions. Hence, young women received a reality shock. To weed out the unsuitable candidates, she introduced the aptitude test.

ELAINE PHILLIPA ORR, OAM, RN, RM, Infant Welfare Certificate, Dip. Ward Management, FRACN. Director of Nursing, RCH 1969–82.[3]

Elaine Orr, the eighth Director of Nursing at the Royal Children's Hospital was a woman of brilliant intellect with an ambition to study medicine. However, she left school in the early years of World War Two and joined the Australian Women's Army Service, attaining the rank of sergeant. She became secretary in the senior command headquarters in northern Australia and, at war's end, was offered a place in the Melbourne Medical School post-war rehabilitation scheme. She opted instead—for personal family reasons—to take up nursing.[4]

She trained at the Ballarat Base Hospital qualifying in 1949 with a string of prizes: General Nursing, Ear, Nose and Throat and Urology. Subsequently, she became Deputy, then Matron of Berry Street Foundling Home in East Melbourne and, in 1958, Deputy Matron at La Trobe Valley Hospital, Yallourn. Elaine pursued her first preference, paediatric nursing, at London's Great Ormond Street Hospital for Children, and on her return to Australia in the 1960s became

Matron at the RCH Orthopaedic Section at Mount Eliza. She held office on the Royal Australian Nursing Federation Council and on the Economic Welfare Committee, where she had enormous influence in achieving salary justice for nurses.

An example of Miss Orr's strength occurred when she was invited to apply for the DON position in 1969 by the Hospital Manager, Mr Dick Feint. She impressed him as someone able to withstand the influence of the deeply entrenched 'old guard' of medical and nursing staff. Miss Orr refused to apply, on the grounds that she wished to have access to the Committee of Management, not to the Medical Director.[5] The Matrons' Association in Melbourne, a powerful group, was well aware of the standoff, advised members not to apply, and virtually boycotted the position.

Eventually, the Hospital caved in and changed the constitutional by-law to accommodate her terms: she would have full access and direct accountability to the Committee of Management. This proved to be a long and successful alliance as changes to nurse education gathered pace in the 1970s and the President, Dame Patricia Mackinnon, became a strong advocate and advisor to Miss Orr on a daily basis.[6]

It was not all plain sailing for Elaine Orr. She encountered many difficulties, arising, she believed, from her denigration by long-serving RCH-trained Senior Sisters who had implied that she was not 'one of them'. This did not alter her determination and she handled the staff diplomatically. Mr Murray Clarke thought Elaine was quite the cleverest woman the Children's Hospital had ever employed.[7]

Miss Orr was clearly on top of the job. Although she suffered intermittently from ill health she did not allow this to interfere with her life and work. She was a gregarious, fun-loving raconteur and gracious hostess. Nevertheless, to first-year nurses initially, she was a remote figure in a big hospital, a little idiosyncratic. Senior nurses valued her presence and insight on ward rounds and, as the years went by, her personal strengths—intelligence, wit, compassion and care for children—became apparent.

Miss Orr had strong views and plenty to say about hospitals, doctors and the administration. She let it be known that she abhorred the impersonal attitude of surgeons engaged in clinical teaching around the bedside. During a stint as a patient herself in hospital she was appalled when her surgeon addressed her as 'the leg'. She was asked: 'How is the leg today?' Outraged, she refused to answer. Any doctor who crossed that impersonal line was likely to receive this treatment. She was quite aware they thought her loud, pushy and brash. Nevertheless, she said, 'it had to be, otherwise I had no voice'. In a memorable incident, she had a fight with Dr Jack Davies in her office at the Orthopaedic Hospital: 'his indecision drove me mad, he procrastinated, he was infuriating about organising the nurses' lectures'. When she threw the roll book at him she thought she had killed him. 'But', she said, 'after that it cleared the air and we actually got on quite well'.⁸

In the 1970s, many traditions and attitudes, the education of nurses, the hierarchical nature and industrial structures of nursing were questioned by sections of the community and thought to be grossly out-of-date. In Elaine Orr's opinion, the administration generally lacked appreciation of the problems in meshing service and education, and a powerful group within the Hospital was not qualified in that area. The curriculum was adult; paediatrics had a very small component (and, according to some, was not always accurate).⁹ During this period, almost all tutors and deputies were non-RCH trainees: Graham Whitbourne, Helen Preece and Cliff Buchanan. Mr Buchanan's appointment as Miss Orr's deputy in 1970, a break with tradition, was highly criticised by the doctors. He came to be accepted because of his attitude, personality and ability.

Miss Orr felt that the hospital was narrow in focus, inbred and lacking in specialist skills. The staff believed that a good paediatric nurse was one who trained at the Royal Children's Hospital and stayed there. She knew that people outside the Hospital would not often vote for Children's Hospital candidates on the various nursing committees because they considered themselves to be a bit apart from the mainstream. There was an element of truth in this, but nurses had not had the opportunities to broaden their horizons; there were limited opportunities for Children's Hospital nurses in Australia. Unless they were prepared to use their own funds for several months, or even years, postgraduate study eluded them.

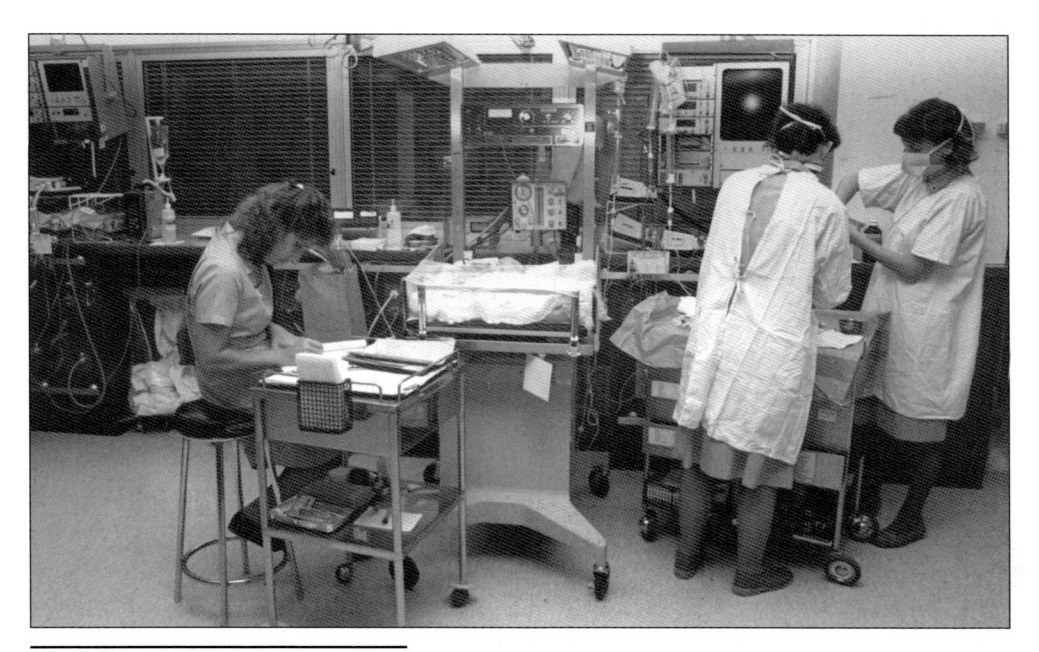

Nurses' mobile work station, ICU, 1970s-style.

The years 1973–74 proved to be a milestone, ending a long drought in the exchange of ideas and training. The Uncle Bobs Club widened the criteria for travel grants and scholarships to include nurses. It became possible for selected trained nurses to move about on study tours, to gain in-service and extracurricular post-basic study.[10] 'To catch up', Miss Orr said, 'I had to send away as many as six senior staff in one year, so arousing hostility among the medical people'.[11]

Rae Anstee successfully completed the infant welfare course and, together with Miss P. A. Miller, undertook the Nursing Administration Diploma at the College of Nursing. In 1977, Heather Telfer, a post-basic Nurse Teacher, Intensive Care Unit nursing course, was awarded a scholarship by the Committee of Management to study intensive care clinical nursing and education. She visited intensive care units in the United States of America, Canada and the United Kingdom and concluded that nursing practice and education in Melbourne Children's ICU were well up with world standards. On her return, after experiencing the bright child-focused facilities in many overseas hospitals, she did, however, find the Melbourne Children's Hospital in the 1970s rather drab.[12]

Advances and new thinking

During the 1970s, an increase in drug-resistant strains of methicillin resistant staphylococcal infection (MRSI) culminated in the opening in May 1980 of a Specialist Isolation Ward. More than twenty-five nurses were withdrawn from other ward areas. The successful establishment of this ward was due to the skill and dedication of Sister Val Duke (Casualty, Nursing officer) and Sister Jeanette Pollock (Infection Control Sister).

The increasing numbers of high-dependency patients needing specialist care, universal in all public hospitals in the 1970s, eventually triggered the changes to the traditional apprenticeship, pre-registration nursing education system. The curriculum of 1,600 hours, implemented on target in 1974, caused chaos for the administration. In 1978, the Royal Children's Hospital changed from a three-and-a-half-year basic nursing education programme (three years in a paediatric setting and six months in an adult setting) to a three-year general programme. This met the requirements of the new curriculum of a general training school and included the new subjects of maternity, gynaecology, psychiatry and public health theory but minimal paediatric nursing. Nurses' lectures were taken in normal working time and students continued to be paid as full-time employees. As predicted, this led to a massive increase in the numbers of nurses required to cover the shifts.

The Royal Children's Hospital embraced the new thinking with seminars and professional meetings. In the centenary year 1970, there were celebrations, seminars, visitors, distinguished guests, scholars and specialists early childhood development and education from around the world. Sister Val Duke arranged the successful Paediatric

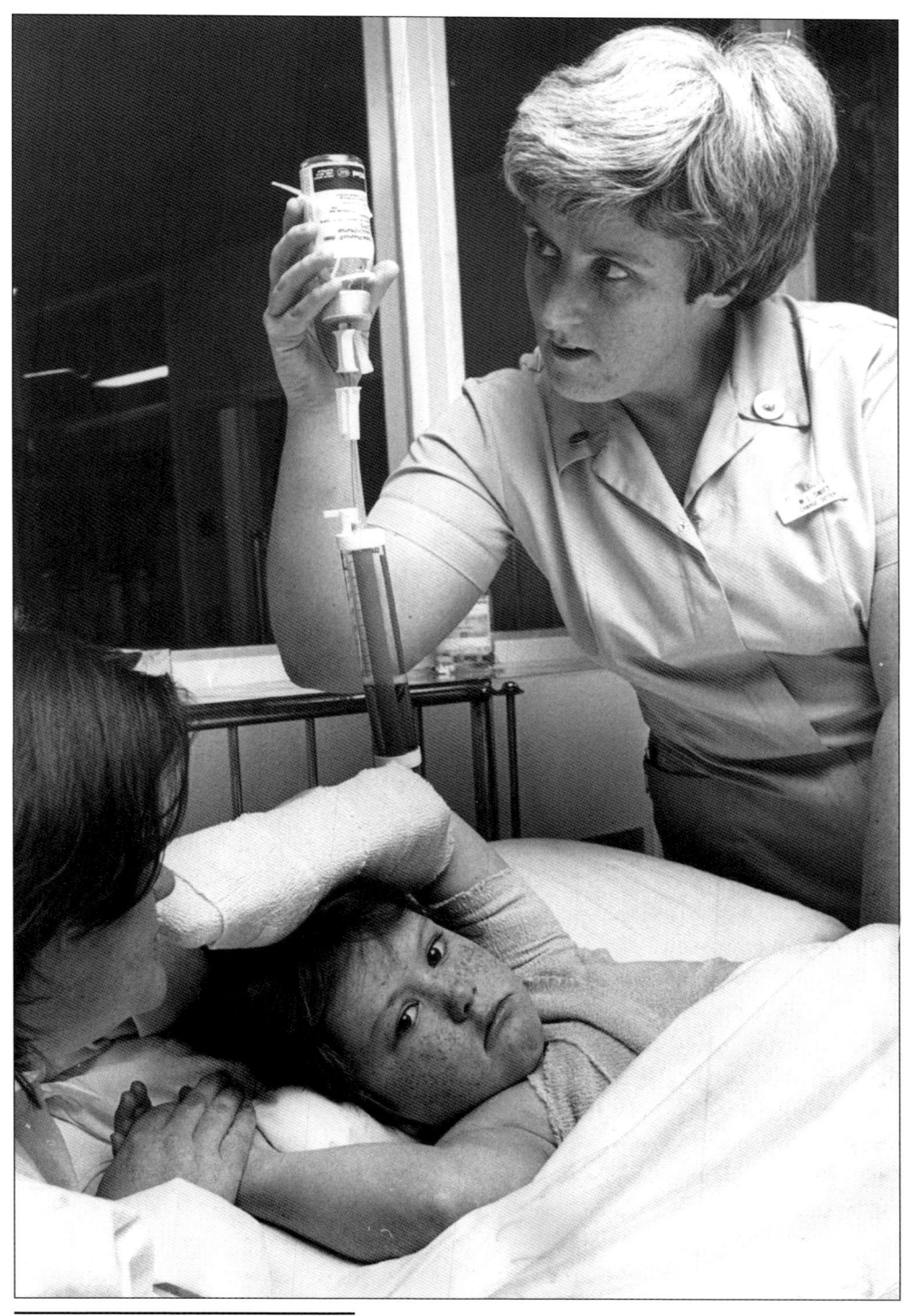

Wendy Swift, Burns Unit, 1970s.

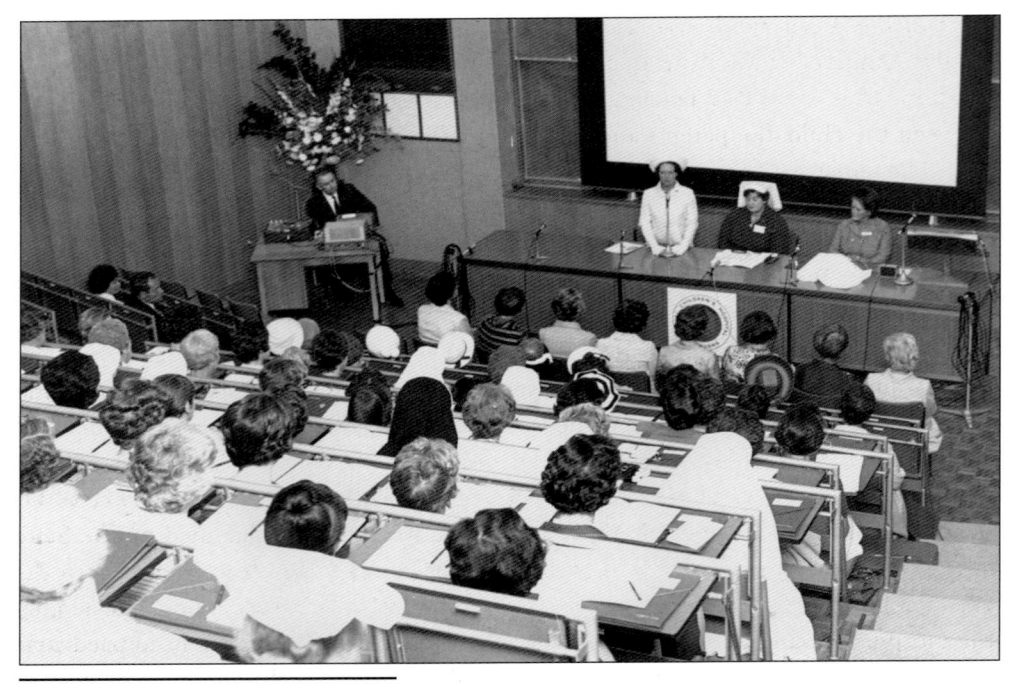

The opening of the Centenary Nurses' Conference 1970, in the Ella Latham Theatre, by Lady Newman Morris (née Sheila Gray, RCH 1936–39).
L–R: Dame Patricia Mackinnon, Director of Nursing Miss Elaine Orr, Lady Newman Morris.

Nursing Conference, attracting visitors from interstate and overseas. This created a greater awareness of the emotional needs of children in hospital. The medical profession, historically focussed on clinical medicine and research, was slow to come to terms with these concepts. Throughout the decade post-basic courses were arranged through Colleges of Early Childhood Development to widen the horizons of child care workers, paediatric nurses, maternal and child health nurses, doctors and allied health professionals.

The International Year of the Child (1979) created a favourable amount of funding for research to study child development, their psychosocial, emotional, cognitive and physical needs. This was a natural progression from the research first begun in the late 1940s and early 1950s in Britain by Dr John Bowlby, commissioned to report by the World Health Organization on the effects of children's separation from their families. His work emphasised the emotional needs of children, and the severe separation anxiety and deprivation, particularly in hospitals and associated institutions.[13] Burton White, Terry Brazelton and Rene Spitz were feted as the new early childhood references, among paediatricians and psychoanalysts, social workers and early childhood specialists studying the longitudinal effects on the first three years of life. Their work was widely publicised: studies of infant temperament and family competency, the role of the father in child development and the rights of children. This created a favourable climate for further research into relationships between the child, the parents and health professionals so commonly accepted today.

The subject of child maltreatment became an important but by no means the major focus of social work in these years. The Hospital's Social Work Department broadened its role when studies into child abuse became public. This was the work of Dr Robert Birrell, OAM, and his brother John, Chief Police Forensic Officer with the Victoria Police based at Monash University, and Dr Dora Bialastock.

Previously, child abuse had been ignored by hospital medical staff; when the initial injuries were healed, the child suspected as a victim was discharged with little or no follow-up. The children returned often. Against advice, Dr Bob Birrell enlisted the assistance of Ward Sisters Elizabeth Fearon and Val Duke to keep a register, while the Hospital strenuously resisted any involvement, largely due to the influence of Dr Vernon Collins. In his opinion, these cases were matters to be handled by the State Social Welfare Department.[14] His argument, until cases began to be referred to the Hospital's Social Work Department, was that parents' rights were being violated, by the Hospital's taking an activist role. Nevertheless, most of the experienced paediatric nurses had very long experience with these children. Miss Kathleen Dawe succeeded Miss Isabel Hodge as the Chief Social Worker in 1962, and became involved in the management of many of the cases of child abuse. Mandatory reporting was thirty years into the future.

The growing recognition of the psycho-social needs of children and their families was the central theme which enabled the professions to respond in a much broader role than the earlier focus of nursing had allowed. For example, the emotional needs of the child and the family in situations of disability, chronic illness and terminal illness, as well as in relation to traumatic injuries such as burns, were all responded to in new ways in the emerging awareness of children's emotional development and the increasingly complex family structures and dynamics. All of these factors had an impact on the way nurses carried out their work and on the knowledge they needed to acquire, and consequently put great burdens on their professional life.

Effects of changes

The New Curriculum for Nursing Training, announced by the Minister for Health, the Hon. J. F. Rossiter, MLA, in 1971, and implemented in June 1974 had repercussions on all hospitals but heightened significance for the Children's as a specialist paediatric hospital.

To train nurses for general registration, there was a responsibility to prepare them adequately to practise in any area, while at the same time maintaining more

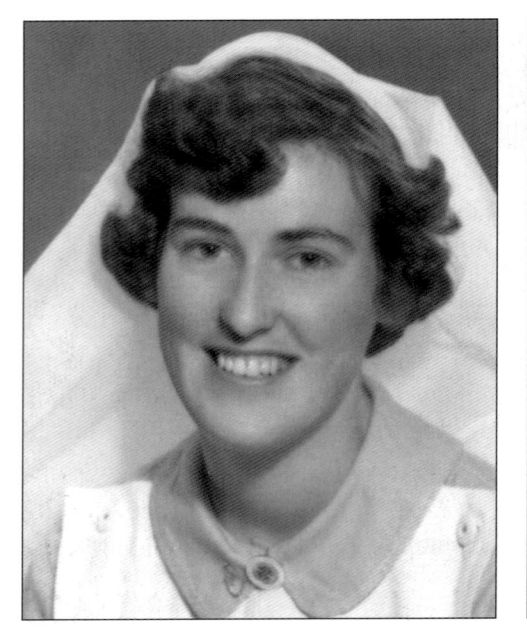

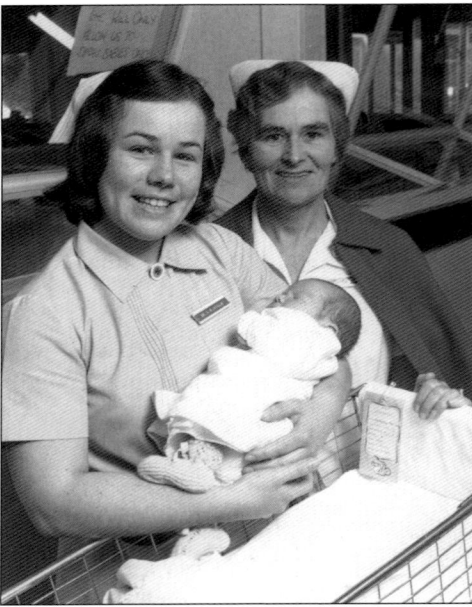

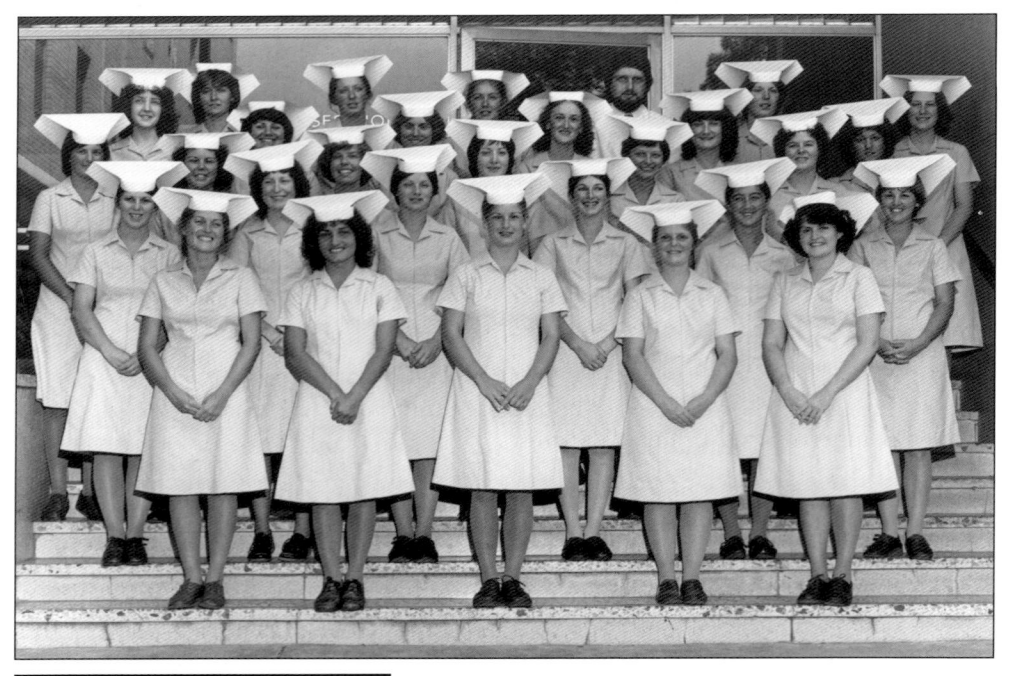

Top left: Joan Nason, Night Supervisor for twenty years.
Bruce Family Collection

Top right: Anne Hardham, top of the State in midwifery, Dandenong Hospital 1976, with her mother, Jennie Coventry (RCH 1946–49).
Hardham Family Collection.

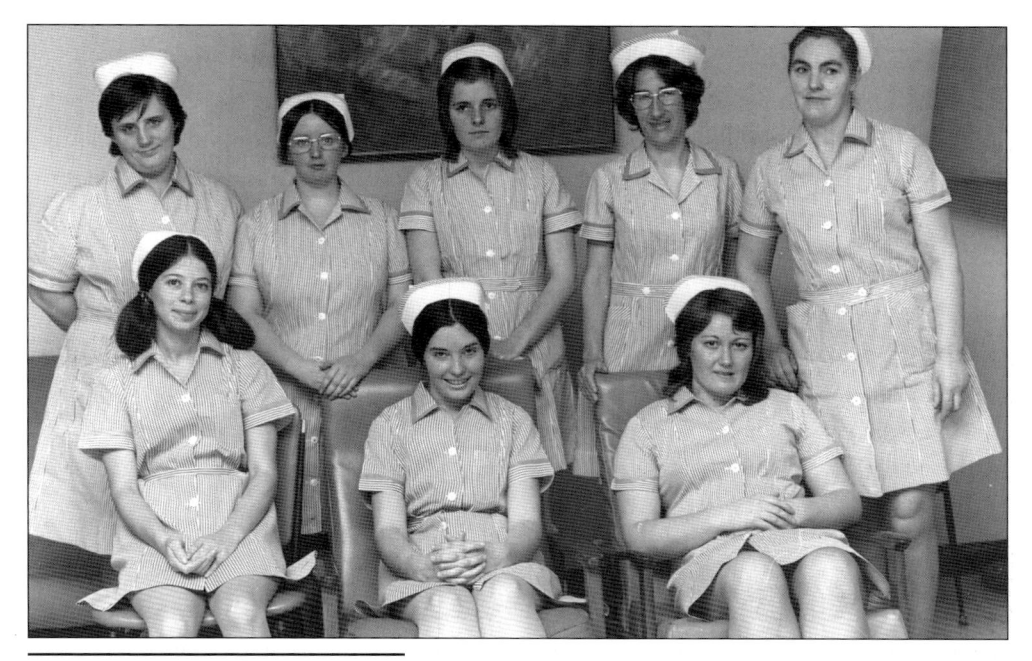

Top: RCH Nursing Aide School, 1970s.
Back L–R: Vivien Gosling, Francine Lancaster, Cathy Farmer, 'S.C.' Elsie Broadbent.
Front L–R: Dianne Pollard, Kathryn Anderson, Lorraine Wiseman.

Opposite bottom: Graduation: 1979. (Names not in order)
Katrina Bamford, Helen Bishop, Jennifer Canning, Marianne Coates, Helen Durkacz, Christina Guaran, Christine King, Neil McGeachin, Amanda McMurtrie, Esselina Mekking (Margaret Adams Prize), Adele Memishi, Nola Millard, Celeste Miller, Margaret Morrison, Leanne Munnerley, Helen Nott, Debra Nunn, Janice O'Callaghan, Jan Palmer, Christine Pollard, Susan Priest, Rosemary Prowse, Catherine Rees, Gwendoline Robinson, Debra Street, Anne Sutton, Deborah Toohey, Leanne Wilkins, Leanne Williams.

complex paediatric nursing skills. Among the many RCH graduates appointed to senior posts in general hospitals were: Elizabeth Jaffray at Woden Valley, ACT, Margaret Playfair, Mavis Greenwood at the Queen Victoria Hospital, Jean Hardham at Williamstown Hospital and Judith Butt (Lady Court) at Princess Alexandra Hospital in Western Australia. The State final examination results proved the efficiency of the programme when, in 1973, Anne Hardham achieved the highest grades in the State.

Elaine Orr believed that a major shift in thinking needed to occur among the long-established staff: undoubtedly a leader in Australia, the Children's was, nevertheless, a general nurse training school in a paediatric setting.

Miss Orr had long suggested modernisation of the uniforms. The distinctions of rank and seniority had hardly changed since the days of Matron Player (1922–47). In consultation with the staff—who thought the emphasis on the length of the uniform to be terribly old-fashioned—the Committee agreed to engage fashion designers including Prue Acton. The nurses generally welcomed the final design, a shorter pale blue uniform without an apron.

By 1969, the veil was out; some persisted, wearing it to ceremonial functions. Only eight out of 138 voted to keep nurses' caps. No one could remember the original function, and all agreed they looked like waitresses. Once again, some agreed to keep this and, for one year, the number of blue stripes denoted the year of training. However, the shedding of the veil was the most significant step in the break with the long tradition, the last bastion of any medieval connection with religious institutions. Interestingly, for the graduation pictures, the veil came out as a symbol of success, 'a badge of office'. On 30 January 1976, Lois Elliott (née Ferguson) was one of twenty-four who graduated wearing the short blue zip-up dress, the fawn stockings and brown lace-up shoes that Lois said, 'were on their last gasp'. As well, they proudly wore their throwaway paper veils.

One of the major changes in the 1970s was the move out of the Nurses' Home. Increasing numbers of girls married, the wages improved and broken shifts ceased. Renting in North Melbourne, Carlton and Fitzroy became a real option and life began to resemble that of college and university students. Increasingly, male nurses took on senior posts, and married women were employed, particularly on night duty. The 'motherly' characteristics of married nurses became readily accepted and, by 1969, twenty-seven were on the staff, night duty being particularly popular among them. The numbers grew throughout the 1970s and Joan Nason (née Joynes), a mother of five, became the night duty supervisor, a position she kept for almost twenty years.

A crèche was established for day staff, limited to children over two years old. Miss Orr noted ten years later that night duty still presented a problem; safe levels of care and supervision could only be maintained by internal rotation of registered nurses and the sporadic use of Agency staff.

In 1971, Miss Orr invited Lola Stokes (née Cumber), a former Children's Hospital trainee and tutor of the 1950s, to start the Children's Hospital's own Nursing Aide School.[15] This highly successful programme taught feeding, bathing and dressing, and small procedures such as giving enemas. The Nursing Aide Scheme led to the State Enrolled Nurses (SEN) of the 1980s.

The shortage of registered nurses was a worldwide problem, and the Royal Children's Hospital found it difficult to recruit graduate staff with specialist paediatric knowledge and secondary skills in areas such as intensive care, psychiatry, and neonatal nursing. The extensions of intensive care and the high patient/nurse ratios required in this unit meant that many skilled staff would be required.

Industrial issues

The President, Mrs (later Dame) Patricia Mackinnon, closely followed the developments of the impending crisis in nurse shortages. The expert State Committees that investigated nursing and the healthcare sector in the 1960s and 1970s provided an important stimulus for change in wages, conditions and education. There was widespread disappointment in the slow implementation of the recommendation of the Commonwealth Committee of Enquiry into the Education and Training of Nurses (the Sax Report, 1978). This was that nurse education and training be moved into the tertiary education system subject to conditions: that tertiary programmes provide adequate clinical experience, that student nurses be given responsibility for patient care, and that the theory and clinical components be closely integrated.

The frustration centred around government procrastination on options for varying the arrangements in existence at the time with regard to the framework of the apprenticeship system—a framework without which hospitals would collapse.[16] For example, at the Children's Hospital, trainee nurses provided 65–70 per cent of direct, hands-on patient care. The remainder of the nurses were administration and teaching staff, Charge Sisters, Staff Nurses and Home Supervisors. The Sax Committee Report recommended upgrading existing hospital schools, regionalising schools of nursing and implementing co-operative arrangements between the hospital-based schools of nursing and educational institutions.

Industrial unrest, perennial staff shortages and an inability to retain students continued. Between 1971 and 1975, an estimated 2,200 Victorian nurses went out of uniform to demonstrate dissatisfaction, while 4,000 off-duty nurses held a protest at Parliament House. Wages and conditions were only part of the problem. Other factors were: disruption to social life (at the Children's, broken and weekend shifts), and the unco-operative and inflexible attitudes by hospital administrators, particularly deputy directors of nursing who were responsible for supervision and rosters.

Hospital work became more complex, with ethical dilemmas, legal complexities and accountability becoming everyday occurrences. Nurses had to know more to accommodate parents from many cultures by learning about their customs and, in some cases, their language. These factors contributed to a re-examination of what paediatric nurses needed to know and what they did.

In 1978, Dame Patricia McKinnon, in consultation with Miss Orr, advised her Committee that the Children's would now make the decision to transfer nurse education from the Hospital to the Colleges of Advanced Education; it was the first hospital in Victoria to do so. So began the process to phase out the Training School.

The end of an era

The decade of the 1970s was notable for resignations, retirements and deaths. Miss Helen Quiney, a Children's Hospital identity, resigned in 27 July 1973, after a period of nineteen years' service including many in administration. Miss Rita Burkitt resigned on 20 July 1973 to take up the role of Matron of Hartnett House, a facility run by the Melbourne City Mission for mothers and babies.

Those who died were Francis Potts, on 11 December 1978, a legend in Outpatients for twenty-two years, and Annie Ida Laidlaw, the first Matron of the Frankston Orthopaedic Hospital, who served for sixteen years and died on 13 September 1978. Elaine Orr retired in 1982 and Mary Patten was appointed Executive Director of Nursing.

MARY PATTEN, RN, BA (Hons), FCNA, Director of Nursing RCH 1982, Executive Director Nursing 1991–95.

Mary Patten trained in the first intake of the Melbourne School of Nursing based at Malvern in 1951. Clinical placements were carried out at three Melbourne hospitals. Miss Patten's affiliation was with the Royal Melbourne Hospital.

Following her training and staff year at the Melbourne, she gained further experience in Scotland. On her return to Australia, she spent many years working as an industrial advocate, as Federal Secretary with the RANF (ANF), and as a representative at the College of Nursing and the Victorian Nursing Council through various committees.[17]

Mary Patten always had a favourable view of nursing at the Children's; she knew that paediatric nurses had to be precise, because with children there was no room for error. However, she thought these nurses were considered a little 'precious'. Many were only allowed (by their parents) to do nursing because they were looking after children rather than adults.

She believed she was appointed to the position because of her non-traditional background and extensive experience in industrial relations. The hospital had lived on the legends of Lucy De Neeve and Vernon Collins for decades and needed a revival. The organisation had been through a difficult time, having lost Australian Council Hospital Standards Accreditation in 1979/80, and her brief to change the nursing structure had many problems. She found most doctors still expected nurses to report to medical staff but she strongly resisted this. With CEO Dr Barry Catchlove, she demanded a more collaborative relationship between doctors and nurses.[18]

Fay Marles, the Commissioner for Equal Opportunity, was called on behalf of the State Government to interview nursing staff and made recommendations to the Minister for Health. This study drew on 228 submissions from Victorian nurses to document the complexity of the doctor–nurse relationship. The findings detailed the role of nurses as medical assistants, devalued to denote subordination, a continuation of the 'handmaiden ethos' to doctors.[19]

Mary Patten recalled a meeting with CEO Barry Catchlove when he was asked if the Senior Nurse should have equal status with the Senior Doctor. His reply was 'Yes'. This became the rule.

She found an entrenched medical establishment, and an elitist nursing hierarchy, partly explained, she thought, by the fact that the Children's was the only paediatric hospital in the state. The slow staff turnover occurred as there was nowhere else to go. Many considered the Children's had rested on its laurels, retaining staff from the old Carlton Hospital who were slow to adapt, and lacked wider postgraduate training and policy development skills. Also, most of the students of the 1980s were better educated and more academic than the 'old school' tutors, some of whom basically started their careers with the Merit certificate or one or two years of high school. Most had been to the College of Nursing and gained affiliation in courses such as administration and teaching and, while they were excellent practical nurses, many were not academically inclined. Some were unable to conceptualise the 'big picture' of nursing, the tremendous changes occurring in the education and health sectors.

Mary Patten caused a tremendous stir at a packed rally of nurses in the Ella Latham lecture auditorium when she said 'adult trained nurses could easily transfer their skills to children without further education'.[20]

She addressed negative responses in preparation for the changeover to tertiary education but met with opposition from a few nurse educators and senior staff of long standing (both inside the Hospital and among past trainees) because of their perception of her lack of clinical experience and knowledge of paediatrics.[21] In their view, paediatric nursing and the understanding of child development was greatly underrated.

Anne Vintiadis, Head of School, 1983–87.

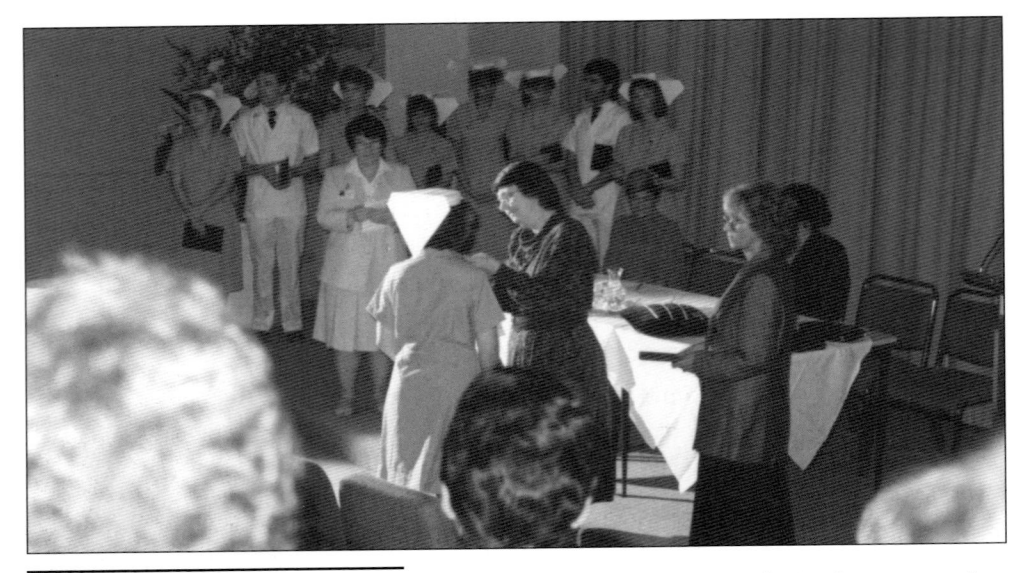

Last graduation, 2 October 1987. Miss Mary Patten, Director of Nursing, presenting the badges.

In fact, the post-basic paediatric course, which had commenced successfully in Carlton and was revived by Val Duke in 1969 to prepare nurses for advanced paediatric nursing, continued until it was transferred in a different form to the University of Melbourne. Later, Beryl Clarke and then Paula Simpson were responsible for the course. The post-basic paediatric intensive care nursing course continued, from its inception in 1974, to educate registered nurses to advanced intensive care nursing skills until it, too, was transferred to Melbourne University. Those involved in teaching were Heather Telfer, Lucy Cuddihy, Marina Tucakic, Jacquie Williams, Kaye Eddy (neonates), Sharon Kinney and Di McKinley. Both courses attracted students from interstate and overseas.

Fortunately, Miss Patten's background experience and education in the industrial and academic world enabled her to overcome these difficulties and begin the process of updating the Nursing School. A Nurse Educator skilled in policy and planning, Anne Vintiadis, assisted by Sue Philpott, was invited onto the staff. Sue developed the adult/paediatric accident and emergency course, which was initially affiliated with the Alfred and Austin Hospitals.

With the collaboration of CEO Dr Barry Catchlove—who also met with fierce opposition to change from the medical establishment—a sympathetic management and the cooperation with the State Health Department, Miss Patten was able to overcome industrial and other issues of the 1980s. The last class of the Mackinnon School of Nursing, named for the three generations of the Mackinnon family, graduated in October 1987.[22]

Unit managers were established in four broad divisions, thus giving equal status to nurses and doctors, something previously unheard of at the Children's Hospital. Ward Sisters became a relic of the past. With the new and flatter corporate structure, the positions of Directors of Nursing and Medicine disappeared in favour of a Chief Executive Officer. The overall responsibility for nursing was allocated to the Principal Nurse, Nursing—Divisional Director of Specialist Services. Lucy Cuddihy was the first person to occupy that position, from 1990 until November 2004.

LUCY CUDDIHY, PhD

Trained at the Mater Misericordiae Hospital, Brisbane from 1969–72.

BA (App. Sc.) Adv. Nursing; Major in Education at Lincoln Institute of Health Sciences, (1982), Grad. Dip. Business Management, RMIT (1994). Midwifery Certificate, Canberra (1973). Premature, Neonatal and Paediatric Nursing Certificate Royal Women's Hospital (RWH) Melbourne, 1977. Family Planning Certificate, RWH 1978. ICU Certificate, RCH 1979. Divisional Director—Specialist Services, 1990–2004.

Responsible for nursing for Cardiac Surgery, Cardiology, Paediatric Intensive Care and the NICU, the Cardiac Unit, the Haemodialysis Unit, Medical Imaging, PETS (Paediatric Emergency Transport Service), Biomedical Engineering, and the Perfusion Service.

Nurses of the 1980s and 1990s believe it was a privilege to be part of Mary Patten's era, for she led nursing in an open-minded and encouraging manner. Laurence Dubourg, a French nurse, owed every success in Ward 6 West to Mary because 'she supported each achievement with trust and added her wisdom when it was needed'. Laurence said,

> I remember facing a disappointment and feeling low. How did she hear about it? She came to my office with her usual smile. I can still see and hear her telling me that I was a 'tall poppy', and that it was a habit in Australia to attempt to reduce tall poppies rather than developing them. She said, 'do not get discouraged' and to persevere and trust myself.[23] Laurence always remembered her words when facing adversity.

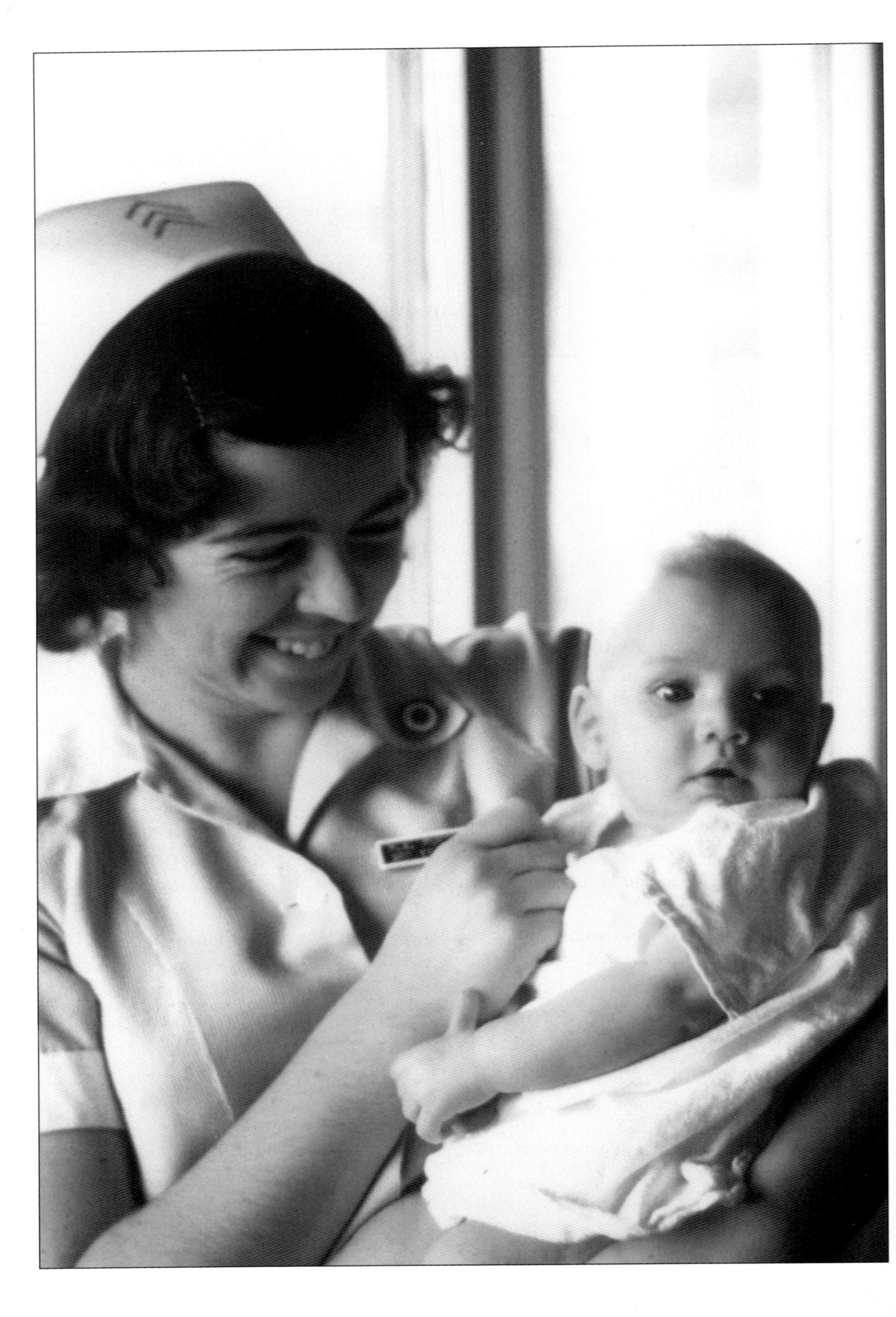

CHAPTER 14

Special Nursing

1970–1987

Advances in medicine and surgery in the last decades of the twentieth century accelerated both the movement towards specialisation and the marked decrease of preventable illnesses. The 1971 Annual Report noted that the three commonest causes of death in infants and children were developmental abnormalities, accidents and malignant diseases.

Developments in cardiac surgery led to an increasing number of survivors among children with cardiac abnormalities, while selective, non-toxic anti-cancer chemicals began to replace other methods of treatment for childhood cancer. The Hospital became more involved in community issues, leading in accident prevention by publicity, education and legislation in the field of burns, poisoning and preventable injuries in the home and in the streets. Nurses have played a major role in community education and care.

From the 1970s, the length of time children stayed in Hospital declined rapidly; in 1980, the average was five-and-a-half days. Coupled with this, the increase over the decade in the number of in-patients from 16,891 to 22,737 followed the trend in large paediatric hospitals throughout the Western world. Patients attending Casualty, General Clinic and Out-patients in 1980 rose to more than 254,881.[1]

James Teasdale and his devoted nurse, 1977.
Teasdale Family Collection.

The changes in Hospital utilisation in the 1970s and 1980s reflected the changes occurring in paediatrics: an increasing number of specialties resulting in the survival of children who may have not previously survived their chronic conditions. There was a greater reliance on medical care and expertise in general, reflected in the disproportionate increase in primary health care given in the Casualty and General Clinic. The numbers of children attending became so large that the Hospital encouraged the growth of primary child care services in outside agencies. This was essential not only for coping with increasing numbers, but, more importantly, for providing adequate services closer to the families' own homes. All these factors presented a challenge to nurses, not only in terms of the specialisation of their work but also in broadening the definition of hospital work to services in the community.[2]

Cardiac, renal and ambulatory services

Janette McEwan first came to the Children's Hospital in 1970 after training at New Zealand's famous Greenlane Hospital, the cardiac centre of excellence and research for the Pacific region, headed by the eminent surgeon, Sir Brian Boyes. Janette had cardiac but not paediatric training. She said: 'It was very hard at first, being sent to ICU when the Cardiac Ward was not busy. There were not as many cases then.'

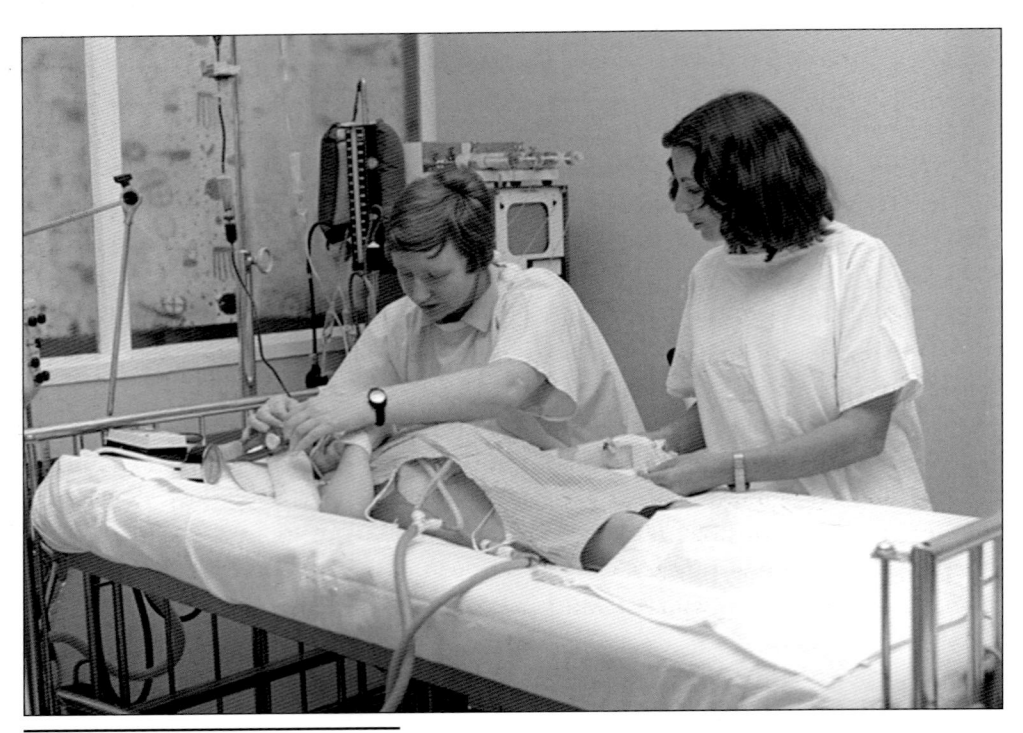

Janette McEwan and Marion Reilly in the Cardiac ICU, 1980.

Janette completed the post-basic intensive care course in 1975. The surgeon, Dr Peter Clarke, a colleague from New Zealand, began at the Children's at the same time as Janette; he was a person she knew and trained with but he left the Children's in 1976. The mid-1970s were difficult for cardiac nurses until a new surgeon was appointed. Cardiac surgery was in the early stages and the success rate was not all that could be desired.[3] Despite the drawbacks, the 1970s were an extremely interesting time.

Some notable surgeons came to the Children's: D'arcy Sutherland from South Australia, Roger Mee from New Zealand and Bill Brawn from England. After a few years, the Cardiac Surgery Unit became very busy and successful. In 1983, Janette moved to Ward 7 East, Medical Cardiac Unit. This became both medical and surgical, with seven registered nurses. In Ward 7 West Neurosurgery, cardiac medicine was also included and staff numbers were increased to allow for high-dependency beds.

From 1980, the surgeon, Mr Roger Mee, built up Unit 7 West to one of the most successful in the world. The Paediatric Cardiac Surgery Unit was designated with responsibility for all paediatric cases for southern Australia, as well as treating patients from parts of Asia and the Pacific. The first heart transplant on a child in Australia occurred at the RCH on 5 October 1988.

The first intensive care nurses dealt more with the surgeons than with the cardiologists. Janette had a pleasant working relationship with Roger Mee and he asked her to move from 7 East to 7 West. A demanding surgeon, he insisted on a team approach in the whole unit, expecting no less than total excellence. This was a high-dependency unit, so staff who cared for patients required superior counselling skills, particularly in assisting the parents of cardiac patients. In 1994, 7 West became the Cardiac Renal Unit.

In 2002, Lee Hughes, one of the first graduates to enter the RCH with the Diploma of Applied Science Nursing (1988) from the Lincoln School of Health Sciences and a Bachelor of Nursing with Honours from La Trobe University (1991), became the Cardiac Renal Unit Manager.

Janette believes some of the team work, values and consideration for fellow nurses from the former training days should be encouraged. The friendships that nurses made with hospital-based training were long-lasting. This is not so evident today. The knowledge base of current nurses is very good but often initially their clinical skills lag behind their knowledge. This situation is, however, being rectified: the annual intake of university graduate nurses from all over Australia is being channelled into a one-year graduate course conducted by the Mackinnon School of Nursing in conjunction with Melbourne University.

Cardiac Transplant Unit and National Centre for Paediatric Transplants

An extension to the Cardiac Unit, the Cardiac Transplant Unit is another relatively new area at the Hospital. Anne Shipp trained at the RCH from 1971 to 1975 and gained extensive experience in coronary care and cardiology intensive care before she was appointed to the position of Cardiac Transplant Co-ordinator in the Cardiac Transplant Unit in 1988. She had been very involved with many of the families and was a most suitable person for their needs. The programme was in its infancy and had then only carried out about eleven heart–lung and seven heart operations. In 1990, Anne became the Co-ordinator for the National Centre for Paediatric Transplants.

The job involved assessment and administration, including helping the families who have come from interstate. Referrals came from various centres throughout the country. Medical staff refer the child, and the family usually stays for at least a week; many of the children are already known to the staff because they have had cardiac surgery in the past. The Hospital carries out cardiac surgery for half the country. Recently, more difficult cases have come from Western Australia which has been included in 'the catchment area'.

Anne acts as facilitator; the patients have physical problems for one of two reasons: either structural or mitral-cardiomyopathy. 'If there has been previous surgery, we are bound to know the child. Children come for a week and do a lot of talking to a lot of people, because transplantation is not a cure. It's a treatment. These kids may not live for more than ten or twenty years and it depends—they may need another one [transplant].' Anne tells the parents: 'You have to get to know us and we to know you. This is aimed at the quality of life, not quantity.' They have to absorb all the information.

Anne maintains her relationship with the family as a resource: 'I am their conduit, resource person and contact to talk it through, to understand what the anti-rejection drugs and the antibiotics do.' Anne admits that the job requires certain personal characteristics: 'It does worry you sometimes; you go through really bad patches. We all do. Children die. Yes, I am there, and yes, it has happened. I am there with the parents. It is a commitment. I don't know if I would be doing this job if I had children of my own.'[4]

Progress in the Burns Unit

When Wendy Swift took over Ward 9 West in 1971, it was a twenty-two-bed Burns Unit. The main causes of injury were hot water and flame burns. When she left in 1992, the ward consisted of an eight-bed Burns Unit with a potential for a further reduction in bed numbers.

Special Nursing

WENDY LOIS SWIFT, OAM, RCH 1963–67

Wendy Swift became the Sister-in-Charge of the Diabetic, Cardiology and Burns Unit 1973–92, and Co-chairman of the Nurses' Training and Recruitment Sub-committee of the International Society for Burns Injuries. Her name became synonymous with burns treatment at the Royal Children's Hospital. At various times she lectured on burns nursing at Mumbai University in India, and in Singapore, and attended international medical conferences on burns practices. Wendy received the Order of Australia Medal in recognition of her service and commitment to burns nursing including her work on Ash Wednesday in March 1983 when she was flown to Warrnambool to set up a Burns Unit. A Churchill Scholarship awarded to Wendy in 1986 enabled her to study burns at children's hospitals in Boston, Massachusetts, and in Buenos Aires, Argentina.[5]

One of the key changes Wendy brought to the care of children with burns was the philosophy that the patient is a child in a family that ultimately also has to cope with injury, pain and disfigurement. Her nursing management involved a great deal of family support and counselling to avoid the psychological damage so often present in the old days when children endured pain and loneliness for months on end, sometimes into adulthood.

In years gone by, one could 'smell' the Burns Ward. The odour of disinfectant hung in the air, children were isolated and the fear of infection was very real. Over the years, improved methods of fighting infection contributed to more natural convalescence of children with burns. The word 'normalisation' became a term used in ward management as wards were shared with both cardiac and diabetic patients, and the children were no longer isolated. Today the burns patients are absorbed into the general ward.

Improved pain management is one of the most spectacular changes since the 1970s. Formerly, when pain relief was far from satisfactory, one of the hardest things to bear was the saline bathing. Many children were given an anaesthetic before a change of dressings.

For twenty years, parents have had greater involvement in their child's treatment, with written information and support groups. There has also been greater liaison with the District Nursing Service, allowing for the earlier discharge of the patient.

Neuroscience nursing practice

Dramatic changes in the clinical care and nursing of children with neurological disorders has been a wonder of the late twentieth century.

Laurence Dubourg came to Melbourne from Paris to begin nursing in the Neuroscience Ward at the Austin Hospital. She trained for her Diplôme d'infirmière (Registered Nurse) at the Assistance Publique, Hôpitaux de Paris (APHP), and at the Hospital Nécker-Vaugirard-Laënnec, Paris, for sick children, in 1978. She came to Melbourne's Royal Children's Hospital in 1989 with extensive paediatric experience in Paris and Switzerland and neuroscience nursing experience from the Austin. She took over the management of the Neurology Ward from a long and outstanding neuroscience nurse, Marge Thomson, who for more than a decade had led Ward 6 West.[6] This author is indebted to Laurence for sharing her memories of the days that followed in Marge's footsteps:

> We were able to gauge how much Marge was admired by a letter of thanks from a doctor who worked one year on Ward 6 West. The letter, in addition to thanking her for the teaching and support she had provided for him and for families, highlighted what he thought was the best about that Ward. He stressed the continuity of care provided for children with cancer, from the time of surgery, through their time of treatment, whether it was radiotherapy, chemotherapy or rehabilitation. Marge Thomson insisted on continuing with the care of children with brain and spinal tumours. Her motivation stemmed from observation that some children transferred to the cancer ward occasionally experienced some incidents that highlighted deficits in neurological nursing. She believed that because of their condition, children could fall out of bed, inhale food or could drift into semi-consciousness from fluid overload. She believed that chemotherapy administration knowledge was easier to assimilate than subtle neuroscience nursing. Hence her commitment to look after these children from diagnosis to their discharge home.
>
> Sophisticated neurosurgical techniques developed further in the 1990s and enabled surgeons to perform extremely invasive neurosurgical procedures of the brain stem. As a consequence, even more precise nursing was needed to prevent further morbidity following surgery.

Laurence Dubourg, 6 West, 1991.

Special Nursing

The nurses must observe even more the subtle development of swallowing problems, absent gag reflex, weak cough, visual problems and hyperventilation. Strategies that become second nature to neuroscience paediatric nurses sometimes elude others. For example, to look for discrete signs such as a weaker or high-pitched cry, a slight decrease in the use of an arm, an uneven smile and or a drooping eyelid. They need to ensure cot sides stay up all the time, to position a pillow on a weak side of the body, to nurse a child on the floor to avoid a fall out of bed, to thicken the food and drinks, and to be wary of a child crying and so prevent increased cerebral pressure.

Today, the children requiring an MRI (Magnetic Resonance Imaging) no longer have to go to St Vincent's Hospital. Nevertheless, they are still required to go to Peter MacCallum for radiotherapy. The treatment sometimes requires forty-five to sixty minutes over a period of six weeks. A very experienced nurse is required to assist, and Wendy Neilson was the anaesthetic escort nurse who took these children to other hospitals. The anaesthetic is administered for forty-five minutes or more if the child cannot stay still, with the specialist nurse escort assisting the anaesthetist to put the child to sleep.

> Wendy made it happen safely and she made it fun, to ultimately try to carry out the procedure without an anaesthetic. Most children would lighten up when she came to take them for the tests; she made it an adventure, not an ordeal. Perhaps it was her constant smiling, her laughter, her bags of tricks, the drawings and surprises. Perhaps it was the stories, accumulated over the years; but it was also her immense knowledge of neuroscience, paediatrics and parenting thus reassuring children and their parents. She wrote information sheets and taught countless parents that radiotherapy can give children a very bad taste in the mouth. Certain soft drinks could hide the taste and she could come back to the ward after a stopover at MacDonald's with a cheerful child thinking 'radiotherapy was like Christmas', after all.
>
> Wendy spent time looking over an unconscious child, watching every detail: the child's breathing and comfort, the arm drifting off the edge of the trolley that needed to be tucked back under the blanket, the warmth of the toes, the droplets of sweat on the forehead, the cough and the tear in the corner of the eye, the alignment of the head and neck, carefully calculated by gauging the thickness of the pillow. She could replace the pillow with a folded towel and cover it with a soft pillow case.[7]

In the 1990s, parents were encouraged to be involved, to help in their child's care, in contrast to previous years when doctors and surgeons preferred parental absence during their Neurosurgical Ward rounds. Night nurses used to believe that parents should go home to sleep and rest and those wishing to maintain a vigil by their child's bed were barred from doing so. Sometimes they slept on the floor of the playroom. Gradually, mothers were allowed to settle a child, breast-feed or do a nappy change. However, it was challenging in the early days when parents questioned overnight care: Why wake a child when he sleeps? Why are the nurses noisy at the nurses' station? Are nurses coming around as often as they should? Eventually nurses and parents settled their differences and parents were allowed to come day and night, but involving them twenty-four hours was a slow process. Nowadays, parents have a lounge room, showering facilities and an overnight bed. Parents are now regarded as clients, enabling them to have a say. One of the key people in this process was Maree Brick, who ran focus groups. Laurence said: 'The parent feedback was positive in such a sad ward. What could have been challenging for ward practices instead became positive and ultimately valuable.'[8]

Ward environments have witnessed modern developments: more colourful surroundings, space and comfort. The nurses minimise the traumatic effects of the children's stay by allowing them to have control over their lives, such as choosing a bed on admission and receiving encouragement rewards when procedures and medications are administered.

The Hospital in the Home (HITH) is a another modern development. Royal District Nursing Services always appeared to focus on adults. Now they assist with paediatric procedures and liaise with the Hospital nurses in the safe co-ordination of discharge programmes and the on-going supervision of teams looking after children at home. Neuroscience is notable for its wide team of neurosurgeons, neurologists, social workers, child development, rehabilitation people and many other allied health specialists.

A key neuroscience nursing development was the establishment of the epilepsy programme. New nursing skills such as video–EEG (electro-encephalogram) monitoring and Ictal isotopic injections (Ceretec®) were developed then. It was a paediatric international first.

Development of the neurological observation chart designed at the RCH (1990) to combine the 'Glasgow Coma Score' and the 'Adelaide Children's Chart' allowed objective reading of neurological observations and recording utilising objective vocabulary. Before this development, observations were based on subjective description of the child's behaviour and activities. Nowadays, the tests and observations are much more precise and can be compared over time.

Rehabilitation, discharge home support services and school integration are attended to in an interdisciplinary manner. Paediatric neuroscience nursing is a precise specialty and the patient's outcome relies heavily on the quality of the nurse's observations and interventions. No piece of equipment can replace the neuroscience nurse.

Oncology and haematology nursing

Mary McGowan came to the RCH in 1978 following her training from 1975 to 1977 at the National Children's Hospital, Harcourt Street, Dublin and then at Stevens Street, Dublin. After visiting Wangaratta, she came temporarily to the Children's but decided to stay after a very brief orientation. She first worked in Haematology and Oncology in Ward 9 East for five years and later in Ward 6 East to the present day.

For Mary, the Royal Children's Hospital was a pleasant, friendly place and the staff was very efficient. However, she was quite surprised at the lack of privacy in those days—there were no curtains around the children's beds. Everything was open. With total parent participation, this policy has changed.

In the past, the scene was not pleasant for oncology patients; there was a lot of vomiting and hair loss. Nowadays there are vastly different treatments; for example, Ondansetron is given to prevent vomiting. While once it was usual to spend most of the day cleaning up, today it would be rare to encounter a child vomiting more than twice a day. With the use of central lines, fluids and treatments can be given, and a lot of the heart-breaking trauma of repetitive procedures is eliminated.

In the beginning, the ward had two registered nurses and students. Supervision was ongoing. Today, graduate nurses have more knowledge but need time to develop communication and practice skills. Previously, Haematology and Oncology were in the General Medical Unit with twenty-six beds. Today, there is one unit and less risk of infection. Much treatment is on an out-patient basis and therefore fewer beds are required.

'Cancer' used to be a frightening word but that has now changed to a large extent. Whereas parents used to feel quite alone and ostracised, today there is much more openness, support and hope for them, their other children and their wider families.

Childhood cancer is rarely an emergency and the whole family needs a great deal of care. The child's long treatment and stay in Hospital takes a toll. It is very emotive and financially draining. Geographically and socially isolated parents can stay at the Ronald MacDonald House and receive a benefit of $150. Those who live less than fifty kilometres away stay for a moderate cost.

Ronald MacDonald House in Gatehouse Street opened in 1986 and made a huge difference. Parents can support each other by talking and swapping stories as well as having a safe place to stay. Previously, the

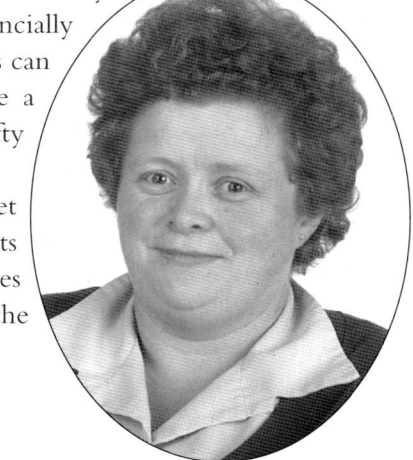

Mary McGowan.

wards had six (parent) beds or lounges and there were far too many who needed to stay and very little space. The office was multifunctional, sometimes used for viewing a dead child. Today, families are much more involved; grandmothers and aunts come into the tearoom and help nurse the babies and young children. There are many parent support groups.

Nurses work out strategies for themselves so that they do not take ward concerns home with them. Staff can become attached to their patients. There is joy when children, sent home for palliative care, return to visit. Children who recover often return years later to introduce their spouses and children.

Many children die at home in their own personal surroundings. The parents of these children receive support nevertheless from the Hospital and the District Nurses. Relationships between nurses and parents build up years after the child has died. The parents are invited back to talk about their child and to reminisce. Someone from the Hospital always attends the funeral.

With the advent of computer technology and databases, calls come in at any time, day or night, particularly for advice for country patients. This saves many trips, alleviates the anxiety of 'what to do' and provides an up-to-date information in changes in treatment. There is also pharmaceutical advice available for the medical practitioner.

Graduate nurses are fully accountable for patient care, unlike student nurses. Postgraduate study days in paediatrics are conducted at Box Hill and Shepparton. Staff members need to have special attributes. Mary asks herself at interview: 'Would I employ this person; will they fit in?' A core of nurses stays a very long time; some travel and return.[9]

Paula Johnson, for example, has worked in the unit for twenty years and still loves her job, while Kaye McNaught stayed for fifteen years as a clinical nurses' consultant. Kaye worked through the stressful times of HIV/AIDS infections in recipients of pooled blood products. She also fulfilled the role of counselling parents and their children with haemophilia.

General surgery

When Ros Willis[10] came to the RCH in 1969, little did she know that she would be staying for more than twenty years in one of the busiest Surgical Wards in the Hospital and serve under four Directors of Nursing: Joan Gendle, Elaine Orr, Cliff Buchanan and Mary Patten.

Roslyn's first ward at the RCH was 5 East as Sister-in-Charge which became Ward 8 West and finally Ward 4 West, General Surgery. She worked with the surgeons Douglas Stephens, Robert Fowler, Durham Smith, Justin Kelly and Ruth Magnus.

The ward cared for children with ano-rectal anomalies, urology and general surgical condition. Patients had diverse conditions, such as spina bifida,

Ros Willis, 4 West, 1990.

hydrocephalus, imperforate anus, Hirschsprung's disease,[11] rectourethral fistula, chronic constipation and hypospadias.[12] Patients often required ileal conduits and bladder augmentations. The staff perfected bladder washout systems, and dealt with the myriad of conditions, and problems involved with working with these children and their parents.

One of the greatest accomplishments during these years was when Ros invented the home bowel washout technique in the 1970s. Developed mainly for spina bifida children, it is now used universally for many conditions of bowel incompetency in children and adults. Known as the 'Willis Home Bowel Washout Programme', it is marketed in countries including the United Kingdom, Israel, Holland, Sweden and Australia. The product became known when Ros presented a paper at a scientific meeting of the Society for research into hydrocephalus and spina bifida at St John's College, Cambridge University, in 1989. Her paper was subsequently published with the proceedings of the congress in the *Scandinavian Paediatric Medical Journal* and the *Australian Nursing Journal*.[13]

The technique of colonic washout is taught to children as young as four while they sit on the toilet. They pass the tube into the rectum and allow a small amount of tap water mixed with ordinary cooking salt so the result is evacuated into the toilet. This procedure can be learnt by very young children in the privacy of their own homes.

Ros had many nurses in the team over the years, including Branka Blatancic as a student in 1984 and then as a registered nurse. Sandy Willis, herself a child patient of Douglas Stephens in the 1950s, later trained at the Children's and became a clinical nurse teacher on the ward and Head of the Nursing School from 1992 to 1995.

In 1994, Ward 4 West became a main ward covering an entire floor, including plastic surgery, burns, urology and general surgery.

Ambulatory paediatrics, community child health and out-patient triage

Throughout the history of the Children's Hospital, Casualty and the Out-patients Department has been the first point of contact for many thousands of children and their families. The old Carlton Hospital department was grossly inadequate and crowded, with few facilities and long waiting times.

From 1970 to 1971, the number of children treated was 46,471 while there were 198,595 attendances to the Out-patients Department. The Hospital served as a

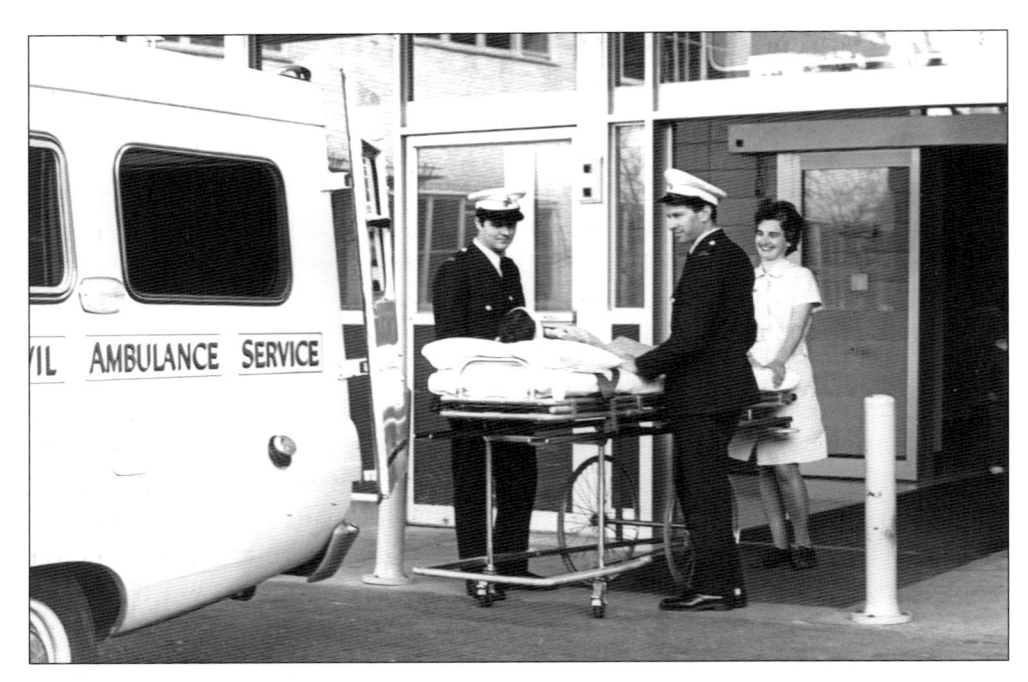

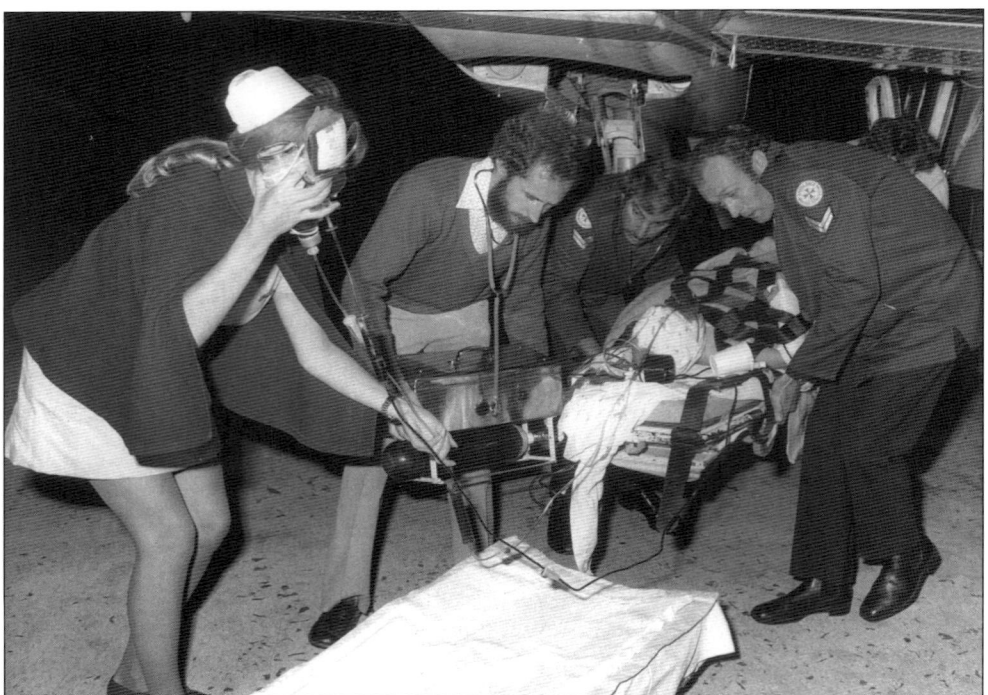

Top: Ambulance Service to Emergency Centre, 1960s. Jane Altmann receiving a patient at Casualty.
Bottom: Modern Air Ambulance service, 1980s.

free general practice, particularly for the northern and western suburbs. Despite the establishment of the universal health system, Medicare, in 1975 as well as community health centres in 1978, the numbers escalated.[14]

Aileen O'Donnell (RCH 1938–42) returned to the Children's in 1963 to become the Triage Enquiry Sister and worked with Dr Una Shergold, a very motherly, caring person with an immense knowledge of paediatrics and community resources for families. Many children presented with psychiatric problems and Dr Shergold referred them to the appropriate clinics. She established the General Clinic in 1953. Sister O'Donnell also handled thousands of telephone enquiries from anxious mothers and referrals from GPs.[15]

All parents came to the Enquiry Sister and very sick children, especially those having convulsions, went to Casualty. Aileen saw first-hand the tremendous problems, the changes and the patterns of difficulty which existed: the large number of migrants, predominantly Italian and Greek at first but, over time, including Spanish, Turkish, Middle Eastern and Vietnamese also. The staff relied on volunteer interpreters, sometimes Chinese nurses and doctors. More often than not, there were none available at weekends. Mr Silvio Proy was employed to co-ordinate an Interpreter Service and the Immigration Department ran a successful telephone interpreter service for some time. Often an older sibling came to interpret for the parents and many times the parents of the child patients waiting in the queue assisted in an emergency.

Other problems, Aileen remembers, were arriving for work early in the morning and finding people already waiting, sometimes from 7.30 am. They came in early hoping to be seen first, but actually waited all day. The first clinics opened at 9 am. By 1974, the Casualty (Emergency from 1983) and Out-patients Departments were clearly overwhelmed. Elaine Orr, the Director of Nursing, spoke 'of the stressful situation for nursing staff when long waiting periods were involved and people of many languages and cultures became distressed and antagonistic'.

A major change came with the treatment of children with thalassemia who were given preference to go into the Special Clinic rather than the Casualty area or the General Clinic.[16]

Dr John Hurst, an experienced general practitioner and Head of the Department, assisted by Sisters Jane Altmann and Valerie Duke in Triage, had, by 1971, succeeded in building a harmonious staff. When he left in 1978, Dr Frank Oberklaid returned with fresh ideas from the position of Fellow in Ambulatory and Community Paediatrics at the Boston Children's Medical Centre where he had specialised in learning difficulties and early childhood development. In 1983, Pam Forsyth was appointed as Nurse-in-Charge of Ambulatory Paediatrics.

The term 'Ambulatory Paediatrics' arose out of the need to differentiate between emergencies and general non-emergency clinical medicine. A programme of education of common childhood illnesses was organised for general practitioners,

Michelle Meehan, RCH Maternal and Child Health Nurse, 1980s.

medical students and nurses, and other community health providers. The local government and state schools, community service providers, pre-school teachers, community health nurses, schools and school medical services, early childhood development programmes, allied health workers, maternal and child health nurses and youth workers all benefited from the rotating programme.

Paediatric Emergency separated from Ambulatory Paediatrics in the mid-1990s. Dr Simon Young and Jan Goudge ran this department. Ambulatory Paediatrics became the Centre for Community Child Health.

Child development received a sharper focus from health professionals. Family function and parent effectiveness could often be assessed at early stages through family counselling and other simple strategies. Community houses and liaison with Maternal and Child Health Services could prevent family breakdown due to isolation and lack of information about community services.

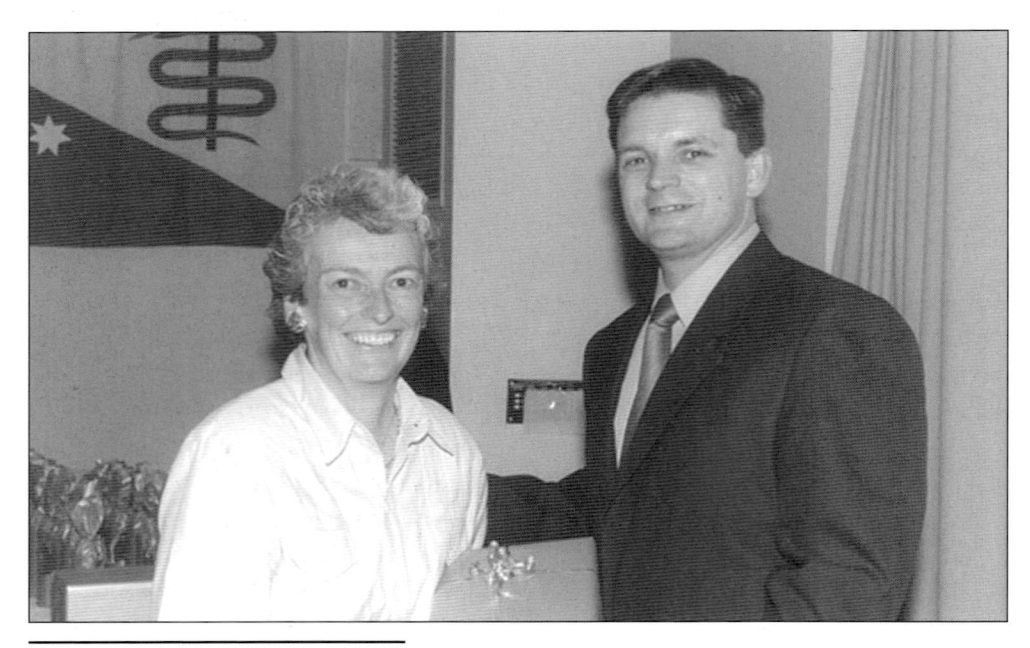

Julia McCoy (RCH 1973), Care Manager for Children and Families for fifth floor Medical, being presented with her 25 years Long Service Award by Phillip Goulding (RCH 1987), Consumer Engagement Officer, 2003.
Photo: Julia McCoy

The general practitioner paediatric training programme of the 1980s was co-ordinated by Dr Geoff Debelle who visited as a paediatric consultant to school medical programmes and early childhood development programmes in the city, suburbs and country Victoria.

The opening of the multi-disciplinary Gatehouse Centre culminated in the Child Protection Unit, co-ordinated by Karen Hogan and headed by Dr Alan Carmichael. Psychotherapist Eileen Anderson, various paediatric assistants and seven social workers worked at the centre, a landmark in services for families in crisis.

Adolescent nursing

The initial mandate of the Children's Hospital was to provide care for babies over two years and young children. At that time, childhood was thought to cease at the age of thirteen or fourteen, the usual age of leaving school. These children were then regarded as adults and their medical conditions were treated in adult hospitals.

By the mid-twentieth century, views of the continuum of human growth and maturation included the adolescent years, when children became known as 'teenagers'. While children with disabilities were cared for at the Frankston Orthopaedic Hospital, others suffering chronic diseases such as asthma, diabetes, cystic fibrosis, neurological disorders and cerebral palsy and complex psychiatric conditions were followed up throughout their adolescence at the Children's Hospital clinics. Improved treatments and the greater survival rate of children from once fatal diseases and disabilities showed that increasing numbers were accommodated in the Hospital side by side with babies and young children. In recognition of the special needs of this age group, an Adolescent Unit was established in Ward 3 East in 1984 within the Department of Developmental Paediatrics.

A series of community consultations with health service providers, schools, the Juvenile Justice Health Service and community services gave the necessary support for a co-operative approach to youth health. A community health nurse who had previously worked in a student health service in America[17] assisted Dr John Court in establishing a referral centre for young people with complex health problems.

For the administration of intravenous antibiotics, the use of long-lines and porta-caths increases the patient's mobility. The focus is to educate the adolescent about their own health care needs and to encourage them to take responsibility for it. CHIPS (Chronic Illness Peer Support) has been established and assists adolescents to understand specific issues related to their needs. The general philosophy is one of normalisation while in hospital, peer group activities, education for personal responsibility and support for those with chronic illness.[18]

The trained nursing staff in the unit combines informality with discipline. Among the nurses who helped build this successful department were Trish Morton, Donna Eade and Robyn Smith.

The Department of Child Development and Rehabilitation

In the 1960s, the crippling diseases of childhood, such as polio and tuberculosis, were almost totally eradicated. A large percentage of children at the Frankston Orthopaedic Hospital suffered from congenital abnormalities: spina bifida, cerebral palsy and muscular dystrophy.

When Frankston closed in 1969, these children were cared for at the Children's through out-patients clinics and, in 1970, the Handicapped Children's Centre was established under the direction of Dr Keys Smith. The function of this centre was to co-ordinate the needs of the children through multi-disciplinary assessment, as in-patients and out-patients; the provision of splints and appliances; and community liaison in the education of carers and teachers, aides and parents as to the needs of the children with multiple disabilities. The Cerebral Palsy Clinic under the leadership of Dr Gooch remained independent until 1979.

To meet the needs and the plethora of treatments for these children required a very large number of specialists from the medical, nursing and allied health professions. Many parents spent days, sometimes months, moving around from one appointment to another in hospitals, clinics and community centres.

The care of children with such diverse needs culminated in 1979 with the establishment of a centralised place of their own, the Chapman Street house in North Melbourne, renovated with the assistance of the Uncle Bobs Club under the directorship of Dr John Court. Since the early days of the Handicapped Children's Centre, new drugs and surgical techniques have improved the life chances and comfort of these children and the well-being and happiness of their parents.

Throughout the 1970s, increased awareness of the rights of people with disabilities led to campaigns towards de-institutionalisation, normalisation and integration. When legislation was enacted for the rights of the disabled, culminating in the *Disabilities Act 1986*, theoretically, this meant that children with disabilities would now be included into mainstream services, schools and kindergartens. For parents with children with profound disabilities, moving out of institutions and nursing homes into mainstream services was a severe test.

In 1987, the Year of the Disabled, in recognition of the specialised nursing needs of children with disabilities and their families, a clinical nursing appointment was created at the Children's Hospital to link the families with Hospital and home, to co-ordinate services and follow-up systems. The Handicapped Children's Centre was renamed the Child Development and Rehabilitation Centre under the direction of Dr Dinah Reddihough and, in that year, Bev Touzel, a Children's Hospital-trained nurse, was appointed to the position of Clinical Nurse Consultant, Developmental Disabilities, later re-classified to the position of Clinical Nurse Consultant, Developmental Disabilities, Child Development and Rehabilitation.

In support of the principles of de-institutionalisation, nurses employed in nursing homes such as Yooralla, Rosine and Moira were replaced by support workers.

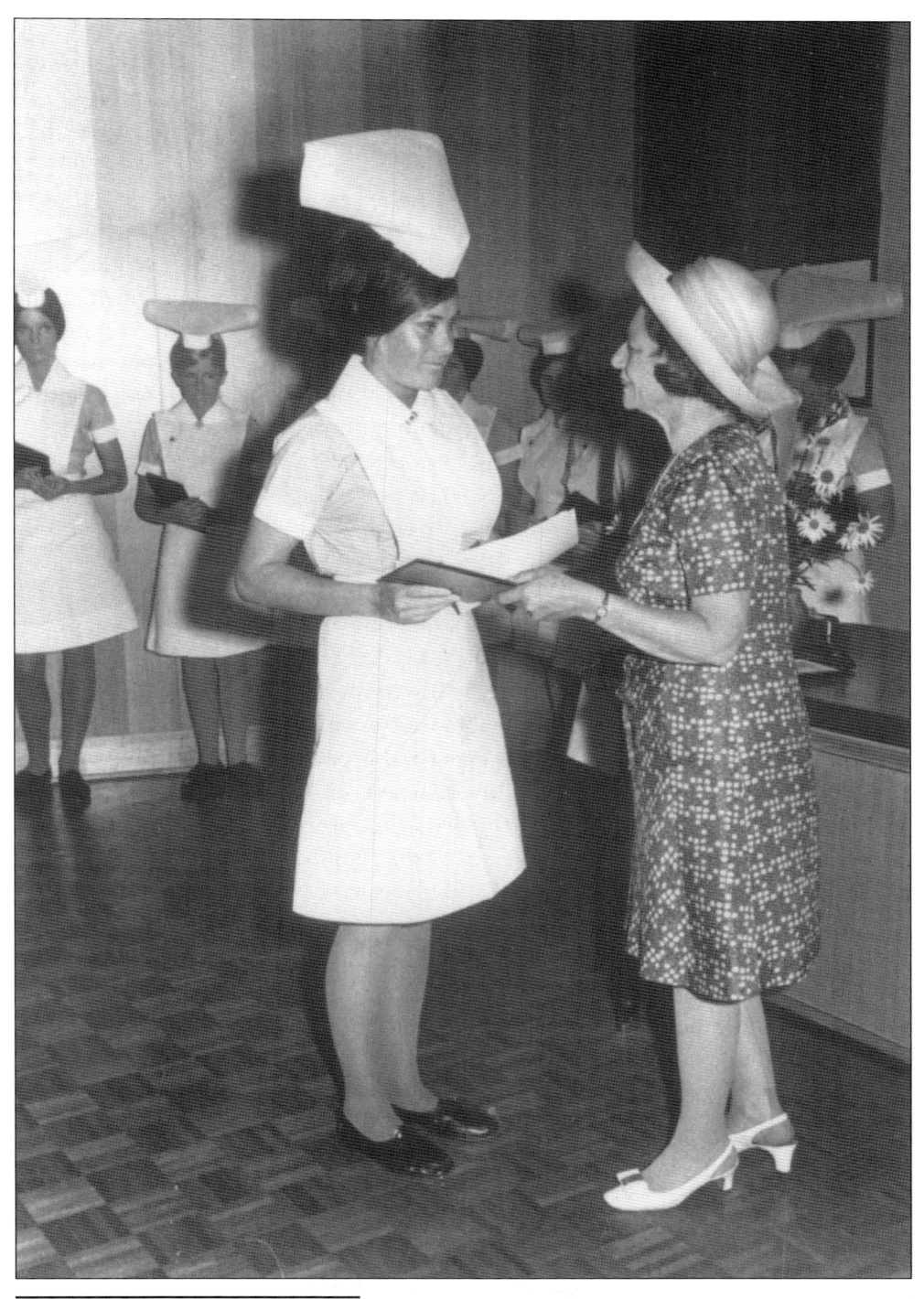

Dame Patricia Mackinnon presents Bev Thorne with the Margaret Adams Prize, 1969.

This resulted in changes in community nursing expertise in the area of disability. While changes in de-institutionalisation were occurring, the growth in scientific knowledge and technical ability was moving rapidly. Thanks to modern medical techniques and services, infants and children with severe disabilities who previously would have died, are now living and growing into adolescents and young adults. In addition to their disabilities, many of these children have associated medical problems that require the services of highly experienced and educated nurses. Children with profound disabilities are totally dependent on others for all aspects of their care. It is not unusual for children to receive their nutrition through gastrostomy tubes and to be administered rectal valium at home.

The majority of children with whom Bev Touzel is involved have cerebral palsy, of the type known as spastic paraplegia, and in addition to being in a wheelchair, they may have intellectual disabilities, epilepsy, scoliosis, hearing and vision impairments, and an inability to communicate verbally. They often have recurrent chest infections, failure to thrive, chronic constipation and social and psychological problems and require tube feeding and oxygen and suction apparatus to maintain them at home. Nurses in the Hospital find the care of these children complex and challenging and they work with families and the community to provide a high standard of nursing care as in-patients and out-patients. Families are more involved in decision-making and more aware of their rights. They seek the best care possible to enable their children to live at home in a supportive environment.

In meeting and adapting to these needs, the nurses and health care workers require not only specialised nursing expertise, but also the ability to critically consider the moral aspects of decision-making. As Bev soon realised, 'these skills encourage reflective thinking with regard to duties and obligations to those entrusted to their care'.[19]

BEV TOUZEL (née Thorne) RCH 1965–68, BA (App. Sci.) Adv. Nursing (La Trobe). MA (BioEth), (Monash), FRCNA.

Winner of the Margaret Adams Prize, October 1969.

Clinical Nurse Consultant, Developmental Disabilities. Royal Children's Hospital 1987 to present.

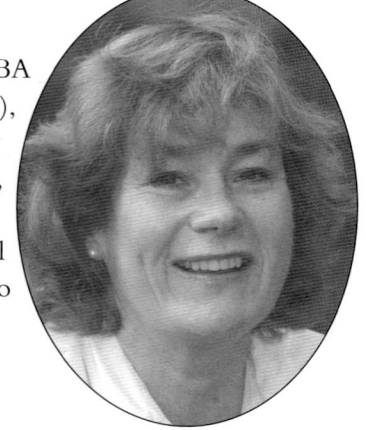

Orthopaedic nursing

Nurses of orthopaedic patients have a constant need to update their knowledge of technology as more major surgical cases are dealt with in the wards instead of ICU. Many procedures involve automatic equipment, for example, the delivery of intravenous fluids, and nurses have to know how to deal with it. There has been a revolution in the treatment of children with scoliosis. No longer do children have halo traction and, with the insertion of Harrington rods, the need for plaster jackets has been eliminated. Modern nurses have allocated specific patients, from admission to discharge; there are no juniors and seniors. Two of the notable nurses in modern orthopaedic nursing have been Cathy Oxnam and Jo Fraunfelder.

The shorter stays and increased turnover, greater parental involvement and increased availability of equipment for home use—for example, car seats for children with congenital dislocated hips—requires a greater use of community resources. These are accessed through Bev Touzel, who liaises with Special Development Schools and organises home help for parents. Children who have undergone spinal surgery now return home with bath trolleys and, after six months, wear hexalite jackets; previously they had a six to nine-month stay and plaster of paris jackets. Those with dislocated hips have less time in traction, resulting in shorter hospitalisation.

A most remarkable development in the Orthopaedic Ward has been the decrease in the numbers of children with spina bifida. The intake of folic acid during early pregnancy has proved to be a triumph for community education and prevention of spina bifida. However, this is offset by an increase in the number of children with cerebral palsy as babies survive prematurity. The result is heavier nursing, requiring increased staff numbers.

The high profile of children with disabilities was largely achieved through the Association for Children with a Disability (formerly the Action Group for Disabled Children), which researched the specific needs of these children. This resulted in raising awareness of this special group of patients in the community. Today, there is much greater involvement of parents through lobbying and a greater awareness of parental needs and follow-up in their children's care. The use of resources such as information pamphlets in the Safety Centre has raised community knowledge.[20]

Cathy Oxnam, 1970s.

Nursing Research Unit (Centre for Studies in Paediatric Nursing)

In 1990, the Centre for Studies in Paediatric Nursing (CSPN) was established at the Royal Children's Hospital with the aim of fostering the development of participatory action research projects among staff.

The establishment of the CSPN was a response to concerns expressed by the senior staff that changes in hospitals had been related to administration and that clinical nursing practice and support of changes was neglected.

Headed by Dr Annette Street, two clinical Nurse Educators, Jeanine Blackford and Andrew Robinson, were seconded from Wards 7 West and 3 West to become Clinical Nurse researchers. Their research focussed on clinical nurse practice, finding out what they did, how they did it, and if they could do it better. However, the CSPN was forced to close in 1993 because of budget cuts.

The aims of the CSPN were to better understand the needs of children and their families, to engage nurses in research and to teach nurses how to conduct research methods suitable to their needs.

As a result of a 1993 paper, 'Moving Towards Empowerment' by Jeanine Blackford and the nursing staff, many changes were made to nursing practice. These related to breast-feeding, resuscitation methods, pain management and the use of pacemakers in children. Andrew Robinson began working at the Royal Children's Hospital at the CSPN for Wards 3 West–3 East and was seconded in 1990 as a clinical researcher. The nursing staff looked at developing effective discharge teaching methods to assist children with orthopaedic conditions when parents expressed a view that support out of Hospital was negligible. The staff also worked on the needs of children with disabilities.

Jeanine Blackford started work at the RCH in 1978 and held a number of positions including Clinical Nurse Teacher for Ward 7 West from 1984. She was seconded to the CSPN in 1990 as a clinical researcher. Sue Pullar was employed in 1990 as the teacher for the critical care nursing programme.

Conclusion

The policies and practices of parental access to their children in hospital have changed a great deal. Parents are much more aware of their rights and accept the need to stay with their child as a normal process. Very few parents these days leave their child alone in hospital.

Some of the most commonly diagnosed diseases where the care and education of parents are essential are cystic fibrosis and diabetes. For these parents, and for those of premature babies, the nurses are on hand night and day to boost their confidence and abilities.

The last thirty years have been notable for the increasing demands in parental accommodation. While at the modern Parkville Hospital, breast-feeding mothers were generally accommodated on the tenth floor, and other parents stayed in Gatehouse Street or slept in the wards. For country parents, accommodation was essential but not always available. Anne Maree Teasdale was one mother who was fortunate enough to be provided with accommodation in the 1970s. On a Saturday in Wodonga, in June 1977, Anne Maree and her husband, Kevin, were enjoying a birthday party for their little daughter, when their four-month-old son, James, became desperately ill. Within the hour, he was in great distress, screaming and drawing up his little legs, his face white and tense. The surgeon at the Albury Base Hospital diagnosed intussusception and referred him to the surgeon, Mr Nate Myers, at the Royal Children's Hospital. The air ambulance was alerted but unfortunately the weather closed in and the baby was transported by road, requiring a police escort through country towns. When they finally arrived, Mr Myers was waiting at the Emergency entrance, 'arms out-stretched'. Anne Maree was whisked up to the tenth floor and made comfortable. Fortunately, she had relatives in proximity to the RCH and stayed there for several weeks. There were difficult times ahead, but after an initial relapse, their baby did well.[21]

Parental presence has obvious benefits: the trauma of parent–child separation is eliminated; even siblings can stay during the day. The unit offers parent education and support, and parents can get adequate rest knowing they can be contacted if necessary. Today, there is a motel-style unit in the front building where parents can stay. Parents from the country who require accommodation for longer periods may stay at the Ronald McDonald sponsored accommodation in Gatehouse Street.

In the 1980s, the Royal Children's Hospital expanded to 500 beds and became a general acute paediatric hospital and paediatric referral centre for Victoria, southern New South Wales, South Australia and Tasmania. Today, the Hospital is the childhood cancer centre for Victoria.

Until 1987, the RCH was a facility for undergraduate nursing education for 1,086 nurses. The Committee of Management determined that, due to changes in requirements for the basic programme, it was not appropriate to continue a general nursing education in a specialist institution. With the closure of the last School in General Nursing in October 1987, negotiations took place with the Victorian Health Department to determine the range of postgraduate and continuing education nursing programmes.

Epilogue

The 125th Annual General Meeting of the Royal Children's Hospital held at the Regent Hotel in Melbourne in 1995 was a significant occasion, marking five generations of care by the Hospital and its people.

In that year, Jan Bell, a registered nurse with a Diploma of Applied Science (Administration), succeeded Mary Patten as Director of Nursing. She was the tenth person to occupy the position, formerly known as Matron, at the Hospital.

The structure she inherited was very different to the previous ones. She was, in effect, an executive member of the Women's and Children's Health Care Network, an amalgamation of the Royal Women's and the Royal Children's Hospitals, which took place on 1 August 1995. The mission of the Network was to improve women's and children's health, to empower staff through a team approach and to put into effect a decentralised management system.

Many people claimed, as they did when the Nursing School closed, that it would never work because the Royal Women's and the Royal Children's were two very different institutions. In 1999/2000, senior qualified nurses were appointed to important positions at the Royal Children's as Divisional Directors, Nursing. These were: Ms Christine Minogue, Community Division; Ms Lucy Cuddihy, Specialist Services; Mr Sean Spencer, Division of Medicine; Mr Phillip Goulding, Division of Surgery; and Ms Chris Best, Division of Neonatal Services. At the Sunshine Hospital, Ms Karen Gibson was appointed to the Division of Obstetric and Gynaecological Services and the Division of Child and Adolescent Services.

There have been many administrative changes in the ten years of the Network. Professor Glenn Bowes, appointed General Manager in 2000, stated that the 'focus is community and teamwork. Health organisations and providers had to have a capacity to respond to rapid and at times unforeseen changes in the health needs and expectations of their communities.'[1]

A new structure of hospital governance was introduced throughout the Victorian public hospital system in 2000 and the Network became Women's and Children' Health (WCH). In 2004, the Women's and Children's Hospitals once more became separate entities. In 2005, the cycle continues with the appointment of an Executive Director of Nursing at the Royal Children's Hospital: Ms Jenni Jarvis, formerly of Westmead Children's Hospital.

Epilogue

The Mackinnon School of Nursing continues its long tradition of excellence, offering education for all levels of nursing staff. The main programmes within the school include a graduate nurse programme for an annual intake of sixty new graduates. There are three educators employed in a full-time capacity and eight clinical facilitators in most wards as clinical support persons throughout the Hospital.

The expectation is that nurses will provide evidence they can achieve set standards in cardio-pulmonary resuscitation, drug awareness assessment and recognition of the sick child. Competency-based learning packages are also available for staff in particular clinical procedures, such as epidural pain relief and patient-controlled analgesia. Computer training is available to Hospital staff. The graduate nurse programme remains a major focus for nurse recruitment and supports registered nurses during their first year in the profession.

The Paediatric Education Centre is an innovative unit within the School of Nursing offering education not only to nurses but also to health care professionals and community groups throughout Victoria. Members of staff additionally assist nurses from other countries to develop and implement paediatric nursing programmes as part of the Royal Children's Hospital International.

All postgraduate nursing education—a child health stream and a paediatric intensive care nursing stream—is conducted through the University of Melbourne. Lectures and educational sessions take place at the Mackinnon School of Nursing, and students rotate through several areas of the hospital for their clinical experience, facilitated by nine Nurse Educators from the University of Melbourne. Nurse Educators and clinical nurses who have joint appointments with the University provide clinical support.[2]

Notes

PART 1 1870–1900
1: FOUNDATION OF A CHILDREN'S HOSPITAL
1   Grace Jennings Carmichael, *Hospital Children: Stories of Life in the Children's Hospital*, George Robertson, Melbourne, 1891, p. 57.
2   Ibid., Ch. 10: 'Night Duty', p. 59.
3   Ibid., Ch. 1: 'A Day in the Wards', p. 5.
4   Ibid., Ch. 10: 'Night Duty', p. 61.
5   *Cyclopaedia of Victoria*, Report of the Founding of the Free Hospital for Sick Children, Melbourne, 1902, p. 428.
6   John Singleton MD, *A Narrative of Incidents in the Eventful Life of a Physician*, Melbourne, 1891, pp. 213–14.
7   Committee of Management minutes, 9 September 1870.
8   *Australian Dictionary of Biography*, Vol. 6: 1851–1890, Bede Nairn (ed.) pp. 129–30.
9   K. F. Russell, *The Melbourne Medical School 1862–1962*, MUP, 1977, p. 47.
10 Geoffrey Serle, *The Rush to be Rich*, Prologue: 'The Years Between 1861–1882', MUP, 1971.
11 Bryan Gandevia, *Tears Often Shed: Child Health and Wealth in Australia*, Pergamon Press, 1976, Ch. 10, p. 79.
12 Ibid., Ch. 10, pp. 79, 82.
13 Annual Report, 1876.
14 Gandevia, *Tears Often Shed*, Ch. 12, p. 104.
15 *Centenary of Nurse Training in Australia 1862–1962*, Royal Women's Hospital, Melbourne, 1962, p. 2 The catastrophic outbreak of puerperal fever at King's College Hospital, London, in 1867, influenced Nightingale's attitude to women and children in hospital; from that date on, she had nothing further to do with midwifery or children. Significantly, the Women's Hospital in Melbourne ceased taking children from 1868.
16 Florence Nightingale, *Notes on Nursing*, first edn 1858, edn consulted: Blackie & Son, Glasgow and London, 1974.
17 *Australian Medical Journal*, 1873, p. 49. From an address against a children's hospital, by Dr Fetherston, President of the Medical Society.
18 By 1901, only thirteen in one hundred women were in nursing, teaching or government and professional services, compared to forty per hundred who remained in personal services as maids and around thirty per hundred in factory work. Tony Dingle, *The Victorians: Settling*, Fairfax, Syme and Weldon, 1984, p. 167.
19 For example, the gin-soaked monthly nurse Sairey Gamp in *Martin Chuzzlewit* by Charles Dickens, 1843.
20 Personal family history known to the author.
21 Singleton, *A Narrative of Incidents*, pp. 213–14.

22 Minutes, 14 November 1870.
23 Andrew Brown-May, *Melbourne Street Life: the Itinerary of Our Days*, Australian Scholarly Publishing, 1992, pp. 107–11.
24 Minutes, 18 September 1871. It was common for straw mattresses to be burnt, particularly during epidemics of diphtheria and typhoid.
25 Jacqueline Templeton, *Prince Henry's: The Evolution of a Hospital*, Robertson and Mullins, 1969, Ch. 12.
26 William Smith, 'On Inter-Cranial Syphiloma', *Australian Medical Journal*, January 1871.
27 *The Centenary of Nurse Training in Australia 1862–1961*, p. 2.
28 Charles West, *How to Nurse Sick Children,* London, 1854. This book was widely read and predated Florence Nightingale's *Notes on Nursing* by five years. Miss Nightingale acknowledged a debt to Dr West's ideas on the hospital care of children. For a critique see: Victor Skretkowicz, *Florence Nightingale, Notes on Nursing*, Scutari Press, 1992. Royal College of Nursing, Great Britain. Acknowledgement: Mr Nicholas Baldwin, archivist at Great Ormond Street Hospital, London, for providing me with access to view the rare original edition of Dr West's *How to Nurse Sick Children*.

2: THE DAWN OF PROFESSIONALISM
1 Rose Vaughan, *Notes on Nursing.* Series 'A' 1886, RCH Archives.
2 Grace Jennings Carmichael, *Hospital Children: Stories of Life in the Children's Hospital*, George Robertson, 1891, pp. 76, 77.
3 Charles D. Hunter, *What Kills Our Babies? A Guide to the Care of Infants*, Health Society, Melbourne, 1878.
4 William Snowball suffered ill health for some years and died on 22 April 1902 at the age of forty-seven at his country home, 'Narracan', near Thorpedale in Gippsland. He left five children: the youngest, Katherine (Kitty), was four years old, the eldest, Jack, fifteen. His wife Maria survived him by only two years. His sons Jack and Eric were killed in World War One, and the remaining son, Tom, succumbed from illness and injuries during World War Two. Katherine was cared for by her guardian, Dorothea Esther Vernon, a former Children's Hospital nurse, at her home in Kew.
5 Minutes, 20 November, 5 March 1879.
6 Annual Report, 1879.
7 Extensive research at the Royal Hobart Hospital Archives has not revealed the presence of Mrs Bellaine. She may have been registered under her maiden name but archival records were destroyed in a fire following a typhoid epidemic in the late 1880s. I wish to acknowledge Cheryl Norris, University of Tasmania School of Nursing, for assistance in this research.
8 Minutes, 19 October 1881.
9 Carmichael, *Hospital Children*, p. 79.
10 Ibid., p. 67.
11 From Dr William Snowball's Casebook 42 studies 1885–87, RCH Archives.
12 Minutes, 25 October 1876.
13 Minutes, 26 May 1888.
14 Carmichael, *Hospital Children*, p. 49.
15 *Report of the Royal Commission into Charitable Institutions 1890*, Minutes of Evidence, PP, LA, Vic. 1892–93 no. 7295 (Bishop).
16 Minutes, 27 April 1887.

Notes

17 Minutes, 21 September 1898.
18 Anthea Hyslop, *Sovereign Remedies: A History of Ballarat Base Hospital 1850s to 1980s*, Allen & Unwin, 1989, pp. 46, 92–101.
19 Details for Sarah Bishop and her son Tom Charles Bishop are from Melbourne General Cemetery Records, MGC TT316. For family details see: Register of Deaths in the District of Bacchus Marsh, Victoria, No. 8389: Tom Bishop died on 13 August 1916. For entry to Australia, see: PRO Victoria, Unassisted Shipping Index of Inward Passenger Lists for British and Foreign Ports 1852–99, Sarah Bishop, Ship: *Champion of the Seas*, March 1857. Shortly before her death, Sarah Bishop managed a hotel for her son in Essendon.
20 Minutes, 29 September 1880.
21 Minutes, 20 February 1878. Buckley of Buckley & Nunn, a rich businessman. Both Mr and Mrs Buckley were on the Committee.
22 Carmichael, *Hospital Children*, p. 54.
23 Main sources of information are the Orbost Historical Society, Mrs Pauline Carmichael Fitzgerald and Mrs Rosemary Cooper, grand-daughters of Grace Jennings Carmichael.
24 *Poems by Grace Jennings Carmichael*, Longmans Green and Co., London, 1895, first edn. In possession of Margaret McInnes, poem: 'Spray of Gippsland Wattle', p. 104.
25 Minutes, 18 December 1889.
26 Minutes, 20 October 1886.
27 Minutes, 30 April 1890. All letters, notes and Minutes (18 December 1889) relating to this matter are in the RCH Archives. Also see: *The Royal Commission into Charitable Institutions 1890*. Martelli, p. 493. 6523.
28 Information from Sally Snowball Rowe, grand-daughter of William Snowball.
29 Carmichael, *Hospital Children*, p. 53.

3: A GROWING WORKFORCE
1   For a full account of Lady Brassey's activities see Marguerite Hancock, *Colonial Consorts: The Wives of Victoria's Governors 1839–1900*, Ch. 11: 'Sybil, Lady Brassey', pp. 226–7.
2   Minutes, 27 November 1895.
3   Minutes, 27 September 1899. Annual Report, 30 June 1900.
4   Grace Jennings Carmichael, *Hospital Children: Stories of Life in the Children's Hospital*, George Robertson, 1891, pp. 53–4.
5   Registers: 16 January 1891–93 to 3 May 1891. One hundred nurses 1897 to 1907. RCH Archives.
6   Children's Hospitals established in Australia: Melbourne (1870), Adelaide (1876), Brisbane (1877).
7   Letter from a subscriber to the *Age*, 6 February 1897.
8   Minutes, 25 March 1896.
9   *Australian Dictionary of Biography*, Vol. 3: 1891–1939, p. 93.
10 For a full description of her career see: Jan Bassett, *Guns and Brooches: The History of Australian Army Nursing from the Boer War to the Gulf War*, OUP, 1992, pp. 53–4. Image from *UNA*, Nurses' Journal, Jubilee Issue 195.
11 Minutes, 11 May 1892.
12 Minutes, 20 April, 11 May 1892.

13 *Australasian Nurses' Journal*, November 1944.
14 Minutes, 7 February 1894.
15 Bassett, *Guns and Brooches*, p. 12.
16 Peter Lempriere interviewed by Margaret McInnes for information about his mother, 1995. Image from David Lempriere Collection.
17 *Just Wanted To Be There: Australian Service Nurses 1899–1999*, Commonwealth of Australia. Ch. 1, p. 13.
18 R. L. Wallace, 'Victorian Nurses in Bulawayo during the Anglo-Boer War', in *The Australians at the Boer War*, Australian War Memorial & AGPS, Canberra, 1976, pp. 249–50.
19 Minutes, 4 August 1897.
20 Minutes, 4 August 1897, 8 September 1897.
21 Annual Report, 1894.
22 Minutes, 22 April 1896.
23 Minutes, 6 September, 1899.
24 *Australian Medical Journal*, New Series Vol. 2, June 1880, p. 274; and New Series Vol. 2, October 1880, pp. 468–70. Also, for an analysis of the ambivalent attitude of the medical profession, see: R. Trembath and D. Hellier, *All Care and Responsibility: A History of Nursing in Victoria 1850–1934*, Florence Nightingale Committee, 1987.
25 *J. K. Watson MD: Edinburgh House Surgeon, Essex and Colchester Hospitals.* n.d.; preface dated 1899, London Scientific Press Ltd, Strand WC, RCH Archives.
26 Minutes, 9 March 1898.
27 Carmichael, *Hospital Children*, 'Special Nursing', p. 71.
28 Annual Report, 1899.
29 Annual Report, 1902.
30 Trembath and Hellier, *All Care and Responsibility*, Ch. 1, p. 11.
31 Royal Commission on Charitable Institutions 6523, 6527, 1890, p. 493.
32 Robert Murray Smith, 'The Children's Hospital: Its Early Life', in Joshua Lake (ed.), *Childhood In Bud and Blossom: The Souvenir Book of the Children's Hospital Bazaar*, Atlas Press, Melbourne, 1900.
33 'Two Visits: A Tale with a Sting' by Mr Punch of Fleet Street, London, in Lake (ed.), *Childhood in Bud and Blossom*.
34 Ian J. Wood (ed.), *A. Jeffreys Wood: Discovery and Healing in Peace and War* (an autobiography edited by Ian J. Wood, son of A. J. Wood), self-published, 1984.
35 Minutes, 25 August 1897.
36 Minutes, 5 June 1893.
37 From the Constance Mary Murray, personal papers held in the RCH Archives.

PART 2   1900–1924
4:   THE YEARS OF MISS PLAYER
1   Edith Dircksey Cowan, MLA, (1861–1932), was the first Australian woman to enter Parliament.
2   Cheryl D. Crocket, *Save the Babies: The Victorian Baby Health Centre's Association and the Queen Elizabeth Centre—The First 83 Years*, Ch. 1, p. 1. Infant mortality was virtually unchanged from the nineteenth century to 1917. More than 8 per cent died within the first year, and in the poor inner suburbs, the chances of an infant's surviving decreased.

NOTES

3   *UNA*, Nurses' Journal, 20 August 1904, p. 83.
4   D. G. Hamilton, *Hand in Hand: The Story of the Royal Alexandra Hospital for Children, Sydney*, John Ferguson, Sydney, 1979, Ch. 3, p. 48.
5   The name of the Australian Nurses Journal, *UNA*, was suggested by its editor of many years, Dr Felix Meyer. It was taken from a famous English poem by Edmund Spenser (1552–99), 'The Faery Queen', in which Una was the lovely lady of the Red Cross Knight who took her wounded lord to a hospital. There, he was nursed back to strength. The motto 'Lenire Dolentum' was adopted by UNA, the official organ of the ATNA, which was set up in 1903. Reference: *UNA Nursing Journal Jubilee Issue, Royal Victorian College of Nursing, 1901–1951*.
6   Elizabeth Lomax, *Small and Special: Development of Hospitals for Children in Victorian Britain*, London, 1996, Ch. 3, pp. 64–5.
7   See R. Trembath and D. Hellier, *All Care and Responsibility: A History of Nursing in Victoria 1850–1934*, Florence Nightingale Committee, 1987, pp. 20, 21.
8   Peter Yule, *The Royal Children's Hospital: A History of Faith, Science and Love*, Halstead Press, 1999, Ch. 2, p. 147.
9   Interview with Mary Wilson by Margaret McInnes and Bronwyn Hewitt, 1993. Transcript and tapes in the RCH Archives.
10   Lyndsay Gardiner, *Royal Children's Hospital 1870–1970*, Chapter X, 102, p. 3.
11   Minutes, 20 May 1909.
12   Minutes, 24 April 1913.
13   Howard Boyd Graham, 'Beacons on Our Way: Some Memoirs of the Children's Hospital', *MJA*, 3 October 1953.
14   Obituary: Hamilton Russell in *UNA*, Nurses' Journal, 1933.
15   Mary Grant Bruce, 'The Least of These Little Ones. Out-Patients', in *The Woman*, Vol. 2, June 28, No. 10, 1909.
16   Trembath and Hellier, *All Care and Responsibility*.
17   For *Nurses' Registration Act 1923*, and various Amendment Bills see Trembath and Hellier, *All Care and Responsibility*. Also, RCH Minutes and Annual Reports.
18   Minutes, 8 October, 1914.
19   Minutes, 28 August 1918.
20   Minutes, 17 May 1917.

5: THE WAR YEARS

1   For the full impact and a social analysis of Australian Nurses in World War One, see Jan Bassett, *The Home Front*, MUP, 1983, p. 45. Also: Jan Bassett, *Guns and Brooches. Australian Army Nursing From the Boer War to the Gulf War*, OUP, 1992, Ch. 3.
2   *Just Wanted to Be There: Australian Service Nurses 1899–1999*, Commonwealth of Australia, 1999, p. 3.
3   Minutes, 10 December 1914. Dr Richard Herbert Joseph (Bertie) Fetherston 1864–1943, GP Prahran, Honorary Women's Hospital (son of Dr Gerald and Mrs Sarah (née Harvey) Fetherston), Women's Hospital, MLA, 1921, BMA (Vic) Pres. 1911, Victoria Militia, 1887, Director General Medical Services Army World War One, August 1914. Based at Melbourne Headquarters initially. F. M. C. Forster, *Australian Dictionary of Biography*, Vol. 8: 1891–1939.
4   Minutes, 1 July 1915. A register of RCH nurses who served in World War One is available in the RCH Archives.

5. Information from her son, David Lempriere. In possession of the author.
6. Bassett, *Guns and Brooches*, Ch. 2, p. 34.
7. John Reid in *Australian Dictionary of Biography*, Bede Nairn (ed.), Vol. 8: 1891–1939, p. 93.
8. No records of nurses under Evelyn Conyers' command are contained in the Archives of the Australian War Museum, Canberra. It has been widely speculated that she did not wish returned nurses to be hampered in their civilian life about events over which they had no control. Many stories handed down also concern fraternisation with servicemen, something that was forbidden, and in at least one case caused demobilisation to Australia.
9. A list of plaques, foundation stones and honour rolls is at the RCH Archives. The list was compiled before the old Hospital was vacated. All of the memorials have been lost or destroyed.
10. *UNA*, Nurses' Journal, Vol. XXI, No. 5, 1 July 1923, p. 85.
11. Minutes, 31 August 1916.
12. From notes by Hilda Lindsay, 'Early Days, World War 1, 1915–1918', RCH Archives.
13. *Herald*, 6 August 1913.
14. Minutes, 10 August 1911.
15. Minutes, 14 December 1911.
16. Minutes, 10 April 1913.
17. Minutes, 20 January 1916.
18. Lindsay notes, 'Early Days'.
19. Minutes, 28 October 1915.
20. Minutes, 4 February 1915.
21. Mary Wilson interviewed by Margaret McInnes and Bronwyn Hewitt, 10 March 1994.
22. From interview notes with Mary Wilson.
23. Minutes, 20 January 1916.
24. Minutes, 10 August 1911.
25. Until the sulphonamides (M&B) came into use during World War Two, it was nearly always fatal in children. In 1944, penicillin was used with some success.
26. *Medical Journal of Australia*, 13 November 1915.
27. Lindsay notes, 'Early Days'.
28. When Kernig's sign is present, it is impossible to extend the leg at the knee joint when the thigh is extended on the abdomen. It is present in the various forms of meningitis.
29. *Age*, 14 October 1915.
30. *Argus*, 13 October 1915.
31. Minutes, 27 July 1916.
32. Minutes, 16 September 1915. Research shows that Hilda Lindsay was a diphtheria carrier.
33. J. H. L. Cumpston, *Influenza and Maritime Quarantine in Australia*, Melbourne, 1919. In November 1918, the Committee advised that the nurses were to be vaccinated against influenza and in January the Children's Hospital Secretary, Mr R. J. Love, was requisitioned by the Australian Government in regard to equipping all Melbourne hospitals to cope with the emergency. Minutes, 28 November 1918 and 30 January 1919.

NOTES

6: WAR NURSES RETURN

1. *Age*, 15 May 1918.
2. Dr W. A. Wood, *Congenital Syphilis and its Prevention*, undated, RCH Archives.
3. Annual Report, 1918.
4. Interview with Jean Hardham by Audrey Grant, 25 January 2000.
5. Information supplied by correspondent (anonymous), 2000.
6. Robert James Love was educated at Scotch College (1898) and took up banking. In 1901 he joined the clerical staff of the Children's Hospital. His exceptional ability in fundraising and in administration quickly earned him promotion to Secretary, and eventually to the first position as Superintendent. In 1922, he was selected by the State Government to be the first Inspector of Charities, a powerful position. Following a trip overseas to study hospital management, he made recommendations to the government for sweeping reforms in all hospital departments. He was influential in the establishment of the allied health industry, particularly occupational health, physiotherapy and dietetics, and recommended massive expansion of nursing and the Nurses' Home at the Children's Hospital. His ideas ultimately improved hospital practice. He became Inspector of Charities (Vic.) in 1923 and was head-hunted to the New South Wales Government in 1925. By then he was reputed to be earning £1,000 at the Children's Hospital; the NSW Government offered him £1,500. He was one of the most brilliant administrators of his day. Acknowledgement: Joyce Druitt (née Lowry), Children's Hospital nurse, 1933–37, niece of R. J. Love (Uncle Jim). Her two cousins were also Children's Hospital nurses: Ivy and Zell (Hazel) Love.
7. Minutes, 30 January 1919.
8. Minutes, 15 May 1919.
9. A. P. Derham, 'Notes on Pneumonic Influenza' with special reference to the epidemic, *Medical Journal of Australia*, 25 January 1919.
10. Notes by Hilda Lindsay, 'Early Days, World War 1, 1915–1918'. Notes in possession of the author.
11. Related to the author by her mother, Alice Lillian Mitchell (née Brown), who remembers as a small child being taken with her mother and carried into the Exhibition Building.
12. W. Hobson (ed.), *The Theory and Practice of Public Health*, Oxford, 1969, 'Influenza', p. 171; Humphrey McQueen, 'Spanish Flu 1919: Political and Social Aspects', *Medical Journal of Australia*, Vol. 1, 1975, p. 565.
13. *Herald*, 3 October 1918.
14. Minutes, 6 January 1921.
15. *Australian Dictionary of Biography*, 1891–1939, pp. 522, 523; *UNA*, Nurses' Journal, January 1957, pp. 4, 5.
16. Minutes, 7 April to 28 July 1921.
17. Minutes, 9 March 1922.
18. Ibid.
19. *Age*, 27 March 1922, 30 March 1922. Newspaper file, RCH.
20. From notes by Nancy McNeil, daughter of Ella McNeil, 2000. In possession of the author.
21. Notes on the meetings of LOFT are in the Sister's Meetings Minutes notebook held in the RCH Archives.

PART 3 *1924–1947*
7: BETWEEN THE WARS
1   Isabel Pilkington, 'Nursing Training at the Children's Hospital, 1932', unpublished notes, 1986. RCH Archives.
2   Patricia May Thorburn, 'My Best Foot Forward, 1923–1932', undated manuscript, pp. 1–15. Copy in possession of the author. Acknowledgement: Margaret Adams (daughter of Patricia Thorburn), Ferndale, WA.
3   Marjorie Allnatt interviewed by Dr Howard Williams, October 1986. Transcript and tape in RCH Archives.
4   Jeanette Pollock interviewed by Howard Williams, 1987. Transcript in the RCH Archives.
5   Marjorie Allnatt interviewed by Howard Williams, 1986.
6   Una Wishart interviewed by Margaret McInnes, May 2002.
7   'A Nurse's Memorial', *UNA*, Nurses' Journal, 1 November 1923, Vol. XXI, p. 179.
8   Minutes, 21 October 1937.
9   Willis Questionnaire, November 2000. This original questionnaire was designed by Sandy Willis and sent out in October 2000. The questionnaires were sent Australia wide and internationally. There was a very satisfactory response. Initially, 33 per cent of 350 replied but more responses came in the following months and sometimes years later. Some, where practical, were followed up with interviews. Many respondents sent supporting letters, memorabilia and photos.
10 Marjorie Allnatt interview, 1986.
11 Notes by Sheila Ferguson (née Gray), 1936–39, 'Anecdotes from Training Days at RCH', undated manuscript. In possession of the author.
12 Contribution by Elizabeth (Betty) Sadlier Chalmers, 2001. In possession of the author.
13 Annual Report, 1938.
14 Interview with Elizabeth Jaffray by Margaret McInnes, Canberra, February 2001. Reginald Webster was Chief Pathologist 1914–47, and the brother of Sister Katherine (Kit) Webster, the Home Sister.
15 Minutes, 19 February 1925.
16 Marjorie Allnatt interviewed by Dr Howard Williams, 1986.
17 Isabel Pilkington, notes, 1996.
18 Jean Hardham interviewed by Audrey Grant, January 2000. Unpublished manuscript. Copy in possession of the author.
19 Jane Widgett Aicheson interviewed by Howard Williams, 1987. Transcript and tape in RCH Archives.
20 Jane Widgett Aicheson interview.
21 Jean Hardham interviewed by Audrey Grant, January 2000.
22 Hope Clarke Ingamells interviewed by Dr Howard Williams, November 1986. Transcript and tape in the RCH Archives.
23 Joyce Druitt interviewed by Margaret McInnes, 22 January 2003.
24 Jeanette Pollock interviewed by Dr Howard Williams, 1987.
25 Jane Aitheson interviewed by Howard Williams, 1987.
26 Gladys McLintock, 'Notes on Nursing', Book 1, February 1927, unpublished, RCH Archives.
27 Annual Report, 1922–23. Dr J. W. Grieve.
28 'Manpower' was created in July 1939 as a compulsory National Register of all males

aged between eighteen and sixty-four. Its purpose was to provide statistics of the labour available in Australia, so as to prevent too many essential workers entering the Armed Forces. By July 1941 more women were being recruited to Manpower and essential industries were restricted.
29   Isabel Pilkington interview, 1987.
30   Ibid.
31   Minutes, 7 January 1926. Also *Victorian Parliamentary Papers* (VPP) 1926, No. 23.
32   From notes in possession of the author, 1955.
33   Sheila Ferguson, 'Anecdotes', undated.

8:   NURSING DISABLED CHILDREN
1   Annual Reports, 1920–39. The number of nurses was never recorded accurately until after World War Two. From the mid-1930s, nursing assistants were employed in the Branches.
2   Bon Winstanley, 'Nursing Days at the Old Children's Hospital', unpublished, 2004. In possession of the author.
3   Today the property is the Mt Eliza Complex for the Aged.
4   *Argus*, 11 April 1930.
5   Notes from the Willis questionnaire, Mary Brodribb, November 2000.
6   Minutes, 20 February 1936; also see notes by Elaine Orr, 1992 Ward Sister Frankston Orthopaedic Hospital 1948–63, Matron 1963–68.
7   Minutes, 19 October 1933, 26 September 1934.
8   Margaret Warr, 'Other People's Children', unpublished, 1986. In possession of the author.
9   Minutes, 14 December 1933.
10   Inez Ferguson interviewed by Margaret McInnes, 26 July 2002. Tape and transcript with the author.
11   Study carried out by R. Webster, Pathologist, during the war, showed that one in three adults visiting the children most likely had a primary tuberculous lesion.
12   Minutes, 13 July 1939.
13   Minutes, 28 October 1937. Dr Douglas Galbraith 1894–1984. Medical Superintendent, Frankston Orthopaedic Hospital, 1935–40, 1948–60. Dr Galbraith was a Scot born in England. He studied at Glasgow and in 1925 became Out-patients physician at the Children's Hospital. After his appointment at Frankston as Medical Director in 1935, he chose as his life work rehabilitation of crippled children. Galbraith had outstanding administration skills and was Chief Rehabilitation Officer to the Australian Army during World War Two.
14   Minutes, 5 March 1936.
15   Anonymous.
16   Minutes, 17 October 1935. These children were 'at risk' from renal calculus.
17   Inez Ferguson interviewed by Margaret McInnes, July 2002.
18   Peg Orford interviewed by Margaret McInnes, July 2000.
19   Una Wishart interviewed by Howard Williams, 27 July 1987. Tape and transcript RCH Archives.
20   Una Wishart interview, 1987.
21   *Just Wanted to be There: Australian Service Nurses 1899–1999*, Commonwealth of Australia, 1999, Annie Ina Laidlaw, p. 72.

22   Manning Clark, *The Quest for Grace*, Viking, 1990, p. 45.
23   Children's Hospital nurses were not accepted interstate until after 1939, when they began a rotation to the Royal Melbourne Hospital.
24   Thyra Thomas (née Watson) and Eleanor Moss (née Peck) were interviewed by Margaret McInnes, 24 January 2000.
25   All reports more than fifty years old of the former Health Department Victoria, Poliomyelitis Division, are at Public Record Office Victoria (PROV).
26   Minutes, 12 November 1936.
27   Warr, 'Other People's Children'.
28   La Trobe Australian Manuscripts Collection, State Library of Victoria.

9:   THE YEARS OF WORLD WAR TWO
1   Committee of Management Minutes, 8 December 1938.
2   Isabel Pilkington, 'Nursing Training at the Children's Hospital from 1932', unpublished.
3   Special Emergency Committee Minutes, 4 September 1939.
4   It was known that German raiders were cruising in Australian waters and Bass Strait very early in 1940.
5   Pilkington, 'Nursing Training', p. 9.
6   Committee of Management Minutes, 1 & 15 December 1938; Annual Report, 30 June 1940; *Nurses' Registration Act*.
7   Letter dated 5 February 2000 from Noel Holcombe (née Heley, RCH 1940–43). In possession of the author.
8   Margaret Warr, 'Other People's Children', 1986, unpublished, Ch. 'The Training Years'.
9   Information provided by Jean Hackett, November 2000.
10   Various Sub-committee Reports, 1938–48, Catalogue No. 80/81.
11   Committee of Management Minutes, 18 December 1941.
12   Special Emergency Committee Minutes, 29 September 1939.
13   Committee of Management Minutes, 4 September 1939.
14   Debra Tout-Smith, 'The History of Burnham Beeches', unpublished manuscript, 1992, p. 57. Mr C. L. McVilly, Inspector of Charities, had also written to G. J. Coles congratulating him on his recent honour bestowed by the King. Letter from C. L. McVilly to G. J. Coles Esq., 2 January 1942, PROV series 423/R1, Box 129, file 1240.
15   Tout-Smith, 'The History of Burnham Beeches', p. 57.
16   Ibid.
17   *Argus*, 15 January 1942.
18   Committee of Management Minutes, 15 January 1942.
19   Interview with Una Wishart, May 2001.
20   Notes provided by Jean Maxwell Barton, August 2004.
21   Notes provided by Nancy Furnell (née Heane), November 2000.
22   Information provided by Beryl Sparks (née Jago), November 2000.
23   Information provided by Alice Charles (née Andrew), November 2000.
24   May & Baker sulphapyridine 693, sulphathiazole 760, and sulphanilamide 125 were the forerunners of antibiotics.
25   Notes provided by Nancy Furnell, 13 November 2000. In possession of the author.
26   Notes provided by Margaret Rogers, November 2000.
27   Information from Jean Maxwell Barton, August 2004.

NOTES

28 Interview with Peg Orford, July 2000.
29 Notes provided by Olive Raymond, August 2000.
30 Una Wishart interviewed by Howard Williams, 27 July 1987.
31 Ivy Flower interviewed by Howard Williams, 1987. Tape and transcript in RCH Archives.
32 Interview with Audrey Bult and Margaret Hosking, September 2004.
33 Notes supplied by Esme Nixon, 16 November 2000.
34 Peg Orford, Willis questionnaire, November 2000.
35 Procedure notes provided by Olive Raymond, 'Day Duties Ward 17', 2000.
36 APC: aceto-salicyclic acid, phenacetin and caffeine, commonly known as aspirin.
37 Peg Orford interview, July 2000.
38 Douglas Hay Scott, Mildred Hainsworth (Tutor Sister, Hospital for Sick Children, Great Ormond Street), *Modern Professional Nursing*, Caxton Publishing, London, first edn 1930, Vol. IV, Section xii, Ch. 3, 'Management of the Child in Health and Disease', 1950 edition. General Editor: Mildred Hainsworth. Acknowledgement: Donation of nursing text books: Valerie Boardman (RCH 1951–55).
39 Pilkington, 'Nursing Training'.
40 All extracts from various Minute Books, 1938–48, Catalogue no. 80/81.
41 Jan Bassett, *Guns and Brooches: Australian Army Nursing from the Boer War to the Gulf War*, OUP, 1992, Ch. 6: 'Coming or Going', p. 112.
42 Allan S. Walker (medical ed.), *Australian Encyclopaedia*, 'World War Two', Vol. 9, pp. 485–6.
43 Betty Westland (née Jeffrey). Married (1) Jack Thompson and (2) Jim Westland. Information provided from the *Packenham Gazette*, Wednesday 2 October 1991. Betty Westland 1913–91. Also Allan S. Walker, *Australia in the War 1939–1945*, Series 5, medical, Vol. 4, 'Medical Services in the RAN and the RAAF: Women in the Army Medical Services', Australian War Memorial, Canberra, 1961.
44 Maureen Minchin, *Revolutions and Rosewater: The Evolution of Nurse Registration in Victoria 1923–1973* (commissioned by the Victorian Nursing Council), Hart Hamer, 1974, p. 40.
45 Interview with Una Wishart, May 2001. Notes provided by Marjorie Tomlinson, OAM, November 2000. Hilda Wash turned sixty in August 1944.
46 Bassett, *Guns and Brooches*, p. 113.
47 Jean Hardham interviewed by Audrey Grant, January 2000.
48 Letter from Isabel Pilkington to Margaret McInnes, 1997.
49 Acknowledgement: by permission of the Newman Morris family, LOFT, Obituary, Lady Newman Morris, 1911–2003. Newsletter, July 2003, Margaret McInnes (ed.).
50 *Herald Sun*, 12 July 2003.
51 From notes by Margaret Rogers to Margaret McInnes, October 2004.
52 Letter from Isabel Pilkington to Margaret McInnes, 1997.
53 Interview with Kate Menzies, October 2001. Notes with kind permission of Janet Leckie (née Menzies). Image from the Menzies Family Collection.
54 *Age*, 10 November 2000, 'A Time to Reflect' by Chris Johnston.
55 Information provided by Joan Wills, Hon. Secretary, Ex-RAAF Nursing Service, 30 November 1996, RCH Archives.
56 Sisters' Minute book, 1950–60, RCH Archives.
57 *Age*, Catherine Margaret Mackenzie. Catherine died on 10 February 2005. Obituary,

1 April 2005. Information from Lucy Mackenzie to Margaret McInnes, 2004–05. Image from the Mackenzie Family Collection.
58 Sheila Krysz (née Mackenzie), Willis questionnaire, July 2001.
59 Information from Judith Lanyon, 22 November 2000.
60 Notes from Marjorie Tomlinson, February 2001.
61 Letter from Esme Nixon, 16 November 2000.
62 Peg Orford, Willis questionnaire, November 2000.
63 Letter from Esme Nixon, 16 November 2000.

PART 4 1947–1962
10: A NEW ERA
1 *Age*, 9 April 1947.
2 Joyce Druitt interviewed by Margaret McInnes, 22 January 2001. Miss Walsh was about sixty when she retired from the Children's Hospital.
3 Dame Elisabeth Murdoch interviewed by Audrey Grant, 30 April 2001. Transcript and tape with the author.
4 Miss Wilson trained as a Mothercraft Nurse at the Presbyterian Babies' Home and completed her General training at the Children's and the Epworth Hospitals in 1937. She remained at the Children's until 1946 with a short break to undertake Midwifery at the Women's Hospital in 1940. In 1947, Miss Wilson undertook a special course in Tuberculosis Nursing at the Austin Hospital and travelled to Canada to observe and work in the Mountain Sanatorium, Hamilton, Ontario. On return to Melbourne, she conducted two courses in Tuberculosis Nursing at the Repatriation Hospital, Heidelberg. From July 1949 to February 1961 she was Senior Sister Tutor at the Children's Hospital. Miss Wilson served on the Victorian Nursing Councils examiner panels for General Nursing (1945–76) and the Nursing Aide Training Committee (from the 1950s to 1976). In 1973, she served on the special Advisory Committee set up by the Whitlam Government to report on all aspects of the care of the aged. In 1968 Miss Wilson became the principal Nurse Educator at Mount Royal Special Hospital for the Aged. She died in 1978.
5 Sophie Brodie was educated at Presbyterian Ladies College and trained at the Children's Hospital 1932–35. She held the positions of Acting Matron of the Victorian Baby Health Centre Association (VBHC) 1945–46; Assistant Matron at the Royal Children's Hospital 1949–52; Matron of the Orthopaedic Section 1952–62 and Principal of the Melbourne Nursing Aide School 1962–67. As a member of the Hospital Matrons Association 1955–75, Miss Brodie appeared on many panels, working committees and examiners representing nursing aides. She died in 1981.
6 Marjorie Green (née Allnatt) trained at the Children's Hospital 1933–37 and gained further experience in the United Kingdom in 1939 as a certified 'Pupil Housekeeper' at Great Ormond Street Children's Hospital in London and as a Child Health Visitor for Wales. On her return to the Children's Hospital, she became Miss Walsh's personal assistant, then tutor in the Preliminary Training School. Her influence spanned a generation of student nurses, many of whom later filled distinguished nursing roles throughout Australia.
7 Dame Elisabeth Murdoch interviewed by Audrey Grant, 30 April 2001.
8 *Australian Dictionary of Biography*, 1940–1980, Lyndsay Gardiner, p. 613. Lucy Sechiari (née Walmsley) married Gerald Alexander Auguste Sechiari on 1 July 1937, at the

Notes

Registry Office, Westminster. This marriage did not last. On January 1953, at Scots Church in Melbourne, she married Josef Anton De Neeve, a Dutch national working as an airlines liaison officer to an Australian airline company. She became active on the Nurses' Board of Victoria (1950–59) and the Royal Victorian College of Nursing (Vice-President 1950–59; President 1959–61) She resigned from the RCH in 1962, and conducted a Nurse Bank Agency for semi-retired nurses from her home in Rathdowne Street, Carlton. She retired to Bali where she died on 19 July 1976.

9. Dame Patricia Mackinnon was interviewed by Margaret McInnes, 5 March 2001. Tape and transcript with the author.
10. Committee of Management Minutes, 10 July 1947. Information provided by Barbara Curwen-Walker.
11. Valerie Duke interview with Howard Williams, 8 December 1987.
12. Mary Hoy, Willis questionnaire, November 2001.
13. Margaret Playfair interviewed by Howard Williams, 27 November 1987. Transcript in RCH Archives.
14. Information provided by Marg Hosking, 16 September 2004.
15. Notes provided by Diana Ramsey, November 2001.
16. Letter from Elizabeth Sadlier to Margaret McInnes, 26 November 2000.
17. Annual Report 1949. Report of the Lady Superintendent, Lucy Sechiari.
18. Contribution from Lorraine Doney and Willis questionnaire, 2002.
19. Isabel Pilkington Baltvilks, secretary to Mrs Sechiari 1949–50, letter to Margaret McInnes, 1997.
20. Nancy Castellan, letter to Margaret McInnes, October 2004.
21. Elizabeth Coombes interviewed by Howard Williams, 27 August 1986. Transcript in the RCH Archives.
22. Jean Cussen, letter to Margaret McInnes, December 2000.
23. Audrey Grant, Willis questionnaire notes, November 2000.
24. From Dr Howard Williams' collection, RCH Archives.
25. Mildred Hainsworth (ed.), *Modern Professional Nursing*, Caxton Publishing, 1950, Vol. 3, 'Tapping–Southey's Tubes', p. 53.
26. Judith Butt (Lady Court) interviewed by Howard Williams, 1987.
27. Personal information from Mr Nate Myers.
28. Kate Harden interviewed by Howard Williams, 16 November 1987. Tape and transcript in the RCH Archives.
29. Barbara Catto interviewed by Margaret McInnes, 13 September 2004.
30. Enid Ingpen, Willis questionnaire, November 2000.
31. Elizabeth Hocking, Willis questionnaire, November 2000.
32. Nancy Hardy (née Hurst), interview with Margaret McInnes, February 2003.
33. From Willis questionnaires circulated among nursing staff who worked with Mr Wakefield in the 1950s.
34. Logan Bow, a type of metal butterfly clip.
35. From Nursing Lecture Notes, Royal Children's Hospital, 1951–55. Provided by Valerie Boardman; H. Douglas Stephens, 'Hare, Lip and Cleft Palate Pre-operation and Post-operation', *UNA, Nurses' Journal*, 1 December 1947, p. 377.
36. Notes by Audrey Grant (née Laugher), RCH 1948–52, November 2000.
37. Notes from Barbara Sutherland (née Clifford), November 2000, RCH 1947–50, A. Jeffreys Wood Gold Medallist 1950, Sister Ward 10 1950s.

38   Jennifer Adam (née Hall), RCH 1956–60, Willis questionnaire, November 2000. Many nurses have agreed with these observations.
39   Personal communication, August 2003.
40   Elizabeth Coombs interview with Howard Williams, 27 August 1986.
41   Phil Thomas (née Richey), RCH 1947–53, letter to Margaret McInnes, 29 June 2000.
42   Notes by Audrey Grant, November 2000.
43   Anonymous.
44   Gwen Coventry, Willis questionnaire, November 2000.
45   Nurses' work record book, 1955, RCH Archives.
46   Nancy Jacobs, Willis questionnaire, November 2000.
47   Notes from Peg Bellair, July 2003.
48   Jane Altmann, Willis questionnaire, November 2000.
49   Ibid.
50   Patricia Pex (née Grieve) interviewed by Margaret McInnes, 29 November 2001.
51   Betty Luke, Willis questionnaire, November 2000.
52   VPP 1951, Vol. 2, Hospital and Charities Commission Report, 30 June, p. 8.
53   Annual Report, Royal Melbourne Hospital, Medical Superintendent's Report, Dr J. H. Lindell, 1945/46; Norman J. Marshall, *The Melbourne School of Nursing, 1950–1963*, The Melbourne School of Nursing Past Trainees Association, 1985.
54   Annual Report, 1954–55, Report of the Lady Superintendent.

PART 5   *1963–1987*
11:   A NEW HOSPITAL

1   Dr John Perry succeeded Dr Vernon Collins in 1960 as Medical Director and Lucy De Neeve's position was restructured from Lady Superintendent of the Hospital to 'Director of Nursing'. This has been interpreted as a deliberate undermining of her considerable influence with the Committee of Management and was a factor in her resignation. She was fifty-eight years old, her financial situation fragile. Superannuation for women was introduced in 1962 and Lucy De Neeve was not offered permanency until 1958. She resigned in May 1962 and stayed on until October—fifteen years to the day.
2   Information from Nance Gooderham (1960–64), Willis questionnaire, November 2000.
3   Elizabeth Coombs interviewed by Howard Williams, 27 August 1987.
4   Elizabeth Jaffray interviewed by Margaret McInnes, January 2001.
5   V. M. Duke (Floor Supervisor, RCH), 'The Perfect Ward' in *UNA*, Nursing Journal, Vol. XIII, June 1965, pp. 185–7.
6   Information from Chris Fautley, Willis questionnaire notes, November 2000.
7   Annual Reports of the Medical Director, Dr John Perry and Joan Gendle, Director of Nursing, 1963.
8   After completing Midwifery at Queen Victoria Hospital and the Infant Welfare Certificate at the Presbyterian Babies' Home in Melbourne, Joan Gendle travelled to Birmingham, England, where she gained the Premature Babies' Certificate. She acquired a Diploma of Nursing Administration at the College of Nursing, Australia. Her career continued with many prestigious posts: Administration Sister at RCH, Ward Sister at Queen Victoria Hospital Children's Ward, and Ward Sister at the King George V Hospital, Sydney. For many years, she was the Theatre Staff Nurse in charge

NOTES

at Great Ormond Street Hospital, London. On her return to Australia, she became Deputy Director of Nursing at Frankston Orthopaedic Hospital, spent seven years as Director of Nursing at Epworth Hospital and was also Matron of the Albury Base Hospital. She retired in 1977.

9 Annual Report of the Director of Nursing, 1963.
10 Elizabeth Fearon interviewed by Howard Williams, 16 July 1987.
11 Dame Patricia MacKinnon interviewed by Margaret McInnes, February 2001.
12 The operation was pioneered by Dr W. Mustard in Toronto, Canada, in 1962.
13 Notes 2001, Anonymous.
14 Willis questionnaire notes, Anne Hardham (née Coventry), November 2000, and interviewed by Margaret McInnes, April 2001. Transcript with the author.
15 Willis questionnaire notes from Dale Craigie (née Hogg), 2001.
16 Peter Yule, Ch. 25: 'Burns Unit and Safety Centre', in *The Royal Children's Hospital: A History of Faith, Science and Love*, Halstead Press, 1999, p. 443.
17 John R. Solomon, 'Paediatric Burns', in *Symposium on Burns: Critical Care Clinics*, Vol 1, No. 1, March 1985.
18 Interview with M. Thomson by Howard Williams, 10 December 1987.
19 Notes from Laurens Dubourg to Margaret McInnes, November 2004. Marge Thompson completed her midwifery at Royal Women's Hospital and, after a stint of four years as a Nurse Tutor, became Charge Sister in Neurosurgery for ten years. She studied computer science at RMIT and began the process of computer storage and retrieval of nursing and patient records. She also put together a nursing *Procedure Manual*, later revised and used to this day. She retired in 1988.
20 Interview with M. Thompson and Joan Gendle by Howard Williams, 10 December 1987, 14 July 1987. Transcripts in the RCH Archives.
21 M. Thomson interview, 1987.
22 Joan Gendle interview, 14 July 1987.
23 Information from Chris Fautley, Willis questionnaire, November 2000.
24 Information from Diana Anceschi, Willis questionnaire, November 2000.
25 Anne Bryan interviewed by Margaret McInnes, 16 November 2004.
26 From an interview by Peter Yule with Mayne Bodycomb (between 1995 and 1997).
27 Committee of Management Minutes, 10 July & 9 October 1958.
28 Minutes, 13 June 1968.
29 Informant wishes to remain anonymous.
30 Anne Hardham interviewed by Margaret McInnes, 31 March 2003. Transcript with the author.
31 Minutes, 7 March & 4 April 1963.
32 The Martin Committee: a federal enquiry into technical education opened the way towards federal funding of basic nursing education. It had become clear to nursing leaders that, if there was to be any major shift from hospital to college education, it would have to come from federal level. For Pat Slater and her colleagues, this was the only way nursing could be brought up to the level of the professions like law and medicine, which enjoyed prestige and status in Australian society. To be united was to have strength, while to have many different systems weakened the cause, the dual system of hospital and college education (as occurred in NSW) was to be abolished. See B. Bessant & J. Bessant, *The Growth of a Profession: Nursing in Victoria 1930s–1980s*, La Trobe University Press, 1991, p. 164.

33   More details in Bessant & Bessant, *The Growth of a Profession*. See also Report of the Committee to the Australian Universities Commission (Martin Report), *The Future of Tertiary Education in Australia*, 2 vols, 1964; Report of the Committee (Ramsey Report), *Nursing in Victoria*, 1970; Report of the Committee of Enquiry to the Tertiary Education Committee (Sax Report), *Nurse Education and Training*, Canberra, 1978.
34   Minutes, 9 July 1964.
35   Willis questionnaire notes, Kathy Smith (née Purcell), 2001.
36   Dr Kestor Brown interviewed by Margaret McInnes, 16 November 2004. Notes with the author.
37   From information received through 350 questionnaires circulated by RCH LOFT, August–November 2000.
38   Notes, Anonymous 2001.
39   Anonymous.
40   Jo Van Valen interviewed by Margaret McInnes, 3 December 2004.
41   *Age*, 'Vietnam War Nurses Fight for Recognition', by Mary-anne Toy, 1 May 1999.
42   *UNA*, Nursing Journal, Vol. LVIV, November 1961, pp. 336–41.
43   Minutes, June to September 1965.
44   Annual Report, 1969. Report of the Medical Director, Dr L. E. G. Sloan.

12: INTENSIVE CARE AND THEATRE NURSING

1   I wish to acknowledge Lucy Cuddihy, Heather Telfer, Doris Flett and Elizabeth Jaffray for talks and notes on ICU, NNICU and other matters discussed in this chapter.
2   Tracheotomy is the operation of opening by incision into the trachea (the windpipe) to prevent asphyxiation in diphtheria and other conditions. The formation of the opening with insertion of a tracheotomy tube, through which the patient breathes, is nowadays commonly called a tracheostomy. Until the 1960s, nurses commonly referred to this as a tracheotomy.
3   Arthur Jeffreys Wood MD, 'Intubation in Laryngeal Diphtheria: Three Case Studies' in *The Australian Medical Journal*, April 1982.
4   Chevalier Jackson of Pittsburgh (b. 1865) in *History of Medicine* by Arturo Castiglioni (*Storia Della Medicina*, first edn Milan 1941), Alfred A. Knopf, USA second edn, 1946, p. 867. Jackson perfected methods of penetrating various remote body cavities so that lesions or foreign bodies could be seen and removed.
5   Doris Flett has written extensively about the history of endotracheal intubation and tracheostomy. The background to the development of the ICU has been researched in conjunction with Doris Flett, Heather Telfer, Elizabeth Jaffray and Louise Blewett.
6   Elizabeth Jaffray, Assistant DON at Woden Valley Hospital, ACT, 1974; Boston Children's Hospital and Duke University Hospital, Durham, USA, 1959–60; Sister-in-Charge, Ward 9 Surgical Children's Hospital, Melbourne, 1960–63; Nursing Supervisor of the ICU/RR, RCH Melbourne 1963–73; DON Woden Valley Hospital, ACT, 1979, until her retirement in 1988. Member of the Institute of Nursing Administration of NSW and the ACT, 1980.
7   Information from the late Mr Nate Myers, 2003.
8   Notes on the development of Nursing in ICU, Royal Children's Hospital Melbourne, are attributed to Doris Flett in conjunction with Elizabeth Jaffray, March 2005. Documents with the author. Doris Flett and Elizabeth Jaffray were interviewed by Margaret McInnes, Canberra, January 2001.

Notes

9   Doris Flett, notes, March 2005.
10   Eileen Morton, Willis questionnaire, November 2000, and further information provided in May 2005.
11   Doris Flett, notes.
12   Ibid.
13   I. H. MacDonald and J. G. Stocks 'Prolonged Nasotracheal Intubation: A Review of its Development in a Paediatric Hospital', *British Journal of Anaesthesia*, 1965, Article 37, p. 164.
14   Doris Flett interviewed by Margaret McInnes, January 2002. Notes by Doris Flett, February 2005, in possession of the author.
15   Acknowledgement: RCH Newsletter, 15 October 2003.
16   Annual Reports 1964, 1972, 1992.
17   Peter Yule, *The Royal Children's Hospital: A History of Faith, Science and Love*, Halstead Press, 1999, p. 480.
18   Dorothy Saunders was born in Bendigo in 1910 of Scottish ancestry. She moved to Melbourne with her parents and completed her education at Firbank, Church of England Girls Grammar School (CEGGS. She began nurse training at the Children's Hospital, including six months in the Surgical Department at the Women's Hospital—a requirement for general registration of Children's nurses at that time. Generations of trainees, doctors and medical students admired 'Dottie', as she was known, for her calm competency. For thirty years she managed a department with deteriorating equipment in dilapidated, obsolete buildings, through the years of World War Two, and the lead-up to the new Hospital at Parkville. She retired in 1974 and died on 1 September 1997.
19   Notes from Anne Bryan (née Holden), November 2004; trained RCH 1967–70. Interview with Margaret McInnes, 19 October 2004. Willis questionnaire, November 2000.
20   Acknowledgement: this information came from Judith Smith, March 2005 (trained RCH 1977–80).
21   Notes from an interview with Siok Chew by Peter Yule, 1997. In possession of author.

13:    TRANSITION TO TERTIARY EDUCATION
1   Anne Hardham interviewed by Margaret McInnes, 31 March 2003. Transcript with the author.
2   From Elaine Orr's notes, 1988. Dr Howard Williams collection, RCH Archives.
3   Obituaries from the *Age*, 17 October 1996 and *Herald Sun*, 9 October 1996. Also, Elaine Orr's notes, 1988. Miss Orr died in Melbourne on 30 September 1996, at the age of seventy-three.
4   From Miss Orr's personal notes, accompanying the interview with Dr Howard Williams, 1985. Elaine Orr was the eldest of eleven children and felt an enormous loyalty to the education of her siblings.
5   Handwritten notes by Elaine Orr, undated. The notes accompany the interview with Howard Williams. Tape and transcript, 24 June 1985 are in the RCH Archives.
6   Dame Patricia Mackinnon interview with Margaret McInnes, 25 March 2001. Notes with the author.
7   Peter Yule, *The Royal Children's Hospital: A History of Faith, Science and Love*, Halstead Press, 1999, p. 415. From an interview with Murray Clarke by Peter Yule, 27 March 1998.

8   Elaine Orr notes, 1988.
9   Information supplied by Heather Telfer, December 2004.
10 Committee of Management Minutes, 18 May 1967. The Uncle Bobs Club was formed in the 1940s by a benevolent group of men who donated a 'bob' from their weekly pay packets for the children of Frankston Orthopaedic Hospital. The fund grew into travelling grants for doctors to pursue research in overseas countries and, in the 1960s, widened to include trained nurses and allied health professionals. Physiotherapists also became eligible for the fund nearly twenty years after it began.
11 Elaine Orr, notes.
12 Personal communication with Heather Telfer, April 2005.
13 John Bowlby, *Maternal Care and Mental Health*, WHO Public Health Papers, No. 14, Geneva, Columbia University Press, 1951; John Bowlby, *Child Care and the Growth of Love*, Pelican, 1953; John Bowlby, *Attachment and Loss*, Vol. 1, 1969.
14 Dr Robert Birrell OAM, from an interview with Margaret McInnes, 10 August 2004.
15 Lola Stokes (née Cumber) interviewed by Margaret McInnes, 1 May 2003.
16 Dr Sidney Sax, Head of the Social Welfare Policy Secretariat, Canberra. Report presented to the Tertiary Education Committee, Federal Government, August 1978.
17 *Who's Who in Victoria*, 2001. Mary Patten died on 13 November 2004.
18 From an interview with Mary Patten by Margaret McInnes, December 2003.
19 Fay Marles, Commissioner for Equal Opportunity. Fay Marles, *Study of Professional Issues in Nursing* to the Victorian Health Minister, February 1988.
20 Information from Heather Telfer, February 2005.
21 Information from Anne Vintiadis, 4 July 2004.
22 The Nursing School was named in 1985 in recognition of the contribution played by three generations of the Mackinnon family: Lady Lauchlan (Emily) Mackinnon, Committee of Management, 1883–1922; her daughter-in-law, Mrs Lauchlan (Hilda) Mackinnon, Vice-President and President, 1922–33; and her daughter-in-law, Mrs Alistair (Patricia) Mackinnon, later Dame Patricia, Committee of Management 1948, President 1965–79.
23 Letter from Laurence Dubourg to Margaret McInnes, November 2004.

14: SPECIAL NURSING
1   Annual Reports, 1970s–1980.
2   Annual Reports, 1970–80. Annual Report of the Acting Medical Director, Dr Keys Smith, 1977.
3   Janette McEwan interviewed by Margaret McInnes, 6 July 2004. For a full account of the development of the cardiac unit, see Peter Yule, *The Royal Children's Hospital: A History of Faith, Science and Love*, Halstead Press, 1999, pp. 454–7.
4   Anne Shipp interviewed by Margaret McInnes, 18 February 2004.
5   Wendy Swift died at the age of fifty, in 1996.
6   Reminiscences by Laurence Dubourg to Margaret McInnes, December 2004.
7   I am indebted to Laurence Dubourg for her extensive notes on her years in the Neuroscience Ward at the RCH. December 2004. Notes with the author.
8   Laurence Dubourg, notes, June 2005.
9   Notes by Mary McGowan to Margaret McInnes, July 2004. Notes with the author
10 Ros Willis trained at Launceston General Hospital, 1959–62. 1963: Midwifery, Camperdown Woman's Hospital, NSW; 1964–66: Private children's nurse, London;

NOTES

1967: Launceston General Hospital Children's and Babies Ward; 1968: Relieving Charge Sister, Camperdown Children's Hospital NSW; 1969–90: Charge Sister RCH, 8 West/4 West, General Surgery–Urology.

11 Hirschsprung's Disease, after Harold Hirschsprung, a Danish paediatrician: characterised by dilatation and hypertrophy of the bowel, usually the colon. First described in 1886, and found in modern times to be due to congenital absence of the nerve cells.
12 Hypospadias: the commonest congenital malformation of the urethra, occurring in one out of 350 males.
13 'Zeitschrift fur Kinderchirurgre' in the *Paediatric Medical Journal of Scandinavia*, 44 Supp. 1 Dec. 1989, pp. 46–7. *Nursing Journal of Australia*, 1989.
14 Dr Howard Williams interviewed by Margaret McInnes, November 1994.
15 Aileen O'Donnell interviewed by Margaret McInnes, April 2005.
16 Aileen O'Donnell interviewed by Howard Williams, 31 August 1987.
17 It is not known who the Community Health Nurse was.
18 From notes provided by Robyn Smith. Notes with the author.
19 From an interview and notes provided by Bev Touzel, 10 February 2005. Notes with the author.
20 Notes from research for the *Mini History RCH 1975–1995*, edited by Nate Myers, published by Educational Resource Centre, RCH, 1995.
21 Anne Maree and Kevin Teasdale interviewed by Margaret McInnes, March 2003.

EPILOGUE
1 Annual Report, 2000/01.
2 Acknowledgement: Dr Maurice Hennessy, Mackinnon School of Nursing.

Appendix 1

PRIZE WINNERS

CHAIRMAN'S MEDAL
(formerly President's Medal, first awarded 1987)

NURSING

1988	Heather Telfer (President's Medal)
1989	Paula Horka
1992	Doris Milliken
	Wendy Swift
1993	Mary McGowan
	Claire Collins
1994	Wendy Neilson
1995	Mary Patten
1996	Rosa Bradilovic
	Jan Bell
1998	Lucy Cuddihy
2000	Judith Smith
2001	Geraldine McDonnell
2002	Peter Tyler (Mackinnon School of Nursing)
2003	Louise Blewett
	Christine Minogue

MARGARET ADAMS PRIZE

The Margaret Adams Memorial Fund is a Trust established by members of the Royal Children's Hospital League of Former Trainees. The purpose of the Fund is to perpetuate the memory of Margaret Adams.

Formerly, a prize was presented at each graduation ceremony. Since the closure of the Nursing School in 1987, the funds are now directed towards nursing research.

A former trainee of the Royal Children's Hospital, Miss Adams lost her life during World War Two, when the hospital ship *Centaur* was torpedoed and sunk off the Australian coast on the morning of 14 May 1943.

The award was made to the graduate voted to be the most outstanding practical nurse in the group who maintained the highest standard of nursing care throughout the three years of the nursing education program.

Margaret Adams was herself an excellent nurse and it is for this reason that the prize was awarded for both practical skills and understanding in the care of sick children.

APPENDIX 1

1960	Margaret Veronica Doherty, Helen Mary Garrett Swanton
1961	Lorraine Ngaire Goodgar, Heather Marie Gome, Patricia Anne Cholerton, Raemonde Isabel Wilde, Kevin Russell Curtis
1962	Beryl Margaret Clarke, Prudence Mary Thomas
1963	Kathleen Sylvia Sutton
1964	Kay Harman, Kheng Hua Wee, Marie Denise Wilson
1965	Marion Dimmitt, Wendy Allan, Glynes Roberts, Elizabeth Goulding
1966	Gwendolyn Chambers, Christine Hill, Glenys Littlejohn
1967	Patricia Dean, Nelly Zybuljak, Lorna Hamer
1968	Elizabeth Johnson, Beverley Thorne, Nolene Fox, Judith Eddy
1969	Teuntje Van Tricht, Robyn Joy McLaren, Elizabeth Bisdee
1970	Elizabeth Thomas, Denise Lesley McDonnell, Janice Winifred Lee
1971	Kathryn Eddy, Valerie Ratten, Dorothy Mary Taylor
1972	Diane Lennon, Judith Robyn Golomb, Julia Margaret McCoy
1973	Jennifer Hailes, Georgina Strachan, Jill Margaret Yeomans
1974	Julie Avent, Bronwyn Madder, Zara Sonenberg
1975	Robyn Poulsen, A. Nevett, A. Ebbels, H. Bradford
1976	Mary Lynne Stewart, Penelope Long, Linda Jurgenstein
1977	Susan Tweedie
1978	Jill Porter, Elizabeth Short, Esselien Mekking
1979	Mr D. Boyes, Yvonne Munro, Barbara Campbell, Annette Eldrige
1980	Merryn Dawn Baird
1981	Jennifer Inch, J. Stapleton, L. Baker
1982	J. Stapleton, L. Baker, L. Donaldson
1983	*name unavailable*
1984	*name unavailable*
1985	*name unavailable*
1986	Dianne Margaret Bennett
1987	Marianne Louise Oliver

THE A. JEFFREYS WOOD GOLD MEDAL

In 1923, Dr A. Jeffreys Wood donated £100 for the establishment of a gold medal to be awarded annually to the nurse who obtained the highest marks in hospital examinations, to the best practical nurse, the kindest to patients and to the most sympathetic with parents.

1923	Teresa Elsie Smith
1924	Ella Grace Robinson
1925	Mary Hannah McCallum
1926	Phyllis Ethel Sheila Murray
1927	Thelma Ada Hooper
1928	Gwendoline Coral Abbott
1929	Catherine Megan Davies
1930	Agnes Nicol Morris
1931	Edna Swift Windsor
1932	Eleanor Annie Green
1933	Isabel Ann Wall
1934	Jean Florence Copland

1935	Madge Mesley
1936	Isabel Mary Pilkington
1937	Catherine Margaret Mackenzie
1938	Gwendoline Mary McHutchison
1939	Clarice Richardson
1940	Kathleen May Hawthorne
1941	Marjorie Hosking
1942	Jean Barry
1943	Ethelwynne Mary Harcourt
1944	Margaret Alison Smith
1945	Margaret Joy Lavington
1946	Sheila Margot Bean
1947	Eveline Brinkworth Ferry
1948	Dorothy Margaret Carter
1949	Rhonda Gwen McCredie
1950	Barbara Clifford
1951	Colleen Margaret Playfair
1952	Elizabeth Ann Lockhart
1953	Nancy Catherine Arnold
1954	Margaret Jane Pollock
1955	Eril Mary Albiston
1956	Wenda May Bond
1957	Margot Noelle Ballard
1958	Judith Lorraine Palmer
1959	Anne Stewart Webster
1960	Elizabeth Wilkinson (née Edelstone-Pope), *Honourable Mention*: Jennifer Hall
1961	Margaret Veronica Doherty
1962	Anne Margaret Sutherland
1963	Beverley Judith Downing; *Runner up*: Kathleen Sylvia Sutton
1964	Beverley Ann James
1965	Kay Harman
1966	Heather Thomas
1967	Robyn Marcia Williams
1968	Elizabeth Robin Hudnott (née Humphrey)
1969	Julie Abbott
1970	Robyn Smith (née McLaren)
1971	Francine Hendrey (née Andrew)
1972	Julie Robinson
1973	Lesley Joan Orr
1974	Ruth Amy Parker (née Stubbs)
1975	Julie Avent
1976	Anne J. Ebbels
1977	Dianne Lawrence
1978	Susan T. Soste
1979	Janet Sasse
1980	Carmel Scott
1981	Mary-anne Dennenmoser

Appendix 1

1982	Amanda Singleton
1983	Jane Reid
1984	Paula Quinn
1985	Judith Glazner
1986	Anna Mifsud
1987	Gabrielle Van Essen

NELL CHRISFIELD MEMORIAL PRIZE FOR PAEDIATRIC NURSING

1967	Kerril Robinson
1968	Julie Abbott
1969	Robin McLaren
1970	Paula Wilson
1971	Carolyn Arnott
1972	Jennifer Spicer
1973	Ruth Amy Stubbs
1974	J. Milligan
1975	Ann Ebbels
1976	A. Cross, J. Tassell
1977	J. J. Scott
1978	R. McCasker
1979	Esselien Mekking
1980	Brenda Lawless
1981	*name unavailable*
1982	D. Greaves

BURROUGHS WELLCOME PRIZE (MATERIA MEDICA)

1972	Kaye Pilley
1973	Leanne Margaret McGregor
1974	C. Moreland
1975	Anne Hall
1976	Mrs J. Bromich
1977	R. Kirkham

CARNATION MILK COMPANY PRIZE (POST-BASIC)

1961	Ruth Marie Butterworth, Margaret Ruth McNeur
1962	Dorothy Millicent Dutton

MURRAY SMITH PRIZES

Awarded annually to those nurses who throughout the year attained the highest marks in the Hospital examinations, and the best ward reports on work and conduct in the wards.

Junior Murray Smith 1st Prize Awards

1946/47	Joan Morris
1947/48	Anne Patricia Johns
1948/49	P. J. Richey
1949/50	Josephine Mary Gregor True
1950/51	Joan Alison Crockford

1951/52	Elizabeth Lilian Strickland, Jean McDonald
1952/53	Joyce Penelope Fancourt Thomas
1953/54	Hilary Clare Cooper
1954/55	Marion George
1955/56	Helen Pennington, Judith Lorraine Palmer
1956/57	Linda Ethelwyn Mills, Anne Stewart Webster
1957/58	Joyce Agnes Neild
1958/59	Lorraine Joy Coutts
1959/60	Beverley Mary Ellis
1960/61	Rosemary Margaret Shaw
1961/62	Kay Harman
1962/63	Phillipa Stott
1963/64	Meredith Kent Hughes
1964/65	Elizabeth Robin Humfray
1965/66	Elizabeth Johnson
1966/67	Nancy Strangio
1967/68	Ruth Stapleton
1968/69	Mary Donovan
1969/70	Lesley Orr
1970/71	Rosalie Brown
1971/72	Julie Avent
1972/73	Leanne Margaret McGregor
1973/74	R. Ruff
1974/75	Rai Anik
1975/76	P. Hall
1976/77	D. Boyes
1977/78	C. Lightbody
1978/79	Suzanne Mansell
1979/80	Jane Reid

Senior Murray Smith Nursing Awards

1946/47	Lois Bridgeborn
1947/48	Mavis Jackson
1948/49	J. Morris
1949/50	Joan Halswell
1950/51	Josephine True
1951/52	Nancy Arnold
1952/53	June Lowe
1953/54	Margaret Pollock
1954/55	M. Joyce Birkin
1955/56	Margot Ballard
1956/57	Brenda Macdougall
	Marion George
1957/58	Laurel M. Palmer
1958/59	Elizabeth Edelstone Pope
1959/60	Margaret V. Doherty
1960/61	Margaret F. Blood

Appendix 1

1961/62	Beverley M. Ellis
1962/63	Beverley M. Ellis
1063/64	Kay Harman, Elizabeth Rodda
1964/65	Elizabeth A. Goulding
1965/66	Gwendolyn Chambers
1966/67	Elizabeth Humfray
1967/68	Julie Abbott
1968/69	Elizabeth Bisdee
1969/70	Francine Andrew
1970/71	Helen Crosby
1971/72	Jennifer Spicer
1972/73	Ruth Stubbs
1973/74	F. Kavanagh
1974/75	Ann Ebbels
1975/76	M. Stewart
1976/77	S. Soste
1977/78	J. Sasse
1978/79	David Boyes
1979/80	Amanda Goy

Appendix 2

GRADUATES OF THE ROYAL CHILDREN'S HOSPITAL SCHOOL OF NURSING

1890–1987

Meticulous care has been taken in this compilation of graduates. All sources have been researched exhaustively from hospital records, the Mackinnon School of Nursing and the Nurses' Board of Victoria. The author is indebted to those who contributed with personal records of their training schools. Therefore no responsibility can be taken for a name or names that may appear to have been missed. Registration did not appear immediately following examination results, but occurred some time after the required time of training. Because nurses were often ill, this could be months, or in some cases years, after time taken off for sick leave was made up.

FIRST CERTIFICATES AWARDED 1890
Carmichael, Grace J.
Danaher, Matilda M.
Goddard, Eleanor
Packenham, Alma
Price, Margaret

1891
Bishop, Sarah A.
Brayshaw, Helena
Collins, Grace
Dean, Eliza
Flack, Alice M.
Hayes, Alice
James, Bertha P.
McLaren, Helen
Ochiltree, Edith F.
Ryan, Mary
Thomas, Maria
Vernon, Dorothea
Wickham, Ada

1892
Donegan, Annie

1893
Argyle, Alice
Collins, Cicely
Hay, Amy
Hines, Frances E.
Rowe, Sophia
Rowland, Annie
Wilson, Elsie S.

1894
Bevan, Emily L.
Conyers, Evelyn A.
Conyers, Louisa F.
Hall, Florence
Kent, Charlotte M.
Laver, Mabel E.
Lonnergan, Annie

1895
Fowler, Blanche
Fysh, Carina
McKechnie, Julia
McKellar, Ada
Palmer, Emily

1896
Anquetel, Roberta
Bailey, Magdalene R.
Bevan, Ida A.S.
Düsser, Minnie
Knowles, Ethel L.
Lempriere, Janie Mc.
Palmer, Hannah D.

1897
Bullivant, Florence
Chapman, Katherine
Fowler, Florence K.
Fraser, Ruby
Lucas, Laurina E.J.
McLuran, Annie
Middleton, May M.
Pulling, Adelaide J.
Reynolds, Ethel S.
Wooton, Edith

1898
Ayres, Christina
Cramer, Constance M.

Appendix 2

Hart, Florence H.
Jaffray, Ethel E.M.
Morey, Marie
Walter, Ella C.
White, Agnes

1899
Greene, Nancy S.
Rooney, Marjorie

1900
Andrews, Susan M.
Appleton, Mary
Armstrong, Kathleen L.
Begg, Laura, J.C.
Blackie, Emma
Burn, Lilian E.M.
Cohn, Ray
Halford, Bertha I.
Lilley, Mary E.
Penney, Annie
Soden, Maud D.
Woodside, Mary C.S.

1901
Callow, Mona L.
Lewers, Eleanor M.
MacCallum, Catherine
Malcolm, Teresa
McKenzie, Grace
Wilmot, Leila M.W.

1902
Ellson, Florence L.
Hurley, Alice C.
Petley, Edith
Warburton, Margaret E.
White, Annie J.

1903
Walter, Hilda M.
Lyon, Jessie M.
Tucker, Elsie
Higgins, Violette H.
Connolly, Evelyn M.
Appleyard, Selina E.

Dobbin, Martha G.
Officer, Isabella D.
Cuthbert, Emma A.
Murray, Constance M.

1904
Tangye, Margaretta M.C.
Nankivell, Constance E.
Vicars-Foote, Helen
Natrass, Phyllis A.
Ingram, Elizabeth H.
Goodison, Constance E.

1905
Elcoate, Florence M.
Gardiner, Annie V.
Kelly, Mary G.
Ick, Helen
Peyton-Jones, M.L.
Mitchell, Mary
Cochran, Muriel
Best, Winifred E.
Walker, Emma M.

1906
Anderson, Enid R.
Baldwin, Emma I.
Bell, Alice
Belstead, Briseis
Bristow, Lorna R.
Hall, May I.
Homan, Helen M.M.
Lucas, Daisy E.F.
Panter, Florence M.
Robin, Ethel May de Jersey
Sproule, Marjorie St. George
Urquhart, Jemima

1907
Beggs, Matilda C.
Cramer, Winifred M.
Dunphy, Sara T.
Halford, Esme
Kenny, Louisa
Lovell, Amye E.
Marshall, Isabel M.
McLellan, Winifred H.

Morris, Constance M.
Peck, Muriel A.
Perry, Bessie
Robison, Evelyn A.
Sherwin, Eva M.
Stevenson, Mary J.L.
Swanton, Dora M.

1908
Beaumont, Jean H.
Best, Kathleen M.F.
Brown, Beryl C.
Gilmore, Elizabeth
James, Harriette M.
Kidd, Ruby G.
Shoobridge, Charlotte M.
Toomath, Ilma G. M.
Topp, Dorothea M.
Watson, Beatrice M.

1909
Aylwin, Dorothy M.V.
Begg, Rosa M.E.
Calvert, Eila I.
Chaffey, Evelyn F.
Gordon, Cecil I.K.
Hall, Edith M.
Hitchcock, Ethel J. deP.
Kennedy, Mary B.
Morris, Kate C.
Nelson, Mabel I.
Smith, Annie
Sproule, Florence St.G.
Yuille, Helen E.

1910
Chester, Edith M.
Cleary, Lucy M.
Glanville, Ella C.
Hayes, Marguerite
Jefferson, Ida G.
Leitch, Margaret
Murdoch, Margaret C.
Parsons, Eva
Richardson, May M.
Scott, Athalie F.
Searl, Alice

Smith, Mora M.L.
Sterling, Helen E.S.
Symonds, Millicent A.
Wilmore, Juliet L.

1911
Dobson, Elise G.
Golden, Helena
Green, Charlotte S.
Hardie, Maud M.
Hart, Ethel
McCausland, Irene
Riley, Olive G.
Roadknight, Muriel G.
Robinson, Muriel V.
Rudd, Ruby B.
Wallace, Mabel I.

1912
Blundell, Madeline P.P.
Fethers, Olive B.
Lockhart, Alice L.
Looker, Fanny M.
MacCallum, Katie E.
Mackenzie, Charlotte A.C.
Roberts, Mary E.
Rogers, Lyla
Slack, Linda M.
Steele, Elfrida A.

1913
Burke, Lalah M.
Cooke, Margaret E.C.
Coom, Grace W.
Payne, Violet M.
Ponsford, Ada T.F.
Willock, Annie W.

1914
Donaldson, Mary B.
Ebeling, Muriel G.
Johnson, Bessie S.
Lindsay, Ina I.
Macartney, Dora L.
Macpherson, Lorna R.
McArthur, Catherine P.
McKenna, Nellie

Moore, Josie S.
Newton, Dorothy J.L.
Newton, Eileen C.K.
Northcote, Doris
Priday, Stella M.
Purcell, Annie W.B.V.
Scott, Susan E.
Stone, Jane H.
Sugden, Edith
Watt, Ruby M.

1915
Bath, Gladys G.
Bishop, Gladys P.
Carter, Hester M.
Hardy, Ada M.
Picken, Marion B.

1916
Alexander, Annie O.
Bristow, Marjorie I.
Butler, Beatrice T.
Campbell, Jean G.
Chenery, Hylda
Clark, Belle H.
Clark, Doris M.
Cummins, Margaret
Johnson, Edith M.
Lowe, Elizabeth L.
McDonald, Isla K.
Nesbitt, Laura C.
Payne, Nancy
Reid, Nellie McI.
Riley, Mary G.
Robertson, Muriel
Rodger, Margaret
Williams, Harriet C.H.

1917
Ambler, Milanie
Archer, Eleanor M.
Belstead, Mabel G.
Beaven, Emily V.
Biggs, Florence A.
Borthwick, Jean E.
Coane, Eileen P.
De Ravin, Christina L.

Graham, Eileen F.
Hudson, Pamela B.
Huon, Ada E.
Laidlaw, Annie I.
McEachern, Emily J.
Miller, Nellie H.
Mitchell, Mary M.
Payne, Nancy
Piper, Sheila Mac.
Taylor, Gertrude M.
Williams, Stella
Wilson, Eileen L.

1918
Brown, Emma L.
Davis, May E.
Johnston, Jean F.M.
Keats, Lucy C.A.
Kemp, Alice J.
Lindsay, Hilda M.
Lugton, May J.H.
Kraefft, Elsie M.
Lyon, Elizabeth I.
MacDonald, Alys R.
MacInnes, Jessie M.
Malseed, Ruby M.
Mathews, Vera M.
Morrison, Mary Mc.
Scott, Lizzie N.
Smart, Helen D.
Tulloch, Jean Mac.
Walford, Gladys

1919
Affleck, Bessie Fraser
Cleveland, Alice C.
Carter, Jessie M.
Dewar, (first name indecipherable)
Green, Jean
Gibbs, Helen
Hill, Gwendolen
Mackinnon, Evelyn F.
Mason, Myra J.B.
McBurney, Marion A.
McCrae, Jane A.
McKenna, Mabel T.

APPENDIX 2

McLellan, Margaret E.
Morton, Dorothy E.
Nieman, Alice W.
Powell, Lucy
Pratt, Elsie M.
Robertson, Mary E.
Skinner, Margaret M.
Stone, Clara C.
Slaughter, Janet P.
Stephens, Elizabeth I.
Stevenson, Dorothy L.
Stodart, Aubrey F.
Stone, Clara C.
Sutherland, Margaret F.
Tatchell, Genevieve E.
Watson, Eleanor D.
Watson, Jessie M.
Wood, Caroline E.

1920
Alsop, Lily
Bristow, Nancye B.
Dodd, Rose M.
Fethers, Hazel
Green, Margaret M.
Hamilton, Agnes L.
Hallowes, Dorothy J.
Lane, Mary A.
Lockyear, Ellis M.
McComb, Rita C.
McKinnon, Evelyn F.
Neil, Margaret
Newnham, Sarah E.
Nieman, Alice W.
O'Rorke, Annie T.
Ormerod, Annie R.
Penrose, Mabel A.
Ramsden, Leila M.
Tadgell, Gladys
Whitford, Ivey M.

1921
Besley, Isabel M.
Beatty, Gertrude O.
Cameron, Catherine A.
Chenoweth, Rachel E.V.
Cooke, Grace M.

Fysh, Marjorie M.
Gaylard, Laura
Hart, Mary
Irvine, Elsie
Jones, Doris M.M.
Malony, Mary A.
Marshall, Agnes
Morris, Margaret G.
Scott, Mary C.
Sutton, Dorothea K.
Tootell, Evelyn M.
Tweddell, Audrey O.
Walsh, Mary S.B.

1922
Blacker, Elsie M.
Bourke, Marguerita K.
Brent, Isabel M.
Gourlay, Doris R.E.
Hardeman, Clarice A.
Hendy, Doris E.
Joseph, Marguerite
Lindsay, Elizabeth I.
McGregor, Adeline M.
Padgham, Emma J.
Powers, Marjorie
Rogers, Jean O.
Sawyer, Marina A.
Scott, Edith L.
Tadgell, Gladys
Tonge, Anna L.
Townsend, Hildergardis C.
Tulloh, Freda G.
Turner, Evelyn M.
Woods, Ethel M.

1923
Bamford, Ella V.
Colebrook, Clara M.
Coles, Vera
Colvin, Jean F.
Hawkins, Ethel B.
Jepson, Eleanor
Loton, Vera
Mason, Doris O.
Newton, Margaret F.
Powell, Laura M.

Richter, Hilda M.
Smith, Elsie T.
Stirling, Margery B.
Travers, Louisa A.
Weber, Irene P.
Werry, Ada

1924
Billing, Miriam E.
Brown, Dorothy O.
Clements, Daisy
Fass, Isabel M.
Fernald, Ethel A.
Flower, Ivy S.
Grant, Eileen G.
Harriman, Maisie I.
Hawkins, Ethel B.
Heath, Ellen
Howell, Ruth F.
Kneebone, Henrietta
Lewis, Muriel M.
Lyell, Doreen M.
McCallum, Sheila M.
McIntosh, Catherine M.
McKenzie, Marion I.
McNamara, Kate M.
McNight, Jean L.
Meldrum, Helen
Milburn, Annie I.
Smith, Frances M.
Steeper, Lorna R.
Theyer, Jean
Toohey, Helen M.
Vidler, Marion
Williams, Florence E.
Williams, Margaret A.
Wright, Elizabeth

1925
Aitkin, Joyce
Carter, Pauline
Davey, Hilda M.
Fitchett, Myrtle
Gilruth, Jean A.
Goff, Doris C.
Graham, Gwendoline M.
Harper, Mary H.

Hunter, Marion A.
Hunter, Shirley S.
Lloyd, Dorothy H.
Lock, Eveline A.
Maddison, Helen E.
McKissack, Frances E.
Macknight, Helen
Norman, Christian
Perretti, Alice A.
Read, Mabel E.
Ready, Ivy E.
Robinson, Ella G.
Scott, Annie
Service, Margeurite A.
Sevier, Enid M.
Skulthorp, Ida A.B.
Smith, Olive M.
Snodgrass, Sybil D.
Twyford, Marie E.F.

1926
Bayley, Ina C.
Black, Ailsa V.M.
Brindley, Bessie A.H.
Broom, Dorothy
Clark, Florence M.
Clark, Marjorie F.
Colquhan, Margaret
Emmerson, Margaret N.
Gibson, Fay
Halls, Doreen M.
Howard, Irma V.
Jones, Dilys F.
Kirkpatrick, Dorothy L.
McCallum, Mary H.
McLeod, Winnie J.
Morrison, Jessie G.
Murray, Phyllis E.S.
Robinson, Lilian
Wade, Dora G.
Webster, Katherine H.
Winter, Lucy E.

1927
Backwell, Lorna L.
Best, Alice E.
Bishop, Evelyn

Bromley, Evelyn M.
Crooks, Nellie S.
Cuc, Mazie E.
Curwen-Walker, Edna C.
Dowling, Nancy C.
Dowsett, Inga M.
Ducat, Alice I.
Harper, Joan H.
Hinchcliffe, Merle D.
Kimber, Vera E.
Lampard, Marion I.
Leaney, Gertrude A.
Lilley, Iris
Luke, Elfrida
May, Helen H.
McCallen, Gladys M.
McClelland, Jessie I.
MacDermid, Janet A.
Moreton, Constance H.
Onslow, Helen M.J.
Phillips, Nancy
Sackwell, Lorna L.
Townshend, Hilda G.C.
Tulloh, Thelma B.
West, Alice E.
Young, Myrtle M.

1928
Abbott, Gwendoline C.
Stuart, Mary L.
Bell, Julia V.
Danders, Phyllis M.
de Belera, Katheryna E.
Finnis, Violette L.
Finkelmeyer, Viola
Fortier, Gwendoline A.
Hall, Iris
Heath, Marie A.
Hooper, Thelma A.
Liddicut, Lillian G.
Liddle, Elizabeth J.
Love, Ivy P.E.
Meredith, Myra A.
Porter, Gwendoline A.
Potts, Isabella
Price, Doris L.
Rossiter, Alison B.

Sandon, Phyllis M.
Silver, Florence
Simpson, Valda
Sloan, Lily A.
Shanks, Margaret B.
Salmon, Clair H.
Utbar, Winifred L.
Wettenhall, Mary F.F.

1929
Anderson, Maude M.
Anderson, Jean
Arthur, Jane W.
Baker, Louise E.
Brindley, Gertrude E.
Brunt, Mary L.
Buchanan, Dorothy J.
Cherry, Margaret I.
Clements, Joyce E.
Darling, Nellie
Davies, Ellinor K.
Davies, Katherine M.
Ditchburn, Louisa F.
Egan, Gertie M.
Fermin, Ellen C.
Fogerty, Marie E.I.
Francis, Annie M.
Halls, Ruby M.
Halls, Oenone M.
Hausewell, Elma L.
Jones, Doris G.
Logan, Eleanor M.
Lousada, Ruth E.
McLintock, Gladys
McLachlin, Mary A.
Matthews, Florence R.
Mills, Christine M.
Morrison, Maggie
Paterson, Irene M.
Potts, Frances F.
Sayle, Edith M.
Scott, Clara E.E.
Sharp, Jean
Tinkler, Amelia S.
Reynolds, Ethel M.
White, Thelma D.

APPENDIX 2

1930
Adeney, Joyce F.
Aicheson, Alison M.
Aisbett, Florrie G.
Aitken, Emma C.
Alexander, Joan L.
Anthony, Dorothy M.
Barlow, Jessie K.
Beaufils, Ada
Buckle, Valerie M.
Buxton, Jessie K.
Chambers, Alice I.
Chesterman, Edna F.
Dawborn, Sheila K.
Deveney, Dorothy M.T.
Evans, Ivy R.
Glynn, Ellen F.
Green, Eleanor A.
Green, Edna F.
Griffith, Florence A.
Griffiths, Dorothy M.
Hunter, Jessie I.
Jeffries, Doris
Love, Hazell L.
Loder, Nellie D.
MacKenzie, Mona
MacDermid, Jean S.
McLeod, Eileen McD.
McLure, Kathleen
May, Patricia M.L.
Miller, Marjorie E.
Morris, Agnes N.
Murray, Jean
Johnson, Eva
Over, Joyce A.
Prendergast, Nell C.
Shattock, Mary A.
Stevens, Gwendoline S.
Storey, Lucy
Threlfall, Kathleen
Utbar, Marjorie E.
Walker, Stella M.

1931
Baker, Eileen M.
Barnard, Nancy C.
Brownlee, Elva W.A.

Caffin, Francis I.
Campbell, Margaret C.
Clark, Betty F.
Coates, Ella
Danne, Dorothy
Faulkiner, Georgina G.
Fearon, Alberta F.
Felstead, Joan V.
Grant, Edna F.M.
Greene, Lorna L.
Harrison, Phyllis G.
Hitchcock, Emily de P.
Jennings, Lily D.
Kain, Mary E.
Leigh, Muriel E.
McKay, Katherine G.
McLaren, Janet A.
Morrison, Rebecca
Nicholl, Sydney E.
Phillips, Ailsa C.
Saunders, Dorothy
Scott, Edna J.
Staughton, Sybil E.
Vigar, Jessie M.
Wallace, Marie W.
Wallace, Norma M.
Wettenhall, Phoebe
Williams, Barbara
Williams, Jean H.
Windsor, Edna S.

1932
Bailey, Edith I.
Brown, Sheila
Bunting, Muriel E.
Dann, Kathleen A.V.
Danne, Nancy
Dossetor, Catherine L.
Falconbridge, Iris J.
Felstead, Elsie M.
Fisher, Eleanor M.
Ford, Nancy E.
Gibson, Florence
Gilbert, Lila
Green, Jean A.
Hardham, Jean B.
Hart, May D.A.

Hayden, Jessie
Hipwell, Patricia
Holmes, Alison M.
James, Lillian M.
King, Irene D.L.
Mair, Mary L.
Martin, Marion L.
Mathison, Annie G.
Meyer, Katherine
Norman, Alma J.
Primmer, Ida May
Richardson, Dorothy M.
Simson, Margaret
Sloey, Patricia M.
Wall, Isabel A.
Walker, Jeannie B.
Williams, Dorothy

1933
Berryman, Lilian
Clarke, Doris M.
Colechin, Dorothy E.R.
Cleary, Phil
Crombie, Annie B.
Cust, Phyllis L.
Drake, Kerin B.
Dunn, Anne V.
Ford, Mary J.
Gason, Harriet P.
Goodwell, Margaret I.
Hannah, Mary R.
Hennell, Elsie M.H.
Holmes, Margeurite
Horman, Alma J.
Irvine, Edith M.
Johnston, Susanna M.
Just, Lillian E.
Keating, Agnes J.
Kimber, Kathleen F.S.
Lamble, Louise M.
Lloyd, Kathleen M.
Lyons, Irene
Maclean, Louisa M.
Malone, Mona L.F.
McLennan, Kathleen I.
Neville, Dorothy F.
Orr, Margery M.

Phillips, Ada M.
Pilkington, Alice M.
Ritchie, Mary A.
Robertson, Alma M.
Russell, Alice F.
Saxton, Zaida M.
Sweeting, Dorothy D.
Turnbull, Patricis M.
Walker, Chola C.
Weir, Gwenyth L.
White, Eva M.
Whitehead, Elva M.
Wigan, Alice F.
Willan, Margaret I.
Wood, Nancy H.G.
Woodyatt, Jean H.

1934
Anstee, Nina F.
Bishop, Nancy G.
Brown, Helen Mac.
Burns, Jean S.
Burns, Netta
Chinnick, Elizabeth A.
Chisholm, Margaret J.
Copeland, Jean F.
Crick, Marjorie L.
Davidson, Alice M.
Elliott, Violet I.
Goldsmith, Joan D.
Graham, Irene M.
Jones, Ruth M.
Levick, Ursula
Miller, Jean A.
Mcleod, Jean S.
Mesley, Madge
Nancarrow, Alma C.
O'Halloran, Mary
Reid, Dorothy M.
Robin, Mary de Q.
Stewart, Mary J.
Thomas, Helen R.P.
Walker, Nellie K
White, Beryl R.B.
Whitfield, Doris M.
Wilde, Elsa H.M.

1935
Adams, Margaret L.
Adamson, Gladys G.
Aitken, Nancy E.
Anderson, Elizabeth A.
Barrow, Nell M.
Brodie, Sophie G.
Bristol, Huia F.
Brownlee, Beryl S.A.
Charles, Eslana E.
Ching, Ethel R.
Cohen, Shirley I.
Colley, Lillian C.
Crocker, Frances M.
Cuthill, Lilian A.H.
Cuttle, Beatrice E.
Dwyer, Elizabeth J.
Finlayson, Florence J.
Frier, Ruth A.
Garden, Wilga M.
Gatehouse, Sheila M.L.
Gellie, Marjorie A.
Gilbert, Eunice E.
Greenwood, Ouida F.
Gregson, Linda J.
Kirchner, Thekla E.
Kyte, Barbara E.
Laing, Nancy T.
Lavington, Margaret J.
Layton, Dorothy
Lindsay, Mary F.
Lochore, Nance E.
McConnell, Edwyna M.
Mitchell, Irma K.
Morton, Josephine E.
Norwood, Gladys W.
O'Brien, Charlotte J.
Parker, Helen M.
Pearce, Sheila R.
Peck, Eleanor M.
Penfold, Joan M.
Pilkington, Isabel M.
Rattenbury, Olive J.
Robertson, Judith S.
Ross, Flora J.
Royle, Patsy R.
Shearer, Jean E.

Stillwell, Jean
Tattersall, Grace E.
Thompson, Mary A.
Vagg, Olga M.
Vigar, Joyce
Watson, Thyra I.
Wilmot, Doris F.
Windsor, Audrey J.
Yule, June E.A.

1936
Ackland, Rhoda B.
Armstrong, Nancy M.
Baragwanath, Dorothy R.
Barrington, Margaret I.
Bautovich, Olga S.
Bechervaise, Ella M.
Bennett, Phyllis T.
Brain, Patricia F.
Brownbill, Constance E.
Butler, Dorothy D.
Carss, Hilda J. Zelma
Clarke, Stella B.
Clarke, Mary C.
Davies, Estelle L.
Dickie, Audrey M.
Engel, Elsie G.
Gallagher, Mary R.N.
Hall, Florence L.
Hogg, Marjorie L.
Hully, Mary K.
Hyslop, Lillian
Jeffrey, May E.
Jackson, Heather
Jones, Brenda J.
Langham, Freda M.
Lowry, Joyce E.
Malseed, Elizabeth E.
Mann, Stella L.
Martin, Betty J.
McArthur, Elizabeth I.
McKay, Jeanette M.
Mcleod, Mary E.
Morris, Nancy H.
O'Donnell, Joan I.
Paterson, Vera G.
Perrins, Nell

Ritchie, Joan A.
Scott, Marjorie K.
Shattock, Betty
Steer, Helen M.
Stockwell, Winifred L.
Trebilco, Jean R.
Troedel, Brenda R.
Walter, Dora A.
Wilkinson, Paula J.
Wilson, Kathleen S.
Young, Elizabeth C.

1937
Allan, Marjorie E.
Allnatt, Marjorie A.M.
Anson, Nancie R.
Avery, Avis G.
Barker, Phyllis J.
Bechervaise, Agnes B.
Bertram, Joan M.
Bourke, Dorothy N.
Burgess, Lottie E.
Chapman, Mary E.
D'Arcy, Flora M.
Dodd, Ilma E.
Eagerty, Nancy M.
Ferry, Mary C.
Flattley, Hester M.
Godley, Mary I.
Gardner, Kathleen C.
Giles, Laurie G.
Graff, Aleda A.
Hoadley, Dorothy
Hogan, Shirley G.
Hollow, Faith
Mackenzie, Catherine M.
McHutchison, Gwendoline M.
Markham, Lily P.
Nice, Gwenneth M.
Oakes, Rhoda J.
O'Donnell, Claire
Plummer, Jean E.
Pollock, Eveline M.
Prentice, Isabelle M.
Rogers, Dorothy P.
Rose, Constance E.

Stirling, Muriel I.
Syme, Jean C.
Vince, Marjorie
Wallace, Margaret F.
Whelan, Eileen M.
White, Muriel G.
Wilson, Beatrice A.
Wiseman, Beryl B.

1938
Boyd, Betty
Buxton, Evangeline M.
Campbell, Harriet B.
Capener, Cecilia E.
Chappell, Zelma E.
Cook, Joan S.
Davis, Lilah E.
Druce, Elsie F.
Dunstan, Catherine E.
Ferris, Pauline H.
Francome, Helen I.
Gendle, Joan M
Grant, Beatrice
Greenway, Rebecca B.
Grover, Margaret
Harbourd, Veronica E.
Hitchens, Irma R.
Horsburgh, Veronica E.
Jobson, Margaret E.
Larmour, Alison M.
Macdougall, Sheila
Mair, Margaret G.
McHardy, J.
McMeekin, Marjorie H.
McNutt, Mabel D.
Miller, Jean A.
Piercy, June M.
Pollard, Agnes J.
Rankin, Jean M.
Richardson, Betty H.
Serpell, Margaret
Smith, Elizabeth C.
Sutton, Lesla
Tolman, Joan M.
Vance, Marjorie
Westley, Mona M.
Woolley, Flora S.

1939
Allan, Marjorie
Anderson, Lorna M.
Andrew, Isabel M.
Barker, Ray M.
Blanshard, Lesla M.
Boone, Joan L.
Brand, Shirley D.
Cole, Marguerite N.
Cowan, Roberta C.
Dawson, Kathleen H.
Doidge, Doris I.
Elvins, Elaine O.
Foster, Myrtle M.
Gray, Sheila K.E.
Griffiths, Nancy M.
Helms, Leslie M.
Holmes, Creslie E.
Howell, Maud M.
Hutchins, Marjorie
Jennings, Joyce F.
Keir, Heather M.
Kellam, Elsie I.E.
Levick, Lois M.
Lornie, Marion F.
Maloney, Theresa E.
Mesley, Joan
Miers, Marjorie J.
McPherson, Constance M.
Nicoll, Marjorie C.
Osborne, Gwenneth
Parsons, Flora M.
Payne, Clara I.
Perrins, Margery M.
Peters, Peggy V.
Pollock, Marjorie I.
Ransome, Elaine M.
Ransom, Mary J.
Richardson, Clarice (Bon)
Robertson, Betty K.
Steel, Frances M.
Stockwell, Margaret E.
Suffren, Beryl L.
Trellicar, Letitia J.
Woolley, Anne S.
Walduck, Betty B.
Young, Joyce C.

1940
Allen, Una
Andrew, Mary D.
Brodribb, Mary E.
Crosthwaite, Marjorie K.
Curtis, Marguerite A.
Cutts, Edith L.
De Bibra, Kathryna E.
Dixon, Lyla J.
Fox, Mona
Gamble, Nance A.
Gordon, Anne S
Hawthorne, Kathleen M.
Heane, Nancye R.
Houston, Elizabeth J.
Howard, Patricia M.
Ievers, Charlotte M.
Livingstone, Frances J.
Lowry, Mary I.
Mackenzie, Lucy G.
McBride, Mary T.
McKay, Eleanor E.
McNamara, Mary D.
Mitchell, Frances J.
Myer, Desiree F.
Oakley, Mary D.
Quiney, Helen E.
Richards, G. Clare
Richards, Gwenyth C.
Schultz, Dorothy
Slater, Patricia V.
Southby, Mary F.
Sullivan, Elsie L.
Vale, Olive H.
Webster, Betty C.
Webster, Olive G.

1941
Anderson, Elizabeth C.
Barry, Jean
Belfrage, Hazel E.
Boyle, Margaret V.
Burgess, Dorothy J.
Cameron, Donella J.
Cameron, Eliza F.
Casey, Margaret E.
Cheeseman, Esme W.

Chipperfield, Joyce E.
Collins, Gwendoline E.
Curtis, M.A. Rita
Daniel, Vivienne B.
Denniston, Winsome E.
Dunstan, Eleanor D.
Findley, Agnes J.
Greenwood, W. Mavis
Gunn, Edith E.
Haebich, Eva F.
Hartley, Minnie H.
Hoadley, Jean
Hosking, Marjorie J.
Hughes, Margaret M.
Kelly, Doreen F.
Kent-Hughes, Elizabeth
Lipsett, Margaret B.
Maloney, Theresa E.
Matheson, Glenda
McCormack, June M.
McIntyre, Patricia
McKay, Elizabeth J.
McLeod, Jean I.
McMeekin, Nancy N.
Moorhouse, Margaret V.
Nancarrow, Jean I.
Norman, Jean W.
Norris, Rayma I.
Nutting, Phyllis E.
Penn, Edith R.
Quiney, Mary P.
Rogan, Thelma G.
Scott, Marjory J.
Schweiger, Joan F.B.
Shannon, Beryl E.
Shaw, Isabella M.
Stichnoth, Ida M.
Thomson, Jean M.
Tipping, Hilda M.
Toohey, Rachel
Webster, Dorothy E.
Wellington, Lesley J.
Wishart, Una M.

1942
Allen, Esme R.
Andrew, Alice

Balmer, Olive G.
Beenie, Margaret I.
Burbury, Barbara A.
Chalmers, Sylvia B.
Clarke, Hope J.
Cootes, Dorothy J.
Craig, Isabel M.
Darcy, Jean L.
Davey, Jean L.
Duncan, Agnes E.M.
Faulkiner, Jean
Gould, Alison E.
Harford, Joyce M.
Harvey, Irene F.B.
Henley, Joyce A.
Hoggarth, Jean H.
Jackson, Margaret J.
Jenkins, Joyce
Johnson, Beatrice M.
Malseed, Marjorie E.
McGregor, Mary
McIver, Isabelle E.
McKay, Muriel L.
McKenzie, Heather H.
Mellor, Joyce
Morgan, Margaret I.
Morgan, Margaret
Norman, Jean W.
O'Donnell, Aileen M.
Parkinson, Joan
Prichard, Margaret M.
Rogers, Grace E.
Royle, Edith B.
Schultz, Adrienne M.A.
Self, Alice E.
Smith, Brenda F.
Snowball, Dorothy F.M.
Tuck, Ethel H.
Warren, Rita C.
Webster, Eva B.
Welch, Nancy L.
Winter-Irving, Flora L.
Wood, Betty L.
Young, Ann
Young, Helen

APPENDIX 2

1943
Air, Iris N.
Adamson, Gladys G.
Allan, Ivy W.
Balmer, Olive G.
Barry, Jean
Breen, Margaret E.
Brumley, Elizabeth V.
Burbury, Peggy R.
Cedergreen, Muriel E.A.
Chalmers, Dorris I.
Cogan, Eileen T.
Daniell, Gloria J.
Dans, Kathleen A.
Davis, Nora P.
Eddy, Clarice
Ewence, Noreen K.
Furphy, Joan M.
Geary, Roma A.
Gordon, Jean M.
Gordon, Lorna M.
Green, Elsie M.
Harcourt, Ethelwynne M.
Hardy, Victoria G.
Hatherley, Anne
Heley, Noel E.
Hollonds, Forsythe H.
Howatson, Susanne S.
Jackson, Dorothy A.
Johnston, Roma E.
Kucks, Estella F.
Keble, Dorothy J.
Langley, Maude A.
Lawrence, Patricia
Lord, Helen D.
Madden, Elizabeth M.
Massie, Josephine D.
Mills, Una H. W.
Moller, Ellen J.
Morrison, Beryl M.
Newton, Ellen E.
Norman, Jean W.
O'Connor, Winifred A.
Ogburn, Margaret V.
Parker, Marjorie L.
Perry, Beth
Radcliffe, Gwendoline J.

Russell, Mary T.
Smith, Valerie
Stilley, Muriel F.
Thompson, Nancy C.
Thompson, Rosalie J.
Warr, Margaret A.
Welch, Barbara A.
Zuppinger, Josephine B.

1944
Anderson, Elizabeth E.
Bale, Wilma J.
Becker, Dulcie E.
Biggs, Helen L.
Bigelow, Betty M.
Brydon, Jean L.
Bulling, Patricia
Butler, Pauline M.
Buxton, Eleanor R.
Carlile, Kathleen M.
Coleman Lawna E.
Connor, Thelma F.
Condely, Hilda M.
Cunningham, Marion M.
Donovan, Clare M.
Evans, Gwenneth M.
Evans, Joyce
Farr, Irene M.
Gilchrist, Gweneth E.
Golden, Ursula M.
Harris, Hilda M.
Hurley, Claire E.
Hyde, Barbara J.
Jardine, Reiva B.
Keirce, Thelma M.
King, Florence I.
Longstaff, Patience A.
Mackenzie, Sheila M.
Marks, Jane M.
Marshall, Irene M.
Mason, Gwenneth W.
Milne, Mary P.
Moore Marjorie C.
Morey, Yvonne M.
Morris, Hilda M.
McCombe, Elizabeth L.
Mackenzie, Sheila M.

Nicholas, Betty
Parkinson, Nancy S.
Patrick, Evelyn E.
Radcliffe, Gwendoline J.
Sanger, Prudence M.
Shoobridge, Mollie J.
Smith, Margaret A.
Steer, Jean E.
Stephenson, Lois M.
Sutherland, Dorothy J.
Tassicker, Norma
Young, Joan
Wasley, Ruth L.
Willmott, Betty K.
Wiltshire, Lilian M.

1945
Aitkin, Nancy E.
Barker, Valerie C.
Beavis, Margery L.
Betteridge, Elsie P.
Borthwick, Kathleen M.
Brearley, Isma M.
Cane, Patricia B
Chalmers, Joan
Cain, Diana J.C.
Coates, Sarah J.
Colclough, Margaret J.
Cunningham, Anthea G.
Dawkins, Ruth I.
Finlayson, F. Joan
Frier, Ruth A.
Gibson, Janet W.
Gregson, Linda J.
Greenwood, Ouida F.
Harrison, Frances B.
Holloway, Patricia P.
Jackson, Barbara A.
Kyte, Barbara E.
Lavington, Margaret J.
Morris, Margaret M.
Morey, Yvonne M.
Morley, Ethel N.
O'Brien, Charlotte J.
McConnell, Edwyna M.
Pearce, Sheila R.
Rattenbury, Olive J.

Robertson, Judith S.
Sartoria, Betty L.
Scott, Jeannie L.
Tattersall, Grace E.
Vagg, Olga Margaret S.
Vigar, Joyce
Yule, June E.A.

1946
Barber, Dorothy J.
Bean, Sheila M.
Bennett, Nada M.
Black, Margaret J.
Braine, Lois M.
Bulling, Patricia M.
Burnell, Lynette M.
Crombie, Jennifer P.
Daniel, Nona
Dare, Olive M.
Forbes, Patricia A.
Hamlet, Patricia E.
Handasyde, Lucy M.
Harding, June
Heginbotham, Ellen M.
Holmes, Katherine J.
Holman, Margaret E.I.
Holloway, J. Annette
Hogg, Dorothy J.
Kelly, Margaret F.
Kelly, Margaret P.
Kennedy, Margaret P.
King, Estelle M.
Lockhart, Margaret L.
Lord, Jessie W.
Morris, Margaret
Morris, Audrey R.
Moylan, Patricia M.
Pederson, Grace M.
Pender, Elizabeth R.
Peters, Olive E.
Reid, Peggie W.
Read, Phyllis M.
Ricketts, Rubena K.
Ross, Flora J.
Seeck, Jean M.
Schofield, Rosemary F.
Stait, Margaret J.

Stainsby, Shirley J.
Tovell, Madeline M.
Turner, Elizabeth W.
Turner, Jeannie M.
Warr, Dorothea M.
Wall, Grace M.
Wiltshire, Mary M.

1947
Allan, Nancy D.M.
Armstrong, Jean B.
Blair, Eva E.
Bridgborn, Lois J.
Brearley, Pauline
Bremmer, Constance L.
Brydon, Margaret E.
Buchanan, Edna M.
Butler, Lorna M.
Campbell, Ruth A.
Clayfield, Frances J.
Cleary, Mary P.
Coleman, Thurka M.
Deacon, Gwendoline M.
Down, Hope W.
Ferry, Evelyn B.
Ferry, Margaret E.
Forham, Joan
Forster, Vivienne
Hayes, Valerie M.
Hooke, Isobel M.
Jago, Beryl H.
Jenkins, Elizabeth M.
King, Lorna F.
Linforth, Esther M.
Lording, Winsome L.B.
Lyons, Patricia M.
Meyer, Muriel M.
McAlister, Elizabeth L.
McConachie, Joan C.
McCormack, Esme B.
Morris, Barbara P.
Morris, Pauline B.
Roberts, Elva M.
Round, Joyce
Secomb, Greta P.
Sewell, Phyllis S.
Scott, Jeannie L.

Shipp, Helen E.
Smith, Meryl
Smith, Cecily T.
Schmidt, Marjorie M.
Stewart, Mary P.
Thompson, Isobel J.
Wallis, Barbara N.

1948
Algar, Mary E.
Alison, Valerie F.
Anstee, Nina M.
Barnett, Barbara
Baulch, Joan E.
Beck, Jean E.
Burke, Eileen I.
Brett, Patricia E.
Bult, Audrey L.
Campbell, Ruth
Carter, Dorothy M.
Casey, Bernice M.
Catto, Barbara E.
Dietz, Nance
Fearon, Elizabeth L.E.
Gould, Katherine J.
Gunter, (first name indecipherable)
Hastie, Bertha A.
Harrison, Diana M.
Heley, Judith
Henty, Ruth A.
Humphries, Gwyneth
Jackson, Mavis B.
Jenkins, Elizabeth M.
Johnson, June Alison
Langlands, Jill
Langlands, Jocelyn I.
Lark, Valerie F.
Lee, Lynette A.
Linton, Elaine J.
Luke, Janet Mary
Mitchell, Margaret Mc.
Mitchell, Margaret G.
Mortyn, June M.
Myers, Kathleen
Maconochie, Joan C.
Reid, Peggie W.

Rogers, Elizabeth L.
Semmens, Annie J.
Schapper, Barbara
Sutherland, Noreen G.
Terry, Joan
Thiel, Edith V.
Truscott, Cecile
Truscott, Gwen
Wettman, Anna J.
White, Violetta M.
Young, Patricia L.

1949
Armstrong, Jennie
Beales, Margaret
Bennett, Diana M.
Bengough, Jean M.
Burgess, Nancye
Burnett, Joan
Colliver, Gwenda
Crosby, Ruth
Crocker, Alison
Cooper, Margaret P.
Doig, Valda M.
Duke, Valerie
Garden, Amy B.
Gay, Linda A.
Glancy, Grace A.
Handley, Patricia M.
Hansen, Elaine M.
Hardwick, Jean D.
Heywood, Vivienne D.
Hooke, Margaret
Hurst, Nancy F.
Harden, Kathleen M.
Jacka, Lorna
Jacka, Joyce
Jaffray, Elizabeth M.
Johns, Anne P.
Joynes, Joan
Kirkwood, Ruth W.
Larritt, Joan E.
Larkins, Dorothy H.
Livermore, Margaret E.
McCredie, Rhonda G.
McCarthy, Gwendoline M.
Lowery, E.

Morris, Joan
Paton, Elaine
Pollock, Jeanette I.
Potter, Elaine S.
Potter, Claire
Powell, Dorothea M.
Quinton, Catherine A.
Sadlier, Elizabeth E.
Shepherd, Miriam
Snowball, Lois M.
Swift, Winifred
Stutterd, Ann
Taylor, Jean M.
Tobias, Lorraine J.
Vinge, Robin
Wilson, Patricia P.

1950
Allen, B.
Burnett, Ursula F.
Burt, Evelyn N.D.
Cain, Peggy M.
Cheetham, Margaret A.
Clifford, Barbara
Clissold, Robina F.
Cousland, Betty D.
Crosby, Ruth M.
Dinning, Dulcie C.
Downing, Elizabeth
Dunstan, (first name indecipherable)
Giddings, Patricia E.
Greaves, Mary J.
Hammett, (first name indecipherable)
Harden, Kathleen M.
Harris, Margaret J.
Hatswell, Joan
Hogben, Wilma G.
Kennedy, Margaret M.
Kennedy, Wilma E.
Lobascher, Elouise Z.
Macquarie, May M.
Male, Maisie L.
Martin, Valerie N.
McCracken, Margaret E.
McGregor, Helen C.

O'Malley, Patricia A.
Playfair, C. Margaret
Porter, Thelma G.
Quinton, Catherine A.
Reid, Elizabeth S.
Roberts, Elva M.
Ryan, Wilma A.
Schulz, Rita V.
Smith, Ruth E.
Thomson, Margaret I.
Threlfall, Gwendoline H.
Uebergang, Patricia M.
Veale, Phyllis L.
Watkinson, Shirley

1951
Akers, Pearl A.
Austin, Jane McP.
Austin, S. Elizabeth P.
Billings, Fay M.
Bland, Betty F.
Borland, Marjorie J.
Buchanan, Frances E.
Butt, Judith
Collins, Marie S.
Curwen-Walker, Barbara
Dahlenburg, Nancy H.
Davis, June M.
Fisher, Alwyn E.
Fitzpatrick, Monica
Fleischer, Rita A.
Goodall, Patricia E.
Granger, June M.
Hitchcock, Caroline J.
James, Sybil T.
Johnston, Helen M.
Jones, Gwenneth M.
Jones, Ivy T.
Kennedy, I. Marjorie
Kiel, Elizabeth M.
Larritt, Joan E.
Lockett, Elizabeth M.
Lockhart, Elizabeth A.
McClelland, Joyce M.
McMaster, Joan G.
Meldrum, June M.
Moffet, Moira B.

Phillips, Laurel S.
Richards, Jean N.
Richey, Phyllis J.
Sartoria, Shirley J.
Scott, Irene M.
Sewell, Elizabeth
Steer, Lynette E.
Strapp, Valerie M.
True, Josephine M.G.
Turner, Margery H.
Wales, Barbara
Wasley, Shirley A.
Watson, Margaret O.M.
Watson, Marjorie
White, Helen Y.
Whitney, Mary B.
Wiber, Margaret A.
Williams, Joyce J.
Wilson, Irene N.
Yates, Judith M.
Young, Florence E.

1952
Altmann, Jane D.
Andrews, Joan L.
Arnold, Nancy C.
Bailey, Doris H.
Ball, Pearl H.
Beaumont, Margaret
Brady, Nancy E.
Bonnor, Lynda J.
Brain, Adele A.
Bramwell, Dorothy K.
Burley, Margaret B.M.
Carter, Helen M.
Christie, Merle E.
Cleary, Shirley M.
Coleman, Beverley S.
Cooley, June P.
Cooper, Pamela T.
Cousley, Margaret E.C.
Cuddy, Rita L.
Cunningham, Rose
Coventry, Florence E.G.
Drake, Nancy C.
Dunkley, June E.E.
Eardley, Margaret J.

Egan, Enid P.
Ford, Irene
Games, Joyce M.
Gillanders, Suzanne V.
Goldie, Gwendoline H.
Goudy, Joan M.
Harrold, Janette
Hesse, Pamela M.
Hubbard, Mary M.
Humphreys, Connie
Hyde, Lois
Johnson, Amy
King, Olive M.
Lamb, Jean M.
Laugher, Audrey M.
Ley, Dawn S.
Levitzke, Enid V.
Ley, Dawn S.
Markham, Shirley R.
Murphy, Margaret A.
Nixon, Joyce G.
Northcott, Gretel
Osborne, Norma L.
Pollett, Barbara R.
Prior, Alison J.
Richardson, Anne L.
Royle, Patsy R.
Russell, Elspeth M.
Salmon, Jane E.
Scarborough, Ruth A.
Smith, Lois Y.
Spicer, Elizabeth L.
Spicer, Elizabeth N.
Telfer, Heather M.
Templeton, Rosanna
Thornton, Suzanne J.
Usher, Jean L.A.
Van Leeuwen, Mary M.
Walpole, Dorothy P.
Weaver, Audrey M.
Webster, Faye C.P.
Whiffen, Lee
White, June B.
Van Leeuwen, Mary M.

1953
Arnold, Nancy C.
Ahearn, Judith M.
Benton, Mrytle R.
Belzer, Una
Browne, Shirley M.
Cumber, Yvonne L.
Barrett, Judith A.
Buntine, Ann J.
Crockford, Joan A.
Brewster, June M.
Doherty, Audrey I.
Downie, Margaret I.
Ellen, Patricia M.
Fenton, Margie
Filleul, Gwenda M.
Gillespie, Alison
Golder, Dorothy J.
Heriot, Beverley
Hore, Jean L.
Hulls, Elizabeth M.
Hurley, Jane
Jackson, Janet H.
Johnstone, Marion E.
Johnston, Beth M.
Lacey, Ruth J.
Lowe, June E.
Longfield, Elizabeth H.
McDonald, Jean
McCall, Margaret G.A.
Mair, Margaret C.B.
Massey, Clara P.
Mitchell, Rosemary
Nicholas, Jennifer R.
Nicoll, Margie F.
Nicholas, Jennifer R.
Prior, Alison J.
Pollett, Barbara R.
Resuggan, Dawn E.
Ross, Lamond D.
Rider, Jennifer J.
Rosa, Lorna M.
Ross, Norma M.
Semmens, Margot R.
Sharman, Thelma I.
Sheperd, Joan A.
Smart, June M.

Appendix 2

Tobias, Lorraine J.
Strickland, Elizabeth L.
Thomson, Margaret I.
Thornton, Suzanne J.
Vagg, Margaret D
Walls, Lois B.
Waterhouse, Margaret J.
Watt, Barbara F.
Webster, Elaine B.
Wheeler, Nan
Wilkinson, Hazel D.
Whitehand, Marion
Wood, Alison M.
Youla, Aileen J.

1954

Barnes, Mary F.
Begg, Ann H.
Brain, Mary E.
Burstall, Judith A.
Butler, Elizabeth F.
Corrigan, Elizabeth J.
Cox, Shirley E.
Cunningham, Barbara J.
Dingle, Betsy
Freeman, Aileen R.
Freeman, Olive J.
Grummet, Joycelyn M.
Harding, Ann B.
Kendall, Beatrice A
Lane, Barbara J.
Langley, Olivia J.
Laycock, Melvie J.
Linforth, Marie E.
Manger, Edna J.
MacLeod, Diana E.
Mackenzie, Eileen M.
McGuiness, Beverley A.
Mitchell, Rosemary
Muir, Margaret
Murfet, Merle C.
Pollock, Margaret J.
Preston, Beryl D.
Strangward, Rosemary
Stott, Shirley I.
Thomas, Jocelyn P.F.
Thompson, Judith A.

1955

Albiston, Eril M.
Alexander, Beatrice B.
Altmann, Frances M.
Baker, Nola C.
Banks, Deirdre M.
Barton, Sonia J.
Berrill, Helen
Birkin, Margaret J.
Bond, Wendy M.
Burstall, Judy
Brennan, Joan L.
Chapman, Mary B.
Chilvers, Jane M.
Colyer, Millicent A.
Cooper, Hilary C.
Darwin, Dorothy J.
Easton, Gwenlyn M.
Gandevia, Marie B.
Giffard-Burgess, Elizabeth C.
Gould, Pamela J.
Gratton-Wilson, Rosamond M.
Hamilton, Patricia
Heard, Eve
Henry, Shirley A.
Hirsch, Etta
Hood, Gloria
Ivey, Margaret R.
Laugher, Lois L.
Liley, June C
Little, Barbara A.
Macauley, Wilma M.
Marshall, Nellie M.
Milliken, Doris M.
Mitchell, Margaret E.
Moore, Valerie J.
Myers, Isabel
Patterson, Lorraine E.
Reid, Marion E.
Riches, Merle
Skene, Barbara R.
Stephenson, Helen M.
Sutton, Barbara B.
Taylor, Valerie
Thompson, Elizabeth A.
Thomson, Marjorie E.
Tilley, Judith M.
Tyler, Barbara H.
Wadds, Wilma M.
Walker, Ann M.
Walter, June M.
Washfold, Gwenda J.
Winch-Williams, Wendy H.

1956

Allen, Valma E.
Ballard, Margot N.
Berryman, Edwina
Bon, Berenice R.
Booth, Jean M.
Brand, Beverley A.
Brothers, Margaret A.
Campbell, Janet S.
Carter, Dorothy J.
Cobbin, Myrna M.
Cowan, Eileen P.
Darwin, Jean
Deery, Nora A.
Down, Marjorie J.
Dunn, Shirley J.
Dunne, Antoinette I.
Farthing, Valma L.
Fitzpatrick, Kathleen
Fox, Noelene E.
Fraser, Dorothy M.
Frizon, Josephine R.
Hart, Pamela J.
Hatherley, Margaret
Hogan, Meryl
Huf, Lynette M.
Hunter, Meriel A.
Jess, Sheila
Kennett, Margaret H.
Kitson, Diana J.
Lodge, Adrienne P.
Lowe, Robin
Matthews, Joy D.
McIntyre, Rhona J.
McKenzie, Pamela E.
Muller, Dawn
Payne, Alice G.
Pearce, Aileen J.
Roberts, Johanna M.

Robertson, Janet N.
Satchell, L. Beverley
Scales, Ethel D.
Smith, Nyree M.
Smith, Wynne M.
Smyth, Marjorie H.
Stark, Yvonne E.
Street, Faith
Strover, Anne C.
Swanson, Dorothy
Taylor, Cecily L.
Tymms, Helen L.
Walker, Judith A.
Walls, Katherine J.
Waterworth, Mary G.
Watson, Isabella M.
Wilson, Judith
Wright, Verna May

1957
Abey, Robin M.
Adey, Helen S.
Allen, Valma E.
Anderson, Jennifer J.
Badkin, Janet
Banks, Cheryl E.E.
Bates, Rosalie A.A.
Berrill, Margaret A.
Brand, Beverley A.
Charlton, Margaret J.
Cox, Aileen M.
Dyason, Jill E.
George, Marion
Gibson, Helen V.L.
Handley, Laurel E.
Harding, Judith M.
Harris, Janet C.
Hart, Pamela J.
Heriot, Alison
Hoadley, Peggy
Holt, Judith A.
Horne-Shaw, Wilma B.
Hunter, Aileen J.
Kearney, Noreen B.
King, Helene M.
Lawrence, Barbara
Lees, Margaret E.

Lewis, Margaret C.
Lindner, Shirley E.
MacDougall, Brenda E.
Macquarie, Shirley
Marriner, Jean E.
McDermott, Eileen P.
McClure, Patricia E.
McDermott, Eileen P.
McEwen, Helen E.S.
McKenzie, Norma R.
McVean, Rachael B.
Mildren, Valma D.
Mitchell, Judith A.
Morton, Annette E.
Norman, Pauline M.
Parton, Margot G.
Perryman, Janice
Petzke, Rosemary J.
Purcell, Beverley E.
Robinson, Helen F.
Rodd, Betty L.
Smith, Kerry V.
Steel, Jeanette D.
Strickland, Margaret E.
Swan, Sally C.
Tonks, Kaye
Tribe, Mary
Tymms, Helen L.
Wait, Mary E.
Webber, Elizabeth M.
Wheeler, Margaret H.
Wood, Judith A.
Woolf, Valerie

1958
Arnel, Valerie J.
Begg, Robin M.
Bon, Lina H.
Cassidy, Dorothy S.
Dixon, Lillian B.
Dyason, Jill E.
Geary, Irene S.
Gibson, Barbara D.
Hall, Margaret R.
Hawker, Marjorie M.
Hayes, Valda M.
Henderson, Jillian M.

Hodgson, Denise T.
Holden, Christine M.
Home-Shaw, Wilma B.
Johnson, Barbara D.
Lake, Judith
Lamb, Lynette M.
Le Masurier, Joan E.
Leontieff, Vera
Littlewood, Sylvia J.
Lloyd, Janet
Lovey, Marita T.S.
Marriner, Jean E.
May, Jeanette
Merritt, Kathleen R.
McNair, Patricia M.P.
McVean, Rachel B.
Macquarie, Shirley
Mills, Linda E.
Morgan, Mary C.
Morton, Eileen T.
Munro, Heather M.
Nance, Marlene
Oldfield, Valda Mae
Oliver, Patricia M.
Palmer, Judith L.
Pennington, Helen W.
Pippard, Margaret E.
Pocknee, Janice M.
Steele, Gabrielle M.
Stokes, Madge L.
Syme, Alice M.
Truscott, Elizabeth
Tucker, Elaine M.
Wait, Mary E.
Wait, Adrienne B.
Williamson, Thelma A.
Williams, Margaret F.
Wilkinson, Janice M.
Wolff, Valerie
Wood, Laurel M.
Woolley, Beverley J.

1959
Aldridge, Rose M.
Anderson, Judith H.
Baker, Helen M.
Boas, Beverley

Bartlett, Dorothy
Canning, Elizabeth M.
Dale, Anne
Eames, Anne
Edelstone-Pope, Elizabeth
Fairley, Rosemary M.
Felder, Joyce M.
Glassock, Barbara C.
Goldby, Gillian M.
Gome, Marlene E.
Green, Elizabeth A.
Harper, Margaret I.
Harper, Patricia
Harris, Faye E.
Hay, Patricia G.
Heywood, Patricia
Hirst, Janice B.
Hudson, Mary
Hudson, Mary E.
Iredale, Anne L.
Jackson, Elizabeth M.
Jackson, Margaret E.
Johannesen, Dawn
Johnston, June M.
Leaver, Margot A.
Lewis, Maureen D.
Lewthwaite, Judith M.
Lindner, Shirley E.
McKaskill, Lesley A.
Martin, Rhonda M.
Patterson, Margaret
Redmond, Jennifer Ann
Reid, Jane E.
Renkin, Wendy A.
Robinson, Lois A.
Ryan, Margaret A.
Sayers, Trilbey
Snowball, Sara A.
Steele, Gabrielle
Sykes, Priscilla J.
Steiner, Patricia J.
Tainton, Dorothy R.
Thompson, Irene E.
Thompson, Valerie J.
Vallance, Teresa F.
Walker, Helen S.
Webster, Trilma J.

Webster, Anne S.
Yeend, Barbara
Young, Beverley L.

1960
Aikin, Susan J.H.
Allan, Elizabeth A.
Booth, Ruth E.
Boucher, Maureen E.
Brady, Mary L.
Buchanan, Faye A.
Chidley, Dorothy R.
Colley, Janet M.
Cox, Pamela J.
Davey, Roseanne V.
Dawson, Shirley A.
Ditterich, Barbara M.
Doherty, Margaret V.
Eastaugh, Lorna A.S.
Ellis, Margaret E.
Farthing, Dorothy M.
Fennell, Lois M.
Grieve, Patricia A.
Goldby, Gillian M.
Hall, Jennifer S.
Hardy, Helen C.
Harry, Margaret L.
Holland, Jennifer E.
James, Elizabeth C.
Jenkins, W. Dawn
Langdon, Valerie
Laughlin, Lorraine
Long, Margaret N.
Mainsbridge, Shirley
McElhinney, Helen F.
McKaskill, Lesley A.
MacLiver, Patricia A.
Meates, Patricia A.
Morriss, Margaret F.
Mottram, Ruby P.
Ng, Oi Yuet
Norman, Judith A.
O'Neill, Elizabeth A.
Pemberton, Annabel
Rieder, Jane
Salmon, Margaret J.
Salter, Frances G.

Shaw, Barbara
Sheehan, Marie T.
Young, Beverley L.

1961
Anstee, D. Rae
Balfour, Margaret J.
Baragwanath, Judith A.
Bartlett, Dorothy M.
Beach, Lorraine A.
Beamish, Heather M.
Beaumont, Ann J.
Blood, Jennifer F.
Bonser, Lauris M.
Bravington, Nora I.
Brown, Margaret J.
Burgess, Jean M.
Caldwell, Anne E.
Curtis, Kevin R.
Davidson, Lynette M.
Dew, Jennifer
Eppinger, Gertruid K.
Frank, Ursula
Fraser, Elizabeth A.
Goldsmith, Janice M.
Goodger, Lorraine N.
Harris, Rae G.
Hughes, Margaret H.
Humble, Vivienne E.
Iu Po Hung, Annie
Kenneally, Maureen
Lawrence, Katherine E.
Lee, Wai Kwan Wendy
Pascoe, Wendy J.
Robertson, Patricia M.
Rumpf, Ann
Smith, Joan D.
Sutherland, Ann M.
Swanton, Helen M.G.
Taggart, Lorraine J.
Tucker, Patricia L.M.
Webster, Julia J.
Wellard, Wendy L.
White, Jennifer N.
Wilde, Raemonde I.
Wilson, Hilda M.
Wooton, Betty A.

1962
Alger, Joyce M.
Allan, Iris E.
Andrews, Elizabeth M.
Ansell, Vivien G.
Beckley, Lorna A.
Belcher, Lynette M.
Berney, Lesley M.P.
Beton, Margaret A.
Boothby, Elizabeth K.
Bradley, Leonie Anne
Burwood, Barbara A.
Chambers, Yvonne J.
Cholerton, Patricia A.
Clarke, Beryl M.
Cook, Kay L.
Corby, Helen
Coutts, Lorraine J.
Cowley, Hellen D.
Downing, Beverley J.
Ellis, Beverley M.
Farrow, Janice V.
Gome, Heather
Gray, Nancy M.
Hammond, Patricia A.
Harkess, Christine
Himing, Judith A.
Humphery, Isobel A.
Humphreys, Elizabeth A.
Johnstone, Shirley M.
Kennedy, Sylvia Grace
Linden, Mary P.
Loorham, Deirdre M.
MacRobert, Anne C.
May, Beverley
May, Jeanette
McLaurin, Mary J
Mealyea, Janet McL.
Moore, Beverley L.
Neil, M. Allison
Newham, Rosemary J.
O'Neill, Elizabeth A.
Ormorod, Lynda E.
Owens, Judith A.
Radford, Ellen P.
Rollason, Barbara J.
Ross, Karin L.

Sanders, Glennys R.
Sanders, Jillian F.
Scott, Jeanette Y.
Siemering, Barbara M.
Sheil, Joan E.
Stabb, Virginia M.
Stewart, Barbara A.
Stabb, Virginia M.
Varly, Barbara
Westerman, Heather R.
Wood, Linda A.

1963
Andrews, Beryl L.
Baldwin, Patricia
Beckley, Lorna A.
Bell, Lynette F.
Begg, Helen M.
Boal, Audrey L.
Boyd, Patricia J.
Boyd, Lynette D.
Brown, Wendy M.
Clark, Sandra E.D.
Conroy, Mary A.
Cucow, Helena
Davey, Barbara M.
Davies, Elizabeth A.
Dunn, Janet V.
Edwards, Noela J.
Evans, Susan M.
Forbes, Carol A.
Garlick, Marilyn R.
Gillespie, Jennifer R.
Grant, Jon A.
Green, Barbara Janet
Halliday, Carolyn J.
Hawker, Ailsa C.
Hamilton, Pamela J.
Harris, Lee C.V.
Holland, Margaret J.
Hardess, Sherrell
James, Beverley A.
Lancaster, Catherine M.
Mason, Heather V.
McGowan, Barbara J.
McKenzie, Lorraine D.
McGowan, Barbara J.

Miles, Laurice E.
Money, Christine M.
Oliver, Nanette
Pannowitz, Robyn M.
Paton, Susan
Patrick, Helen P.
Paxton-Petty, Georgina K.
Ralph, Valerie M.
Reid, Margaret F.
Rogers, Patricia E.
Runnalls, Doreen M.
Rutherford, Janne
Seamons, Gwenda
Shaw, Rosemary M.
Simmons, Patricia J.
Stephens, Beverley K.
Stott, Phillipa B.
Street, Nance P.
Sutton, Kathleen S.
Thomas, Prudence M.
Thompson, Ellen I.
Van Valen, Johanna
Wilkin, Marjorie I.
Wollmer, Beveley J.
White, Helen K.

1964
Andrews, Dorothy A.
Bamford, Lesley A.
Banks, Sandra R.
Beck, Lynette J.
Bolles, Helen J.
Broinowski, Dorothy M.
Bullock, Noeline M.
Cake, Olwyn A.
Carmody, Judith A.
Carter, Valerie Joan M.
Chegwin, Joan I.
Clayton, Barbara C.
Crockett, Margaret J.
Dear, Margaret M.
Dixon, Wendy
Duxson, Valerie P.
Eadie, Elisabeth J.
Edward, Carol A.
Erlanger, Marianne
Evans, Sandra L.

Appendix 2

Fallu, Leonore (Lea)
Follett, Margaret V.
Goldsbury, Mary J.
Goodman, Marjorie E.
Harland, Judith E.
Harman, Kay
Holt, Margot W.
Hughes, Helen M.
Hughes, Nancy H.
Hutton-Jones, Alison
Hyland, Barbara M.
Johnson, Anne L.
Lardner, Susan D.
List, Margaret A.
Lloyd, Joyce A.
MacNaughtan, Gabrielle M.
Maddocks, Susan E.
McLean, Beverley L.
McNutt, Beverley F.
Peacock, Joyce E.
Prentice, Eleanor S.G.
Priest, Judith L.
Roberts, Judith A.
Rodda, Elizabeth D.
Stokes, Marlene J.
Terrill, Diane L.
Thomas, Beatrice M.B
Titshall, Margaret Ana
Wee, Kheng H.
Weir, Mary J.
Wong, Choon Y.
Woods, Beryl F.
Yates, Eunice A.

1965
Allan, Wendy E.
Anderson, Judith G.
Baxter, Pamela C.
Bhatt, Harcharan K.
Blyth, Helen P.
Brideson, Denise R.
Burke, Rosalind M.
Campbell, Jennifer
Clearson, Shirley M.
Crutchfield, Janice M.
Dale, Jennifer J.
Dimmitt, Marion L.

Ditterich, Anne R.
Duncan, Catherine B.
Fidge, Helen R.
Ford, Marie
Fowler, Diana F.
Foxwell, Kay F.
Gordon, Veronica B.
Haebich, Aurelia E.F.
Halliday, Wynette L.
Hann, Shirley D.
Hill, Lois A.
Hobday, Mary F.
Holland, Helen
Jayes, Jennifer
Jurk, Imas H.
Lambourn, Jennifer A.
Lehmann, Judith E.
Letheby, Carol A.
Love, Jillian M.
Lowcock, Stephane J.
McClelland, Yvonne J.
McElhinney, Alison J.
McKenzie-McHarg, Robin G.M.
McLean, Beverley L.
McRae, Glennis M.
Meehan, Lynette M.
Murphy, Sandra M.
Murray, Sandra M.
Nash, Beverley A.
Noall, Jillian V.
Nolan, Judith F.
O'Dell, Rosemary A.
Oxley, Treena E.
Parish, Clare E.
Roberts, Glynes J.
Robertson, Ann C.
Scales, Lynette J.
Siggins, Gillian M.K.
Steel, Pamela M.
Stott, Philippa B.
Sturtz, Josephine M.
Thong, Swee Kam
Traill, Margaret M.
Treleaven, Roslyn H.
Wilson, Marie D.
Yip, Choon L.

1966
Aitken, Margaret N.
Blewett, Kathleen L.
Bouchier, Barbara C.
Bram, Ruth
Bruce, Wendy J.
Cardwell, Suzanne M.
Carroll, Sandra J.
Chambers, Gwendolyn J.
Chambers, Merlyne L.
Chandler, Pamela J.
Cram, Helen A.
Cronin, Mary J.
Davis, Ruth B.
Daws, Berris J.
Dean, Pamela J.
Driver, Elizabeth P.
Fleming, Janette
Frew, Helen M.
Gibson, Dianne R.
Gordon, Dorothy
Goulding, Elizabeth A.
Hill, Christine K.
Howell, Patricia M.
Hutton, Margaret A.
Irwin, Suzanne J.
James, Evelyn J.
Kelly, Dawn E.
Kent Hughes, Meredith
Lind, Bernadette E.
Love, Elaine B.
Mahon, Lynette J.
McLennan, Diane L.
Miers, Jennifer E.
Moon, Carole A.
Moore, Rosalind J.
Morley, Ruth L.
Morris, Jennifer
Munro, Nancy P.
Pang, Si Yan
Parker, Marion
Parkes, Sandra D.
Peddie, Anne M.
Powne, Morag S.
Purbrick, Helen M.
Reed, Diana F.
Robinson, Helen

Robinson, Kerril A.
Rolfe, Jillian K.
Rollason, Barbara J.
Rumsey, Diane
Sadler, Ruth I.
Smith, Helen P.
Spicer, Helen M.
Summons, Laraine
Swift, Wendy L.
Thomas, Heather
Thompson, Lesley D.
Thompson, Yvonne E.
Wilson, Margaret H.
Wilson, Susan B.
Wiseman, Joan V.
Young, Carole J.
Young, Elizabeth A.

1967
Belcher, Gaye M.
Beltran, Rosita
Bodkin, Carol A.
Boughton, Jillian R.
Bride, Helen J.
Broderick, Helen A.
Browne, Lynette E.
Carmody, Margaret P.
Carr, Janet H.
Chappell, Wendy J.
Crook, Patricia M.
Damman, Gertruida A.C.
Dean, Joyce M.
Dean, Marianne W.
Dean, Patricia A.
Dickson, Noel J.
Duncan, Rosemary K.
Fitch, Elizabeth W.
Fowler, Jane D.
Gardner, Vivienne D.
Gladstone, Marilyne A.
Gower, Heather E.
Greaves, Jeanette N.
Greenlees, Beverley R.
Grzemski, Erika
Hamer, Lorna M.
Hansen, Merryl A.
Harris, Alice J.

Haussegger, Pamela K.
Hawkes, Gail L.
Hayes, Patricia V.
Hearty, Anne
Hollowood, Susan P.
Hudspeth, Elizabeth J.
Humffray, Elizabeth R.
Ippel, Janneke
Jennar, Kathleen F.
Johnson, Anne E.
Jones, Jennifer A.
Jones, Robyn M.
Kelly, Jean M.
Lamb, Margaret H.
Leitch, Stephanie J.
Lennox, Christine A.
Leonard, Carol R.
Littlejohn, Glenys J.
Lukies, Lynette M.
Maughan, Jennifer
McColl, Marilynne A.
McMillan, Monnalyna
Menzies, Janet C.
Millar, Prudence J.
Neilson, Karen M.
Onslow, Jane E.
Ooi, Boon See
Paul, Ruth
Peace, Judith M.R.
Philippe, Robin S.
Podger, Rosemary A.
Puser, Mila M.T.
Raleigh, Janice M.
Rhys-Jones, Meryl A.
Rogan, Helen M.
Russell, Glenda M.
Salmon, Rhonda J.
Shadforth, Susan E.
Sheehan, Judith O.
Smalley, Jillian R.
Starr, Kaye L.
Stephenson, Joyce M.
Taylor, Ruth
Van Rompaey, Margaret S.
Walker, Jeanette
Walters, Suzanne T.
Webster, Robyn D.

Widmer, Catherine A.
Williams, Robyn M.
Wong, Wendy J.
Wood, Susan A.
Wright, Margaret M.
Zybuljak, Nelly

1968
Abbott, Julie E.
Allison, Dorothy L.
Anderson, Jayne F.
Atkinson, Susan E.B.
Baker, Helen M.
Barrand, Andre V.
Bennett, Susan E.
Bonython, Robyn D.
Bowden, Diane J.
Braithwaite, Susan G.
Brideson, Patricia M.
Carman, Alison G.
Ciddor, Pamela E.
Clements, Diane M.
Coombs-Shapcott, Carolyn
Freedman, Prudence
Doyle, Sheila M.
Eagle, Frances E.
Eddy, Judith K.
Edwards, Terri A.
English, Judith M.
Etheridge, Janice L.
Farley, Margaret A.
Fox, Nolene M.
Frampton, Diane L.
Freitag, Cheryl C.
Giblett, Judith M.
Glynn, Patricia
Gray, Deborah J.
Gregg, Jennifer J.M.
Grose, Carol J.
Gunn, Jean N.
Hamilton, Meredith A.
Hewett, Anne L.
Hope-Campbell, Georgina W.
Hose, Julie M.
Johnson, Elizabeth
Johnson, Joanne S.

APPENDIX 2

Jones, Robyn F.
Jorgensen, Ann L.
Lee, Roselie
Littlehales, Bronwen M.
Mackenzie, Jill
McAllister, Susan R.
McKay, Dorothy E.
McKenzie, Heather
Middleton, Helen S.
Morgan, Wendy G.
Moyle, Delwyn J.
Murgatroyd, Helen J.
Murphy, Elizabeth P.
Parkinson, Elizabeth E.
Paterson, Heather A.
Pearse, Judith E.
Pearson, Juliette C.
Pincombe, Helen M.
Poulter, Margery A.
Power, Pauline
Prokopavicius, Brigitte
Pygall, Janice M.
Ramsey, Norma E.A.
Ramsey, Sharon G.
Reid, Erika F.
Salmon, Rhonda J.
Sanders, Gayle C.
Sherlock, Pauline A.
Small, Glenys R.
Smith, Roslyn M.
Smith, Penelope K.W.
Snow, Patricia
Thorne, Beverley A.
Tomkins, Beverley J.
Tooher, Judith A.
Trinca, Hilary J.
Tyzack, Winifred R.
Van Efferen, Magdalena H.
Van Staveran, Maria
Wassilieff, MArgaret
Wills, Marjorie A.
Wilson, Rae A.
Winter, Heather G.
Woods, Helen J.

1969
Anceschi, Diana M.

Arnold, Helen M.
Aston, Kathleen J.
Bachelor, Ruth E.
Ballantyne, Lynn C.
Bishop, Julie A.
Bode, Leila J.
Bremner, Judith A.
Charles, Vicki
Chrisp, Dorothy A.
Cole, Susan
Colwell, Julie M.
Coombs-Shapcott, Carolyn
Coutts, Jocelyn M.
Craigie, Dale
Crow, Elizabeth A.
Dalton, Jo-Anne M.
Davis, Marie R.
Dinsdale, Margaret J.
Dolamore, Catharine H.
Donovan, Robyn G.
Dubbeld, Wypkjen
Esler, Adrienne M.
Faragher, Jennifer D.
Finch, Barbara K.
Foley, Margaret L.
Ford, Linda
Fothergill, Lorraine M.M.
Fulton, Margaret J.C.M.
Gillies, Roslyn E.
Hunt, Julie A.
Keen, Christine L.
Lambie, Linda C.
Lamond, Sue S.
Linke, Margaret J.
Macdonald, Marion F.I.
Maynard, Robyn J.
McKenzie, Margaret
McLaren, Robyn J.
Miethke, Joan M.
Murphy, Helen P.
Mowacki, Kay L.
Ord, Florence M.
Ord, Michelle
Orford, Anne L.
Paton, Margaret G.
Payne, Gillian M.
Philistin, Diane K.

Pincombe, Helen M.
Prater, Avis I.
Radcliffe, Janet H.
Russell, Glenda M.
Rydel, Doris N.
Sawrey, Kay L.
Smith, Margaret J.
Smith, Roslyn M.
Stone, Margaret A.
Strangio, Nancy V.U.
Swan, Kaye N.
Thorne, Beverley A.
Trannore, Maxine P.
Unmack, Robyn
Van Staveren, Maria J.
Van Tricht, Teuntje H.
Walsh, Karen F.
Watts, Margaret A.
Way, Lynette J.
Welch, Lynette J.
Whitelaw, Prudence S.
Williams, Margaret F.
Willis, Anne B.

1970
Andrew, Francine M.
Andrews, Mary L.
Barraclough, Leigh E.
Barton, Christine M.
Beckingsale, Mary L.
Bell, Helen M.
Bisdee, Elizabeth
Biss, Joan M.
Black, Laurel J.
Bower, Susan N.
Brown, Lynette J.
Byatt, Kathleen J.
Cations, Catherine G.
Cotton, Mary E.
Crain, Diane E.
Desborough, Joan
Dickie, Jocelyn D.
Doran, Gayle F.
Edwards, Beryl F.
Edwards, Kathleen A.
Elms, Denise L.
Friend, Jennifer R.

Gee, Margaret R.
Gibbons, Kaye H.
Hall, Patricia M.
Hallgrem, Janice L.
Hassold, Betty L.
Hayes, Gabrielle D.
Hempenstall, Catherine A.
Henderson, Carol A.
Holmes, Judith K.
Holmes, Robynne G.
Hughes, Christine M.
Irwin, Susan E.
Jaboor, Anna M.
Johnston, Brenda M.
Knapton, Patricia A.
Lee, Janice W.
Liang, Mun Heng
Lyon, Diana M.
Mallock, Patricia
McNeilage, Jillian
Meehan, Michele
Millar, Heather
Moran, Helen M.
Mortimer, Winifred A.
Perry, Janice M.
Petersen, Gloria J.
Phillips, Jan S.
Phillips, Marion J.
Plenderleith, Jennifer M.
Porter, Judith L.
Roberts-Thompson, Jane S.
Royce, Josephine L.
Ryan, Glenda M.
Simpson, Lillian J.
Smith, Dianne
Smith, Elizabeth M.
Smyth, Dianne
Stanton, Marcia K.
Stapleton, Ruth G.
Thomas, Elizabeth
Uhe, Lorraine E.
Underhill, Hilary N.
Vucinic, Vera
Weddell, Carole G.
White, Maureen C.
Whitehead, Kay E.
Whitford, Judith M.L.

Williams, Denise H.
Wilson, Paula M.
Withington, Catherine A.
Wynn, Susan E.
Yole, Pamela J.

1971
Arnott, Carolyn J.
Austin, Margaret H.
Baker, Merridee D.
Bartlett, Suellyn
Black, Pamela C.
Blaine, Barbara A.
Brien, Anthea M.
Burris, Jan M.
Conn, Nerida J.
Craig, Christine
Crosby, Helen M.
Crothers, Judith E.
Dahl, Jeanette F.
Davey, Barbara J.
Delaney, Mary F.
Dickers, Jennifer A.
Dillon, Mary R.
Donahoe, Genevieve M.
Donovan, Mary P.
Eddy, Kathryn J.
Evans, Judith M.
Finley, Jane L.
George, Kristine A.
George, Susan E. S.
Halbert, Carolyn
Harris, Susan M.
Healey, Helen O.
Holden, Elizabeth A.
Holten, Susan D.
Houfe, Mary E.
Houston, Elizabeth M.
Hunter, Kay
Ingram, Pamela A.
Jaboor, Pamela
Kern, Maria H. J
Lamont, Gail C.
Lethbridge, Sally A.
Lord, Jennifer A.
Manuel, Elizabeth M.
Matthews, Louise M.

Mayo, Elizabeth L.
McCabe, Helen C.
McGavin, Virginia K.
McGrath, Patricia
Melrose, Lesley J.
Meenan, Loretta A.
Morley, Carol A.
Newman, Judith C.
Pellas, Julie E.
Revill, Suzanne J.
Roach, Sharyn A.
Robinson, Julie D.
Rolley, Glenda J.
Rolls, Geraldine E.
Russell, Marilyn A.
Thomson, Kay T.
Sloan, Joan C.
Smith, Janice J.
Stevens, Margaret A.
Taylor, Dorothy M.
Traynor, Joanne M.
Vowles, Margaret M.
Wade, Valerie R.
Watson, Heather F.
White, Deborah F.
Wilks, Dearne P.
Williams, Jennifer R.

1972
Altmeier, Robyn J.
Ashmore, Judith R.
Bartlett, Julie-anne
Baxter, Gayle L.
Beach, Dawn J.
Berrisford, Judith A.
Blaine, B.
Brown, Pamela J.
Burke, Margot M.
Burtt, Annette J.
Campbell, Janet F.
Cochrane, Helen M.
Cook, Dianne M.
Cooke, Beverly J.
Cotter, Patricia M.
Dickens, Meredith M.
Duke, Alison M.
Edwards, Cheryl A.

APPENDIX 2

Enever, Dianne L.
Ferguson, Elizabeth A.
Firth, Sally R.
Foley, Jennifer Y.
Fotheringham, Angela M.
Fowler, Helen P.
Frankland, Robyn K.
Goldsworthy, Faye M.
Golletz, Susanne R.
Goodger, Alyson P.
Gyngell, Kathleen E.
Holmes, Denise C.
Hoskin, Robyn L.
Hunt, Jillian G.
Kearton, Janet M.
Kodre, Rita
Langdon, Kathlyn M.
Lennon, Dianne M.
Livermore, Marien J.
Madder, Bronwyn J.
McConchie, Andrea M.
McLean, Rowena E.
McLeod, Robyn H.
Meagher, Rosalie F.
Menzies, Judith A.
Mitchell, Ann M.
Mitchell, Sheridan A.
Moon, Glenda L.
Morone, Susanne C.
Moss, Gail
Murnane, Maureen F.
Neill, Caroline D.
Notman, Glenda L.
Orr, Lesley J.
Perry, Suzanne M.
Pontin, Sandra L.
Ratten, Valerie J.
Robertson, Ruth H.
Ronay, Barbara C.
Ruwoldt, Helen M.
Scott-Mackenzie, Susan W.
Skitt, Joanne E.
Smith, Jennifer H.
Spierlings, Patricia W.
Taylor, Merryn B.
Thomas, Edna A.
Thomas, Susan P.

Watson, Heather J.
White, Deborah
White, Gaylene A.
Whitford, Carol A.
Williams, Dianne M.
Wright, Sally E.
Yarwood, Lilian C.

1973

Arthur-MacDonald, Jeanette
Auty, Wendy M.
Baker, Linda M.
Barry, Leonie B.
Barrie, Susan M.
Bartram, Diane E.
Beckingsale, Janet
Beecham, Merle J.
Bokor-Farkas, Winifred
Bottomer, Jill S.
Brewer, Ann
Brown, Rosalie Y.
Bryce, Catriona W.
Carlisle, Winifred A.
Carr, Rhylla C.
Cawdle, Michele A.
Chick, Suzanne E.
Conroy, Jennifer E.
Cook, Jeanette A.
Cooper, Judith A.
Coventry, Anne N.
Cowden, Judith A.
Cranston, Anne E.
Crowe, Gwenda A.
Crowley, Meryl F.
Davies, Beverly G.
Davis, Anne E.
Diffey, Heather
Doherty, Susan M.
Downey, Jennifer S.
Finley, Shirley A.
Fletcher, Pamela M.
Foreman, Christina J.
Gadsden, Jennifer J.
Gayer, Susan V.
Gordon, Anne M.
Graham, Anne
Hailes, Jennifer A.

Halls, Mary O.
Hanlon, Barbara J. A.
Hardisty, Ann C.
Hewett, Margot J.
Hocking, Sally M.
Holmes, Barabara G.
Hosking, Cheryl A.
Johnston, Lesley M.
Kelly, Ann M.
Kennedy, Lynne M.
Lagula, Paz
Lane, Margaret
Macdonald, Prudence L.
MacDowell, Beverley I.
MacRae, Islay M.
Marshall, Helen J.
McCoy, Julia M.
McDonald, Jeanette
McEwan, Robyn
McKenzie, Margaret A.
McKinley, Janet
McMahen, Anne B.
Menzies, Susan M.
Mullan, Ann
O'Neill, Wynne E.
Panczyszyn, Janine M.
Parkinson, Diane M.
Philp, Susan M.
Purves, Katherine J.
Read, Ann F.
Rogers, Nancy E.
Scott, Suzanne M.
Sims, Leona M.
Smedley, Pamela J.
Smith, Deidre J.
Smith, Janice H.
Smith, Jennifer D.
Spencer, Beverley J.
Spicer, Jennifer E.
Strachan, Georgina R.
Swan, Bernice E.
Tamblyn, Susan M.
Teh, Bee Lee
Watkins, Bronwyn A.
Wilson, Meryl F.
Wright, Catherine A.
Yeomans, Jill M.

1974
Aird, Heather A.
Allen, Sheryl A.
Anderson, Janette L.
Andrew, Jennifer M.
Armstrong, Jane L.
Avent, Julie C.
Bain, Lynette A.
Bainbridge, Robin M.
Baker, Cheryl M.
Bourne, Robin J.
Boyd, Jennifer N.
Bransgrove, Annette J.
Bromley, Ann C.
Brosnan, Kathryn M.
Clarke Michelle
Clee, Joy Elizabeth
Cramond, Elspeth J.
Crockett, Rosemary A.
Daniels, Penelope A.
Doran, Helen M.
Duncan, Gaye M.
Dunn, Barbara G.
Eason, Judith
Eccles, Catherine J.
Edwards, Diedre F.T.
Everitt, Marilyn I.
Farrant, Susan J.
Fitzgerald, Dianne T.
Franklyn, Pauline A.
Goode, Dianne N.
Hale, Janet C.
Hanger, Anne J.
Howden, Kay L.
Hughes, Denise A.
Jackson, Kathleen
Jarvis, Yvonne L.
Jung, Heather E.
Kavanagh, Freda A.
Kay, Monica C.
Kee, Elizabeth I.
Kelly, Maureen G.
Lamb, Sue
Leach, Karen D.
Lewis, Marilyn E.
Long, Gail M.
Madder, Bronwyn J.

Martin, Heather J.
McCann, Yola L.
McDowell, Beverley I.
McGeoch, Margaret
McKay, Erica H.
McKenzie, Sue
McLeish, Barbara A.
McNulty, Maree J.
McPhee, Fiona N.
Meager, Rosalie F.
Menzies, Susan M.
Millar, Robyn G.
Milligan, Johanne M.
Morshead, Elizabeth A.
Newnham, Sally L.
Osborne, Ruth E.
Parish, Lynette J.
Paton, Alethea J.
Pilley, Kaye L.
Porter, Cheryl A.
Power, Christine M.
Prater, Janice E.
Pryor, Alison L.
Radzimirski, Josephine E.
Reilly, Anne E.
Robertson, Elizabeth M.
Rowley, Diane
Roydhouse, Heather J.
Ryan, Colleen T.
Schubert, Ann V.
Sillett, Penelope M.L.
Sims, Leona M.
Sonenberg, Zara L.
Stubbs, Ruth A.
Sutherland, Linda Joy
Swan, Kathryn A.
Tann, Pamela
Taylor, Annette J.
Thornton, Heather
Tom, Jennifer C.
Uvira, Hana
Van Langenburg, Yvette
Wagner, Patricia M.
Waites, Ernesta A.
Walker, Margaret L.
Westwood, Anne M.
Wettenhall, Alison M.

White, Janet P.
Whyte, Heather
Williams, Gabrielle T.
Williams, Margaret
Williamson, Patricia
Winn, Karen M.
Wraith, Pauline M.
Yeo, Noeline M.

1975
Abbott, Katrina J.
Amor, Julie M.
Anderson, Robyn K.
Armstrong, Alison J.
Barrie, Anne C.
Bence, Rowena C.
Billing, Barbara E.
Blandon, Madeleine M.
Bolles, Helen J.
Brant, Jennifer R.
Bristow, Jillian
Brown, Katherine A.
Browne, Viva E.
Campbell, Sandra M.
Christie, Kathryn I.
Coburn, Jane E.
Coggins, Alison R.M.
Conley, Vivien G.
Conway, Kathleen A.
Cummins, Monica J.
Darling, Sue E.
Davis, Debra L.
Day, Judith M.
Denison, Donna M.
Docking, Janice E.
Duffy, Maria T.
Ebbels, Anne J.
Emerson, Cheryl A.
Farrell, Glenys L.
Fenton, Robyn L.
Firth, Sally, R.
Francis, Donna-Lee
Francis, Susan G.
Gale, Pamela M.
Griffiths, Robyn A.
Hatton, Heather R.
Henderson, Margot G.

Henson, Janice
Higgins, Judith F.
Hope, Linda N.
Horton, Lynette J.
Houghton, Denise A.
Howard, Wendy M.
Hunt, Pamela M.
Hurrell, Julie
Jenkinson, Denise M.
Johnson, Karen A.
Kneale, Susan P.
Kupsch, Wendy H.
Law, Alisa C.
Lee, Dianne P.
Lewis, Catherine J.
Linpinski, Veronica S.
Liston, Pauline M.
Macans, Inese R.
Marshall, Jillian B.
Marshman, Wendy J.
Martin, Heather J.
Matthew, Sharyn L.
Mazur, Dianne E.
McConvill, Anne C.
McGregor, Leanne M.
McKew, Mary R.
Morgan, Diana H.
Morone, Suzanne C.
Mott, Lyndall C.
Murphy, Margaret E.
Nedza, June M.T
Nevett, Anne N.
O'Keefe, Colleen E.
Panczyszyn, Janina M.
Palmer, Ann L.
Palmer, Ruth A.H.
Patterson, Dianne P.
Perry, Judith A.
Perry, Catherine L.
Petronella, Anna M.
Pickard, Lynette S.
Pritchard, Barbara J.
Rodell, Christine A.
Romanis, Janet L.
Rose, Debra A.
Shanahan, Kathryn M.
Shaw, Lyndsey J.

Shipp, Anne T.
Simmonds, Vivian J.
Smith, Anne C.
Stone, Dawn M.
Taylor, Helen J.
Taylor, Wendy M.
Tyson, Margaret A.
Varga, Mary T.
Wallace, Marion E.
Wait, Christine
Warmington, Robina M.
Weir, Robyn
Whitelaw, Andrea G.
Widdison, Annette J.
Wilcox, Dianne E.
Worden, Margaret A.

1976
Alcock, Lynette J.
Allan, Donna M.
Anguey, Edna M.
Archer, Catherine C.
Arney, Susan J.
Baldwin, Dione H.
Bannister, Carol A.
Barr, Sally A.
Baruta, Maria A.
Bedgood, Cheryle M.
Begg, Elizabeth A.
Beswick, Kim E.
Bickford, Gail M.
Bonuda, Edna M.
Booth, Joanne L.
Boutcher, Vivienne M.
Bouvier, Deborah J.
Boyd, Susanne H.
Brabham, Jennifer R.
Bradford, Helen P.
Brant, Jennifer R.
Britten, Wendy J.
Broadhurst, Dianne O.
Brown, Katherine A.
Bruce, Julie L.
Burrows, Judith N.
Butler, Wendy J.
Cameron, Ann
Cantle, Karin M.

Carmichael, Heather S.
Carr, Joanne M.
Chalmers, Jane L.
Chambers, Cheryl L.
Ciancio, Fernanda
Clancy, Annette M.
Cordy, Glenda
Corrigan, Helen J.
Cousins, Elizabeth N.
Darling, Sue E.
De Lean, Corinne C.
Dingjan, Astrid J.E.M.
Elliot, Lois
Ferguson, Lois
Fitzgerald, Louise M.
Fleming, Susan K.
Frances-Williams,
 Gariad M.I.
Francis, Helen E.
Freckleton, Barbara A.
Gapes, Vivienne B.
Glare, Suzanne J.
Gould, Kathryn M.
Grant, Janet E.
Grieg, Kim E.
Gunawardana, Sandra W.
Harcourt, Karen J.
Harrison, Gayle L.
Hawkins, Anne T.
Heaton, Susan M.
Hodgkinson, Angela R.
Hunter, Jillian M.
Hunter, Maureen T.
Hutchinson, Kerri M.
Ivers, Suzanne W.
Kent, Lynette M.
King, Christine E.
Kupsch, Wendy H.
Lamont, Linda M.
Langshaw, Sheryle A.
Lauricella, Sheryn M.
Lehmann, Alma R.
Long, Penelope J.
Madigan, Robyn J.
McInnis, Ann V.M.
Miles, Gail M.
Milton, Helen L.

Moreland, Carolyn A.
Morgan, Eleanor C.
Morone, Suzanne C.
Natoli, Lynette V.
Nymeyer, Theresa M.
O'Sullivan, Monica M.
Overton, Robyn G.
Parsons, Linda M.
Pate, Rosemary J.
Paton, Janet N.
Perkins, Sandra C.
Prosser, Jennifer L.
Reid, Margaret A.
Rendle-Short, Johanna
Rice, Raelene J.
Richards, Alison M.
Rodgers, Carol E.
Rodgers, Judith K.
Ross, Carol G.
Ryan, Jacqueline A.
Shaw, Leanne J.
Shirley, Jeanette A.
Smith, Jennifer A.
Spinks, Diane P.
Stevenson, Anne E.
Stewart, Mary L.
Tassell, June W.
Taylor, Christine R.
Taylor, Wendy M.
Teasdale, Susan J.
Thomas, Sheryn M.
Twomey, Janette
Ward, Pamela J.
Watson, Catherine L.
Watson, Linda M.
Whelan, Jennifer L.
Wilcox, Dianne E.
Wild, Jennifer J.
Wilkins, Susan K.
Young, Leonie A.

1977
Ackland, Robyn A.
Amon, Karen
Barker, Marjorie L.
Baxter, Ruth A.
Beddome, Nola J.

Bennett, Anne C.
Berrisford, Susan J.
Boswell, Linda C.
Broardhurst, Dianne
Burgess, Jennifer A.
Burn, Karen L.
Campbell, Ann F.
Cheffers, Robert M.
Clark, Philippa J.
Clemance, Moira
Corcoran, Adele M.
Cossens, Rae L.
Craig, Gariad M.I.
Crawford, Wendy A.
Crow, Janet E.
Csik, Susan E.
D'Arcy, Lynette M.
Davidson, Judith D.
De Vaus, Wendy E.
Delaney, Marianne P.
Drew, Dorothy, C.
Drysdale, Janine P.
Eckersley, Gillian S.
Ellis, Rosemary A.
Feeney, Annette M.
Feery, Roseanne
Follett, Glenda R.
Gamble, Lynne A.
Garrett, Deborah A.
Geary, Susanne B.
Goodman, Judy L.
Gray, Alexandrina M.
Guille, Denise H.
Haig, Janet A.
Hall, Anne M.
Hards, Kathleen M.
Hayes, Bernadette M.
Hegarty, Pamela A.
Herbert, Kay M.
Hester, Margo A.
Hirsh, Priscilla S.
Hodgins, Elizabeth A.
Hodgkinson, Angela
Inglis, Elizabeth D.
Jane, Robert B.
Jess, Kathleen M.
Joseph, Ammini

Jurgenstein, Linda L.
Kelly, Paul J.
Killa, Christine H.
Laird, Denise J.
Lawley, Julie C.
Lawrence, Dianne E.
Lithgow, Roslyn N.
Lo, Po Kuen
McDonell, Deborah A.
McGregor, Denise H.
McKenzie, Karen A.
McManis, Sharon L.
McMillan, Edith B.
Morgan, Kerry E.
Munro, Birgit I.
Nankervis, Karen E.
Noonan, Sharon E.
Northwood, Helen E.
Padongwej, Sivaporn
Palmington, Lynne M.
Parks, Dianne M.
Patten, Mary T.
Plum, Lynette A.
Pump, Jennifer K.
Punshon, Susan M.
Reith, Patricia M.
Robinson, Geoffrey D.
Rocke, Philomena L.
Rodgers, Glenys C.
Rodgers, Judith K.
Sadlier, Jennifer J.
Scott, Jennifer J.
Senior, Dianne J.
Shaw, Anne M.
Sheyne, Dorothy C.
Short, Catherine J.
Small, Linda D.
Smith, Carolyn A.
Sneddon, Robyn I.
Stead, Robyn R.
Stone, Julie A.
Storer, Wendy A.
Street, Susan E.M.
Strijbos, Rosemary A.
Sutherland, Linda J.
Tanner, Michelle G.
Taylor, Jill

Taylor, Susanne E.
Tippett, Anne C.
Topp, Robyn F.
Tweedie, Susan M.
Vacar, Elaine M.
Valeriano, Erlinda
Van Nooten, Joanne
Vanderheiden, Joy C.
Waldschmidt, Monica
Wraith, Jennifer
Young, Belinda J.
Young, Judith A.

1978
Adams, Desmond J.
Adams, Jeanette L.
Adams, Lynne M.
Auld, Deborah M.
Barlow, Wendy A.
Barnes, Helen I.
Bowden, Dianne J.
Boynton, Judith S.
Braidie, Helen L.
Brereton, Helen F.
Brewster-Webb, Warrick G.C.
Bristow, Jillian
Broom, Melva J.
Brown, Susan M.
Burchell, Karen M.
Burrows, Jennifer L.
Cleary, Gail V.
Cooke, Debra I.
Coonan, Therese I.
Day, Suzanne E.
Druhan, Lindy N.
Dunk, Elizabeth L.
Eason, Jill L.
Edge, Helen
Edge, Jennifer A.
Ferguson, Claire E.
Findlay, Sheryl L.
Francis, Lorraine J.
Fraser, Sally-Anne E.
Gardner, Ann M.
Garratt, Susan H.
Gray, Ann S.

Haggarty, Catherine J.
Hall, Patricia J.
Higgs, Deborah J.
Hocking, Joy E.
Hunter, Fiona J.
Hutton, Janece M.
Iveson, Susan L.
Jenkins, Debra L.
Kelly, Michelle I.
Kerr, Merrilyn A.
Kirkham, Rhonda J.
Kuyper Harteloh, Yolanda C.
Lefoe, Maree P.
Lyon, Michelle J.
Lui, Deborah J.
MacDonald, Julie A.
Maplestone, Ann C.
Marshall, Alison J.
Mashiter, Jannine E.
Maxwell, Jan E.
McCasker, Rhonda L.
Medley, Lynette A.
Middleton, Christine A.
Middleton, Dianne E.
Millen, Gayle J.
Murray, Janine
Ogrizovic, Danica
Peacock, Eileen P.
Pellas, Toni M.
Peters, Madeleine T.
Porter, Jill E.
Powell, Heather A.
Pritchard, Robert G.
Purbrick, Mary A.
Purcell, Patricia A.
Radojevic, Dushka
Richardson, Elizabeth A.
Riley, Jennifer J.
Ritchie, Ingrid M.
Robertson, Elizabeth P.
Ross, Barbara A.
Ryan, Helen M.
Sartori, Colleen J.
Short, Elizabeth L.
Shuttleworth, Heather M.
Smolarek, Celina A.
Soste, Susan T.

Spicer, Sandra J.
Stanistreet, Sally A.
Stephenson, Lesley A.
Strachan, Lynette J.
Summers, Pauline M.
Thomas, Merran C.
Thomas, Susan E.
Treseder, Ruth D.
Turner, Janine M.
Vine, Lesley R.
Virgona, Jenny M.
Ward, Cheryl D.
White, Rosemary A.
Wilkinson, Linda J.
Worland, Elizabeth J.
Youlden, Catherine M.
Young, Angela V.

1979
Allen, Julie A.
Anderson, Kathryn M.
Bamford, Katrina J.
Begg, Linda J.
Bell, Christine R.
Bishop, Helen L.
Boal, Janet
Bolton, Sharon A.
Bounds, Julie A.
Boyes, David R.
Brendel, Sabine
Brereton, Susan L.
Brolon, Marie T.
Burke, Carol A.
Cameron, Fiona C.
Camilleri, Gayleen M.
Campbell, Barbara A.
Canning, Jennifer M.
Cavanagh, Robin C.
Chilton, Wendy G.
Clarke, Valerie E.
Cleland, Julie A.
Coady, Elizabeth A.
Coates, Marieanne
Considine, Julianne E.
Craig, Carolyn D.
Davis, Vickie A.
Durkacz, Helen J.

Ebbels, Sue A.
Edmonds, Glenys J.
Eldridge, Annette H.
English, Kerryn M.
Farmer, Beverly A.
Farrington, Anne E.
French, Edith J.
Geddes, Janette E.
Gladstone, Melanie T.
Goy, Heather C.
Gray, Sandra C.
Grigg, Sheridan J.
Guaran, Christina M.
Harrison, Leonie E.
Hayes, Grace E.
Heard, Michelle M.
Heinz, Kathryn J.
Howden, Jane M.
Juvonen, Anneli M.
Keeling, Sharon L.
Kelly, Deborah G.
Keogh, Cathryn E.
Kilpatrick, Dallas M.
King, Christine R.
Kirby, Carolyn A.
Lange, Jennifer W.
Leiper, Beverley J.
Lillis, Karen N.
Macdonald-Johnson, Vicki D.
Mackenzie, Christine A.
Mance, Joanne L.
Manley, Robyn J.
Marshall, Kathleen R.
McConchie, Debra J.
McGeachin, Neil A.
McGuire, Beverley H.
McKay, Jane A.
McKendry, Julie A.
McKenna, Joanne C.
McLaughlin, Bernadette
McLaws, Suzanne P.
McMurtrie, Amanda J.
Mekking, Esselien C.
Memishi, Adele
Millard, Nola G.
Miller, Celeste M.

Millman, Glenda M.
Morrison, Margaret L.
Morrison, Michelle
Morrow, Andrea L.
Morton, Prudence M.F.
Munn, Kerry D.
Munnerley, Leanne C.
Murphy, Jennifer H.
Murphy, Nola M.
Neale, Jennifer A.
Nott, Helen T.
Nunn, Debra M.
O'Callaghan, Janice M.
O'Halloran, Carmel F.
O'Keefe, Jane A.
Palmer, Jan R.
Parker, John E.
Pawsey, Lynne
Peel, Debra V.J.
Phelan, Grace E.
Pollard, Christine J.
Priest, Susan J.
Prowse, Rosemary J.
Rees, Catherine A.
Rhynehart, Theresa A.
Riordan, Joy H.
Robinson, Gwendoline A.
Rowe, Ruth M.
Sasse, Janet
Scott, Carmel
Semerak, Jill A.
Shaw, Karen P.
Shapcott, Jennifer B.
Slopak, Jennifer A.
Speed, Prudence M.
Smith, Judith A.
Snellen, Marinda
Stone, Pamela A.
Summerbell, Deborah J.
Sutton, Anne L.
Sutton, David F.
Thomas, Gail M.
Toohey, Deborah J.
Vanderree, Elizabeth M.
Vanthoff, Lisa J.
Virgona, Catherine M.
Walsh, Bernadette M.

Wilkins, Susan K.
Wilkins, Leanne, J.
Williams, Leanne D.
Wright, Nerida J.
Yates, Gayleen M.

1980
Anderson, Fiona J.
Baird, Merryn D.
Barnes, Carlene J.
Bayly, Elizabeth L.
Beggs, Ann E.
Begley, Shani E.
Bolton, Sharon A.
Braham, Lynette
Brown, Julie
Bucknill, Catherine A.
Callaghan, Elise A.
Campbell, Christina J.
Carroll, Patricia C.
Christie, Davina
Chilton, Wendy G.
Connelly, Frances E.
Cordell, Anne M.
Crawley, Helen
Crompton, Leanne F.
Darcy, Valerie A.
Davies, Meredyth J.
Denison, Anne I.
Dennemoser, Mary-Anne T.
Dodd, Carmel P.
Elliott, Robyn H.
Fuller, Catherine A.
Gardner, Christine J.
Goy, Amanda G.
Greet, Cheryle
Griffiths Jennifer L.
Guyatt, Rosalind E.
Hatzigeorgiou, Fotios
Hook, Marisa J.
Howden, Karen A.
Hulland, Robyn A.
Hyams, Debra
Jenner, Leonard J.
Johnston, Pamela F.
Johnstone, Jenny M.
Kerr, Cathryn M.

APPENDIX 2

King, Carolyn L.
Lawless, Brenda P.
Lechelt, Gabriele C.
Lee, Amanda M.
Lewis, Janine L.
Lightbody, Christine A.
Lingham, Julie V.
Marion, Yvonne L.
Martin, Wendy L.
Massey, Belinda J.
McLean, Patricia L.
McKendrick, Robyn E.
McMahon, Helena
MacDonald, Lynette R.
McIntosh, Anne M.
Mackenzie, Jeanette A.
Mills, Kym C.
Mitchell, Janet C.
Mitchell, Myra E.
Mullins, Karen E.
Munro, Yvonne E.
Murray, Heather J.
Nelson, Lesley A.
Ng, Lean Chang
Peel, Suzanne J.
Robinson, Fiona C.
Semerac, Jill A.
Seres, Elizabeth
Serle, Sharon T.
Short, Margaret H.
Smith, Judith A.
Sommerville, Maree T.
Stewart, Jennifer A.
Suttie, Fiona M.
Tan, Keng Csee
Thomas, Julie A.
Thomson, Leanne F.
Torney, Sharon L.
Treble, Diane E.
Waring, Suzanne M.
Williams, Jennifer A.
Williams, Rozelle M.
Wright, Susan E.

1981
Adams, Christopher L.
Allan, Kerry S.

Allard, Angela J.
Anastasios, Vasssiliki
Azzopardi, Rita
Balfour, Rhonda B.
Barnden, Jeanette
Birrell, Christine S.
Boyes, Kim C.
Brook, Karen J.
Buckingham, Heather M.
Bunting, Joanne M.
Byrne, Heather J.
Cahill, Marie T.
Carr, Jennifer M.
Clarke, Christine A.
Coad, Anne M.
Connell, Jeanette M.
Conzelmann, Lynette M.
Dean, Jayne M.
Durant, Dianne L.
Evans, Noeline M.
Everill, Serena J.
Fitzsimmons, Mary M.
Garner, Helen M.
Glascott, Joanne H.
Gork, Christine M.
Grundy, Susan M.
Guest, Robyn J.
Hahn, Katrina M.
Hayes, Deborah J.
Holland, Beverley
Hughes, Elizabeth L.
Inch, Jennifer K.
Johannesen, Julie A.
Kuhle, Suzanne
Leppien, Christine M.
Lynch, Felicity M.
Macdonald, Sharyn J.
Mansell, Suzanne J.
May, Elizabeth A.
McFadzean, Annette Y.
McGregor, Leanne M.
McKay, Colette A.
McKenna, Sonya L.
Meeking, Jan C.
Melville, Bronwyn
Mercer, Fiona
Mitchell, Amanda J.

Morrison, Kaye A.
Mullins, Charlotte
Murphy, Catherine G.
Murray, Julie M.
Nischwitz, Dagmar
Oliver, Kaye M.
Payton, Jan M.
Pearson, Julie E.
Pelly, Karen B.
Pollock, Belinda M.
Proposch, Leonie J.
Purcell, Kathleen M.
Rigby, Helen M.
Sear, Tracey L.
Sheers, Janette M.
Shelley, Melinda J.
Sloan, Jane E.
Stapleton, Jane C.
Suttie, Fiona M.
Sudholz, Anne M.
Vallance, Jeanette A.
Waddell, Debra A.
Walsh, Helen P.
Wilkins, Christine A.
Wilkinson, Fiona M.
Winton, Karen J.
Woods, Dianne J.
Young, Mary-Anne
Yule, Vanessa

1982
Acevedo, Jorge G.
Ansems, Belita
Avasalu, Linda M.
Baulch, Margaret A.
Barber, Pamela M.
Barker, Loretta M.
Barnacle, Bronwyn E.
Barry, Susan L.
Bliszczyk, Elzbieta
Bossel, Janine A.
Breen, Mary-ann
Brendel, Sabine
Brown, Carole E.
Carney, Joanne F.
Cassar, Kathryn G.
Charter, Joanne R.

Clarke, Carole D.
Clarke, Warren A.
Clayton, Merrilyn, L
Charles, Elizabeth M.
Coghlan, Margaret E.
Cousins, Rachel A.W.
Cousland, Helen M.
Cowles, Victoria A.
Cox, Jacinta M.
Cross, Janelle M.
Crouch, Roslyn S.
Crouch, Tracey J.
Donaldson, Lyn M.
Doery, Hilary J.
Dunlop, Lisa A.
Ellis, Lisa G.
Emmett, Rhonda J.
Finemore, Maureen E.
Fisher, Coral J.
Gacs, Elizabeth M.
Godbold, Raymond G.
Gozens, Lyn
Greaves, David
Hanger, Juliana T.
Howell, Kerrie A.
Ireland, Leonie H.
Johnson, Anne M.
Keating, Helen
Laffin, Jennifer A.
Lamont, Joy A.
Lepp, Julie M.
Maddison, Christine M.
McKellar, Sue G.
Menzies, Lindsay
Mills, Rhonda J.
Newman, Lindy A.
O'Donnell, Wendy H.
Pearson, Julie E.
Phillips, Linda J.
Potter, Caitlin J.
Quanchi, Andrea C.
Preston, Gail M.
Reid, Jane L.
Rouch, Susannah D.
Russell-Browne, Julianne C.
Russo, Amanda
Seres, Elizabeth

Scott, Carol L.
Singleton, Amanda J.
Short, Margaret H.
Smith, Jane E.
Smith, Andrea C.
Standish, Julie A.
Stevenson, Jennifer C.
Steiner, Caitlin
Stubbs, Rosemary
Topsom, Melanie A.
Vine, Cheryl-Anne
Wallace, Kerrie E.
Wall, Jennie Mc.
Walsh, Kaye M.
Webster, Kathryn K.
White, Linda M.
Williams, Robyn J.
Wilkins, Kerrie-Anne
Wilson, Anne
Vaanhold, Leonie M.
Yarnton, Kim A.

1983

Anderson, Kaye L.
Ashley, Karen A.
Barrow, Julie R.
Beilharz, Ingrid K.
Belfrage, John M.
Bell, Karen E.
Bish, Roslyn M.
Bodinnar, Jeanette C.
Bradbury, Jennifer L.
Broadbent, Jennifer M.
Brophy, Clare T.
Brown, Lee-Anne
Butler, Carolyn E.
Cannington, Cheryl A.
Carr, Mary K.
Carter, Catherine J.
Chamtaloup, Paula M.
Chirnside, Sarah J.
Clarke, Catherine M.
Colbert, Amanda J.
Coleman, Paloma
Cook, Jacqueline J.
Curzon, Julie-Anne
Dagiandas, Ekaterina

Date, Margaret L.
Davis, Margaret C.
Daymond, Carlene A.
Dean, Gregory P.
Dean, Caron F.
Donker, Maria J.
Douglas, Claire M.
Dunn, Wendy J.
Egerton, Yvonne C.
Farrington, Leah M.C.
Finn, Penelope S.
Franke, Kaye C.
Glen, Pauline D.
Gordon, Jane-Ellen
Greve, Lisa J.
Guilieri, Rosemary J.
Hahn, Rita A.
Hargrave, Rosemary E.
Hay, Frances A.
Hayes, Elizabeth A.
Hopkinson, Kim
Horch, Irma G.
Huelsebus, Ruth U.
Johnson, Darleen J.J.
Johnston, Andrea R.
Johnstone, Julie A.
Kelly, Margaret A.
Kent, Jenny McK.
King, Susan M.
Kingston, Anne P.
Kueter-Luks, Susanne J.
Lane, Catherine M.
Laundy, Karen A.
Lawrence, Ruth M.
Lewis, Leanne T.
Maher, Caroline A.T.
McCosh, Janet M.
McDonald, Susan
McGawley, Patricia A.
McKeon, Margaret A.
McLennan, Elisabeth M.
McNab, Catriona J.
Menzies, Alexander R.
Meyer, Jillian R.
Murphy, Barbara I.
Murray, Catherine E.
Naismith, Jennifer A.

APPENDIX 2

Nguyen, Thi Cong Dung
O'Connor, Stephanie J.
O'Donohue, Julie A.
O'Shea, Kim P.
Paris, Rosa S.
Pelly, Tracey M.
Phillips, Susan C.
Quinn, Paula M.
Rajamany, Ramasamy
Rayner, Gail E.
Reid, Anne
Reiper, Ruth E.
Renkin, Jennifer E.
Reynolds, Tracey H.
Rice, Debbie J.
Rodda, Rowena I.
Ryder, Paul R.
Sampson, Julie K.
Sayers, Joanne M.
Scott, Sherie K.
Shaw, Christine A.
Smout, Pauline A.
Spry, Penelope A.
Stares, Jennifer D.
Stewart, Janelle S.
Szondy, Catherine E.
Teasdale, Carolyn E.
Torry, Helen S.
Trump, Christine R.
Verstraeten, Michelle T.
Wishart, Lynette J.
Woodward, Julianne M.
Worland, Helen M.
Wotley, Catherine J.

1984

Adams, Janine M.
Adamson, Tania
Anglim, Genevieve
Anthony, Kathryn L.
Atkins, Janice H.
Bailey, Anne M.
Bald, Sara A.
Bale, Helen E.
Ball, Barbara N.
Barker, Simone-Lea
Basham, Maree

Beed, Sara A.
Besley, Fiona K.
Bicknell, Kathryn A.
Bos, Beatrix I.
Boyle, Judith A.
Brearley, Megan J.
Brown, Alison J.
Bruce, Susan G.
Boustead, Suzette G.
Caldecott, Kaye M.
Caspersz, Fleur T.
Charlesworth, Diana M.
Charlwood, Glenis
Clarke-Jones, Jennifer A.
Coleman, Brendan A.
Conron, June E.
Cox, Megan
Crobie, Elizabeth A.
De Keyzer, Karen A.
Devereux, Louise A.
Drummond, Michele D.
Dyer, Cheryl E.
Dyson, Sue L.
Eva, Tracey
Fitzroy, Elizabeth M.
Foley, Lisa J.
Fulton, Janet L.
Gohler, Anette P.
Graham, Heather C.
Green, Anna L.
Green, Lorraine S.
Grenfell, Jan L.
Grima, Anne C.
Harris, Gayle J.
Hausler, Helen M.
Hawkins, Catherine M.
Haywood, Katherine
Hosking, Greer C.
Hutchinson, Carolyn J.
Ives, Kerrie A.
Janes, Heather E.
Jeffrey, Jennifer M.
Jennings, Karyn L.
Jones, Robyn L.
Kane, Leah M.
Kendall, Susan T.
Kennedy, Susan E.

King, Jennifer M.
Knichala, Diana R.
Kokas, Susan
Land, Jillian E.
Lau, Wai Ling Nancy
Lee, Merinda J.
Lia, Terance G.
Lingard, Phillipa A.
MacCurrach Fiona J.
Marshall, Helen M.
Martin, Wendy J.
McCallum, Sarah J.
MacDonald, Julie M.
McFarland, Susan A.
Mitchell, Janine F.
Montague, Suzanne
Moreland, Tracey J.
Nicholson, Louise M.
Phillips, Wendy E.
Pryor, Sally J.
Radobuljac, Branka A.
Redmond, Joanne M.
Reed, Anne L.
Revell, Linda
Rodgers, Felicity M.
Saville, Dianna J.
Stoyles, Sally E.
Thomas, Elizabeth J.
Thorn, Dierdre
Tilley, Caroline E.
Waite, Ruth M.
Walsgott, Catherine M.
Webb, Nicola J.
Whitlock, Leanne M.
Wignell, Colette E.
Wright, Leonie P.
Young, Robert J.

1985

Antonie, Terri-Anne
Armstrong, Lyndel L.
Bailey, Michelle T.L.
Baker, Jennifer H.
Barnacle, Katherine A.
Baulch, Karen L.
Bence, Gabrielle J.M.
Bennett, Georgina P.

Bernardi, Vera J.
Bobadilla, Estrellita B.
Bridges, Susan
Burns, Katrina J.
Buttery, Anne M.
Byrne, Carolyn
Byrnes, Marguerite L.
Campbell, Susan M.
Casserley, Ann M.
D'Ambra, Marcelle L.
Davies, Karys W.
Dearnaley, Celia A.
Dooley, Amber T.
Duff, Linda A.
Ellingford, Joanne
Gault, Barbara H.
Gilmour, Delwyn J.
Glazner, Judith A.
Green, Barbara F.
Harkins, Andrea L.
Haywood, Paula V.
Hearn, Elizabeth A.
Henderson, Heather
Holdenson, Anna K.
Holland, Lynda G.
Howell, Trudi A.
Hunter, Susan L.
Ickeringill, Jacinta M.
Jordan, Sally A.
Kanthardis, Despina
Kemp, Kathryn L.
Lie, Petrina M.
Ling, Debra A.
Lord, Debbie L.
Low, Vivienne
Lunt, Carolyn A.
Malone, Kathleen M.
McKemmish, Shelley L.
McCulloch, Judith M.
McGregor, Elaine M.
Mifsud, Anna C.
Miller, Kathryn M.
Mills, Bernice A.
Murphy, Sharon M.T.
Murray, Andrea
Parigi, Michelle R.
Petrini, Joanne L.

Pirie, Ian D.
Pittorino, Lydia A.
Prudon, Marina J.
Read, Marie-Anne
Reichelt, Marion
Riddell, Julie A.
Riley, Kim P.
Sainsbury, Louise
Sampson, Tanya J.
Scerri, Caroline A.
Shalders, Tricia A.
Sicherdick, Susan J.
Silva, Melissa J.
Simon, Michelle L.
Smith, Edwina J.
Solomon, Dianne M.
Soulsby, Mary T.
Stafford, Elizabeth A.
Tellus, Denise A.
Thompson, Jenelle R.
Thorp, Carolyn L.
Topsom, Sarah L.
Turnour, Louise M.
Van Rijn, Catherine M.
Veber, Frank M.
Weybury, Lisa J.
Webster, Elizabeth M.
Wieland, Susan C.
Wilson, Lorey M.
Witt, Robyn A.
Wood, Penelope Mac.

1986
Airey, Michelle A.
Allans, Marisa L.
Armstrong, Lyndel L.
Baxter, Brigid Ann
Bellin, Sara L.
Boag, Jane M.
Botheras, Kay E.
Bennett, Dianne M.
Bortolot, Caterina
Brady, Anthony J.
Brooks, Lisa Anne
Brown, Rosemary H.
Browning, Megan E.
Burnett, Jillian R.

Casley, Melissa J.
Cleary, Pamela R.
Coleman, Moira J.
Constantine, Tracey A.
Dickison, Karen L.
Dignum, Lisa J.
Dow, Martin P.
Dudycz, Anna
Eddy, Wendy E.
Egert, Katherine E.
Evans, Lynne M.
Fitzgerald, Elizabeth A.
Foley, David C.
Galloway, Lynda J.
Gibbs, Bronwyn E.
Grace, John R.
Guzys, Angela T.
Henley, Julie E.
Hine, Trilby E.
Hopgood, Andrea S.
Johns, Michelle E.
Jokic, Ruza
Joyce, Nola A.
Judge, Judith E.
Lawson, Suzanne J.
Leavey, Joanne T.
Leevers, Jon K.
Long, Marita T.
Lovett, Robyn L.
Mackie, Julie C.
McDonnell, Anne M.
McGregor, Josephine M.
McLennan, Nicole L.
Mills, Jennifer A.
Mills, Helen C.
Mullens, Anne M.
Mulqueen, Jacqueline
Newton, Anne E.
Nosiara, Tania J.
O'Hehir, Linda J.
Patterson, Sandra L.
Pearce, Esther E.
Pitkin, Michael J.
Posselt, Michelle A.
Purchase, Jennifer D.
Quinton, Simone A.
Reiter, Sylvia D.

Reynolds, Kylie E.
Ridgway, Jennifer A.
Rigby, Christine M.
Rivett, Kristin M.
Ryan, Maree J.
Setalo, Victoria
Sexton, Jennifer M.
Slykhuis, Renae L.
Streefkerk, Kerryn A.
Soanes, Clare M.
Spotswood, Christopher
Stevens, Catherine S.
Stevens, Gary C.
Stewart, Wendy K.
Thomas, Fiona L.
Veitz, Bernard
White, Helen P.
Widdison, Bernard D.
Wilson, Sandra D.
Woulfe, Anne-Marie
Young, Michael K.
Zeglinas, Agnes
Waugh, Jacqueline S.

1987
Barnard, Helen V.
Bibby, Michelle P.
Bolton, Fiona K.
Brick, Maree B.
Cahill, Catherine M.
Condello, Vincenzo N.
Cook, Bruce A.
Corbett, Sharon D.
Davey, Kym L.
Dawson, Penelope J.
Dee, Louise M.
Delcore, Anna M.
Dorling, Eliza I.
Downey, Kaylene J.
Eccles, Elizabeth R.
Fischer, Mark A.
Foley, Nicola P.
Forgas, Wendy K.
Freidrich, Letizia
Goulding, Nicole C.
Goulding, Phillip A.
Grant, Melanie T.

Gretton-Watson, Sally
Hoare, Mary J.
Humphreys, Julie E.
Johnson, Lynda K.
Kearins, Tracey A.
Kelly, Sarah J.
Lane, Carolyn A.
Lindros, Sally E.
Mander, Bradley P.
Moller, Helen Lisa
McGenniss, Kerryn G.
Olney, Sandra S.
Oliver, Marianne L.
Palmieri, Franco
Privitera, Vincenzo
Shaw, Susan
Shea, Leanne K.
Singleton, Debra M.
Smith, Tracey N.
Spencer, Sean M.
Tyler, Stuart B.
Truong, Boa Lan (Tracy)
Van Essen, Gabrielle
Viney, Melissa M.
Wilson, Debbie G.
Wood, Alexandra M.
Wright, Jennifer A.

Select Bibliography

Newspapers
Argus
Age
Sun News Pictorial
Herald
Royal Children's Hospital newspaper files 1900–1970s

Royal Children's Hospital Archival Records
Minutes and Annual Reports 1870–1987
Nurses' Registers 1890s–1963
Nursing Administration records 1963–83
Nurses' Records 1940s–1987 held at the Mackinnon School of Nursing
Sisters' Committee Minute book 1928–32

Journals
Australian Medical Journal (AMJ 1890–94)

Medical Journal of Australia (MJA 1950s)

UNA, the Journal of the Royal Victorian Trained Nurses' Association (RVTNA) 1901–33. Thereafter, the Journal of the Royal Victorian Branch of the Australian Nursing Federation (ANF Vic).

Nurses' Board of Victoria (NBV)
Record Books of the Royal Victorian Trained Nurses Association 1901–18.

Registration records of the NBV 1924–87.

Articles
Bruce, Mary Grant 'The Least of these Little Ones', *The Woman*, 28 June 1909.

Godden, Judith 'The Founding of Nightingale Nursing in Australia 1868–1884' in *Australian Historical Studies,* Number 117, October 2001.

Graham, H. Boyd 'Beacons on our Way—Some Memories of the Children's Hospital' in *Medical Journal of Australia*, 1953, Vol ii, p517.

Hunter, Charles D. 'What Kills Our Babies? A Guide to the Care of Infants' in *Health Society*, Melbourne, 1878.

Macdonald, Colin 'Harry Douglas Stephens, Herbert Hewlett and Some of their Colleagues' in *Victorian Historical Magazine*, August 1962, p274.

Select Bibliography

Southby, Robert 'The Colonial Child' in *The Journal of the Royal Historical Society of Victoria*, 1951.

Webster, M.E. 'The History of Trained Nursing in Victoria' in *Victorian Historical Magazine* xix 121, 1942.

Books

Abel-Smith, Brian *A History of the Nursing Profession*, Heinemann, London, 1960.

Ballarat Base Hospital Annual Report 1887–1988, School of Nursing Centenary 1888–1988.

Bassett, Jan *Nursing Aide to Enrolled Nurse—A History of the Melbourne School for Enrolled Nurses*, Melbourne School for Enrolled Nurses, 1993.

Bessant, Judith & Bessant, Bob *The Growth of a Profession—Nursing in Victoria 1930s–1980s*, La Trobe University Press, Bundoora, 1991.

Burnett, F.M 'The Natural History of Communicable Diseases' in *The Theory and Practice of Public Health*, 2nd edn, W. Hobson (ed.), London, 1965.

Cannon, Michael *Life in the Cities*, Thomas Nelson, Melbourne 1975.

Crocket, Cheryl, D. *Save the Babies: The Victorian Baby Health Centres' Association and the Queen Elizabeth Centre—the first 83 years*, Arcadia, Melbourne, 2000.

Cumpston, J.H.C. 'The History of Diphtheria, Scarlet Fever, Measles and Whooping Cough in Australia, 1927' in *History of Poliomyelitis, Tuberculosis and Meningitis*, Commonwealth Department of Health, 1960.

Dormandy, Thomas *The White Death—A History of Tuberculosis*, New York.

University Press, Washington Square, New York, 2000.

Durdin, Joan *They Became Nurses—A History of Nursing in South Australia 1836–1980*, Allen & Unwin, 1991.

Galbally, Ann *Redmond Barry*, MUP, 1995.

Gandevia, Bryan *Tears Often Shed: A History of Child Health and Welfare in Australia*, Pergammon Press, 1978.

Gardiner, Lyndsay *Royal Children's Hospital, Melbourne 1870–1970*, Royal Childrens's Hospital, 1970.

Goodman, Rupert *A Hospital at War*, Queensland Bunurong Press, 1983.

Huxley, Elspeth *From Nightingale to Now. Nurse Education in Australia* Nicholson & Wiedenfield, London, 1975.

Hyslop, Anthea *Sovereign Remedies: A History of Ballarat Base Hospital*, Allen & Unwin, 1989.

Inglis K.S. *Hospital and Community—Royal Melbourne Hospital 1848–1958*, MUP, 1957.

Jaggs, Donella *Neglected and Criminal: Foundations of Child Welfare in Victoria* Phillip Institute of Technology Centre for Youth and Community Studies, 1986.

Jalland, Pat *Death in the Victorian Family*, OUP, 1996.

Kosky, Jules & Lunnon, Raymond J. *Great Ormond Street and the History of Medicine*, Granta Editions, Cambridge, 1991.

Lake, Joshua (ed). *Childhood in Bud and Blossom. A Souvenir Book of the Children's Hospital Bazaar*, Atlas Press, 1900.

Lewis, Myles, *Melbourne—The City's History and Development.* Published for the City of Melbourne, 1995.

Lansdown, Richard *Children in Hospital—A Guide for Family and Carers,* OUP, 1996.

Lomax, Elizabeth *Small and Special: The Development of Hospitals for Children in Victorian Britain,* Wellcome Institute for the History of Medicine, London, 1996.

Minchin, M.K. *Revolutions and Rosewater: The Evolution of Nurse Education in Victoria 1923–1973,* Hart Hamel, 1974.

Mitchell, Ann M. *The Hospital South of the Yarra. A History of Alfred Hospital, Melbourne, from foundation to the nineteen-forties.* Published by the Alfred Hospital, Melbourne, 1977.

Paterson, Helen *5.30 Nurse—The Story of the Alfred Nurses,* History Books, 1996.

Russell, Lynette R. *From Nightingale to Now—Nurse Education in Australia,* Harcourt Brace Ivanovich Ltd, London, 1990.

Russell, K.F. *The Melbourne Medical School 1862–1962,* MUP, 1977.

Sayers, C.E. *The Women's Melbourne—A History of the Royal Women's Hospital* (The Lying-In). Published by the Royal Women's Hospital, 1956.

Serle, Geoffrey *The Rush to be Rich—A History of the Colony of Victoria 1883–1889,* MUP, 1971.

Serle, Geoffrey *The Golden Age—A History of the Colony of Victoria,* MUP, 1977.

Smith, J. (ed) *The Cyclopedia of Victoria,* the Cyclopedia Co., Melbourne, 1903.

Smith, G. Russell *In Pursuit of Nursing Excellence—A History of the College of Nursing 1949–99,* OUP, 1999.

Tames, Richard *Florence Nightingale,* London, 1989.

Trembath, Richard & Hellier, Donna *All Care and Responsibility—A History of Nursing in Victoria 1850–1934,* Florence Nightingale Committee, Australia. Victorian Branch, 1987.

Twopeny, Richard *Town Life in Australia,* Penguin, 1883 (1976 edition).

Williams, Howard *From Charity to Teaching Hospital.* Self-published, 1989.

Yule, Peter *The Royal Children's Hospital—A History of Faith, Science and Love,* Halstead Press, 1999.

Vellar, Ivo *The Doers—A History of Surgery at St Vincent's Hospital, Melbourne 1890s–1950s,* Publishing Solutions, 2002.

Government Reports and Parliamentary Papers

The Victorian Year Book 1889–90, Census data 1851, 1861.

Progress Report on the *Royal Commission upon Public Health,* PP, 1889, Vol 2, No. 27.

Report of the Board of Public Health 1890–91, PP, Vol 6. No.197.

Victorian Parliamentary Papers (VPP), Vol ii, No 45, p17, 1927. Robert James Love, 'Hospitals and Other Philanthropic Institutions and Organisations: Notes and Recommendations as to Hospitals'.

Index

Italic page references indicate photos and/or captions.

a'Beckett, Dr William 17, 23, 24
abused children 234, 281
Adams, Margaret 130, 172, *173*, 173–4, *174*
Age (newspaper) 50, 88, 102, 103, 117, 186, 189–90
Ahearn, Judy 188
Aicheson, Jane 123, 125
Alfred Hospital 8, 35, 70, 71, 74, 75, 91, 96, 99, 100, 102, 144, 221, 247, 265, 275, 288
Allan, Elizabeth 212
Allen, Una 248
Allnatt, Marjorie 116–17, 119, 121, 125, 127, 128, 130, 186, *187*, *188*, *194*, 213
Altmann, Jane 216, *302*, 303
ambulances 136, *136*, *302*, 311
amenities for nurses 35, 82, 86, 161, 196, 241, 284
Anaesthesia Department of 253, 257, 259, 262
anaesthetics 10, 185, 203, 204, 207, 208, 234, 253, 266, 295, 297
Anderson, Kathryn 283
Anderson, Eileen 305
Anstee, Rae *266*, 278
antibiotics 185, 202, 207, 211
antiseptics 10, 71
appendicitis 207, *270*
Argus (newspaper) 8, 17, 69, 90, 93, 135, 137
Arnold, Meg 239
Arthur, Jane 150, 160
Ashton, John 17
Auldist, Alex 235
Austin Hospital 197, 265, 288, 296
Austin, Catherine 13, 51, 70
Australasian Nurses' Journal 52
Australasian Trained Nurses' Association 79
Australian Army Nursing Service (AANS) 51, 52, 53, 69, 79, 80, 81, 98–9, *99*, 170, 171, *171*, 172, 173, 174, 275
Australian Army Nursing Service Reserve 79
Australian Medical Journal 8, 14, 57
Australian Nursing Journal 231–2, 301
Auxiliaries 73, 87, 120, 127, 135, 150, 153, 189
awards/prizes: Margaret Adams Prize (offered by LOFT) 173, 174, *283*, *307*; Chairman's Medal *264*; Nell Chrisfield Memorial Prize 243, *273*; Florence Nightingale Medal (offered by Red Cross) 178; Arthur Jeffreys Wood Gold Medal 103, 105, *220*, *273*

Baby Health Centres 97, 102, 103, *104*, 105, *106*, 248, 250
Baby Wards 66, 87, 96–7, 121–2, 123, 128, 129, 150, 154, 156, 161, 162–3, 198–9, 208, 209, 244 (*see also* Princess May Pavilion, 'Save the Babies' Appeal)
Bail, Mrs 13, 17
Bamford, Katrina 283
Barlow, Maud 40
Barnett, John 205
Barry, Sir Redmond 18, 31, *33*, 38
Barton, Anne 161
Barton, Jean Maxwell 160–1, 163
Beavis, Margery 181
Belfrage, Hazel 150, *156*, 160
Bell, Jane 124
Bell, Jan 312
Bellaine, Mrs 25–6
Bellair, Peg (née Mitchell) 216
Belstead, Mabel 77, 82
Bennett, Dr Annie 82, 91
Bennie, Dr Peter 74
Benton, Myrtle 188
Best, Chris 312
Bevan, Ida 37, *54*
Bialastock, Dora 281
Birrell, John 281
Birrell, Dr Robert 281
Bishop, Dr Frank 235
Bishop, Helen 283

Bishop, Sarah Anne (née Gove) ix, 18, 25, 34, 35, *36*, 36, *37*, 40, 43, 55, 59–60, *61*, 67
Black, Dr Joseph 17, 23
Blackburn, Nurse 36
Blackford, Jeanine 310
Blatancic, Branka 301
Blewett, Louise 262, *263*, *264*, 266
blood transfusions 122, 169, 181, 203, 262, 267
Board of Public Health, Report of Dr Robertson (1918) 93
Bodycomb, Mayne 241
Boer War 53–3, *53*, 87
Bon, Berenice 215
Bond, Helene 274
Bond, Wendy 235
Booth, Eliza 35
Boston Children's Hospital (USA) 229, 303
Bowes, Professor Glenn 312
Bowlby, John 280
Boyle, Edith 156
Brain, Adele *194*, *201*
Bram, Ruth 243
Brassey, Lady Sybil 45–6
Brawn, Bill 293
Brearley, Pauline 209
Brereton, Kate 235
Brian, Barbara (née Morris) 162, 209
Brick, Maree 298
Brighton Convalescent Cottage ix, 38, 43, *54*, 54, 77, 82, 86, 112, 144
Bristol, Huia 160
Broadbent, Elsie 283
Brodie, Sophie *129*, 130, *174*, 186, 227
Brodribb, Mary 136
Bromby, Dr 12
Bromby, Eliza 12
Brooks, Lady Violet 219
Brown, Dr Kester 244, 247, 262, 270, 271
Brown, Sheila *see* Newman Morris, Lady Sheila
Bruce, Mary Grant 73
Bryan, Anne 241, 268, 270
Buchanan, Cliff 268, 277, 300
Buckley, Mars 36
Bullen, Dr 84
Bullivant, Florence *47*, *48*

Bult, Audrey 155
Burbidge, Gwen 169, 221
Burkitt, Rita 286
Burn, Hilda 55
burns nursing 85, 161, 163, 205, 207–8, 210, 234–5, *279*, 291, 294–5, *295*
bursaries 218, 273
Butler-Walsh, Mrs
Butt, Judith (Lady Court) 200, *255*, 283
Buxton, Mary 250

camaraderie, and trainees 117, 118, 160–1, 162, 165, 186, 216–17, 240
Campbell, Janet 215
Campbell, Dr Kate 236
Campbell, Dr Neil 267–8
cancer nursing 200, 202, 291, 296, 287, 299, *299*, 300
Canning, Jennifer 283
cardiac nursing 16, 150, 160, 202, 205, 233, 246, 253, 254–5, 257, 259, *269*, 270, 271, 291, 292, *292*, 293, 294, 295
Carmichael, Dr Alan 305
Carmichael, Grace Jennings 3, 23, 28, 34, 38, *39*, 39–40, 43, *61*
Carruthers, Miss 168
Casey, Lady Maie 186, *189*
Casey, Peggy 156
Castellan, Nancy *194*, 197, 210
Casualty Ward 85, 195, 198, 202, 205, 206, 210–12, 233, 234, 255, 257, 258, 291, 292, 301, *302*, 303
Catchlove, Barry 270, 287, 288
Catto, Barbara *see* Smith, Barbara
Centre for Studies in Paediatric Nursing (CSPN) 310
Centre Ward 32, *66*
cerebral palsy 305, 306, 308
certification/testamonials 11, 38, 43, *48*, 48, 59, 61, 75, *75*, 86
Chalmers, Doris 150, *159*, 160
Chalmers (née Sadlier), Elizabeth 195, *219*, 250

375

Chambers, Mrs 4
Chan, May 269
Charles, Alice 162–3, 167
Cheatley, Joan 155
chest diseases 112, 150
Chew, Siok 270
Chipperfield, Joyce 156
Chirnside, Annie 13
Chirnside, Isabella 13
Chrisfield, Nell 230, 243, 243 (see also awards/prizes)
Christmas celebrations 125, 181, 192, 220
Clark, Hope 123–4, 135, 145
Clark, Manning 145
Clark, Mrs 4
Clarke, Beryl 288
Clarke, Lady Janet 13, 18, 24, 70
Clarke, Murray A. 208, 234, 276
Clarke, Dr Peter 293
cleft lip and palate 205–6
Coates, Marianne 283
Cobbin, Myrna 215
code of conduct, nurses' viii
Cogan, Sister 230
Cole, Dr Hobill 103
Coles, Mrs 158
(Australian) College of Nursing (formerly RVTNA) 102, 130, 222, 242–3, 278, 286
Colley, Janet 212
Collier, Miss 138
Collingwood Dispensary 4, 5, 9
Collingwood Gas Company 14
Collins, Claire 270
Collins, Dr Vernon 118, 167, 170, 195, 196, 197, 208, 210, 229, 231, 281, 286
Colquhoun, Dr John 137, 138
community nursing 248, 250, 291, 292, 304, 305, 306, 308, 309
conditions of work (see also illness, industrial issues): hours worked 11, 17, 26, 29, 38, 43, 50, 58–9, 69, 85, 88, 97, 103, 130, 143, 154, 196, 238, 285; leave entitlements 69, 98; wages 11, 18, 26, 50, 52, 55, 76–7, 97–8, 103, 114, 115, 130, 161, 248, 285
Convalescent Cottages see Brighton, Hampton, Sherbrooke
Conyers, Evelyn Augusta 50–1, 51, 52, 74, 80–1, 106
Cook, Nurse 106
Coombes, Elizabeth 197–8, 210, 211, 229
Corrigan, Elizabeth 188

cortisone 199
Cottage Bush Nursing Hospitals 103, 151, 250
Court, Dr John 306
Court, Lady Judith see Butt, Judith
Coventry, Gwen 213–14
Coventry, Jennie (née Armstrong) 273, 282
Cuddihy, Lucy 262, 264, 288, 289, 289, 312
curricula for nursing 242–3, 264, 265, 277, 278, 281
Curtis, Kevin 270
Curtis, Rita 156
Curwen-Walker, Edna 116
Cussen, Jean 198, 217
cystic fibrosis 234, 305, 310

Danaher, Matilda 55, 56, 77, 86, 106
Daniel, Vivianne 156
Davey, Rosanne 212
Davies, Dr Ellice 82
Davies, Dr Jack 276–7
Davies, Estelle 111
Davis, Dr John Bunnell 9
Dawe, Kathleen 281
day surgery 271
De Neeve, Lucy see Sechiari De Neeve, Lucy
death of a patient, nurses dealing with 29, 83, 123–4, 161, 162, 163, 180, 200, 203, 213, 217, 234, 245; parents dealing with 162, 180, 210, 213, 234, 267
Debelle, Dr Geoff 305
dehydration 162–3
Denman, Lord 82
depressions, economic, and nurses 26, 46, 52, 55, 112
diabetes 160, 198, 295, 305, 310
diarrhoea 66, 123
Dickens, Charles 11
diphtheria 8, 28, 31, 82, 85, 96, 161, 163, 201–2, 233, 254, 255
Directors of Nursing (DONs) see Matrons
Disability Act 1986 306
Ditterich, Barbara 212
Doble, Miss 138
domestic staff 86, 90, 100, 165
domestic work, and nurses 11, 16, 26, 28, 36, 38, 40, 54, 56, 84–5, 97, 122, 128, 130, 159, 161, 165, 165, 167, 168, 205, 213, 229, 269
Drake, Margaret 194
Drury, Mick 150
Dubourg, Laurence 289, 296, 296, 297, 298
Duffy, Mrs 72, 76, 84
Duke, Valerie 231, 232, 250, 251, 278, 281, 288, 303

Dunne, Shirley 268, 270
Durkacz, Helen 283
dystentry 8, 16, 199

Eade, Donna 305
eczema 198, 199
Eddy, Kaye 288
education, and nurses: see awards/prizes, examinations, graduation, Mackinnon School of Nursing, Nursing School, Preliminary Training School, post-basic/postgraduate education, study leave, tertiary education
Edward Wilson Surgical Pavilion 82
Edwards, Mrs 65–6
electrolytes 180, 199, 202
Elizabeth Ward 32, 38, 45
Elliott, Lois (née Ferguson) 284
entry fee, and trainees 69, 97–8
entry tests, and trainees 273–4, 275
epilepsy 298, 308
ethical dilemmas 268, 285
Ettershank, Mrs 20
examinations 46, 57, 100, 101, 102, 128, 131, 154, 156, 178, 214, 232, 243

Factory and Shops Act (Vic.) 58
Fairfield Hospital 52, 74, 89, 96, 221, 255, 258
Farmer, Cathy 283
Fautley, Chris 232
Fearon, Elizabeth 197, 230, 271, 281
Feint, Dick 276
Ferguson, Inez 138–9, 141–2
Ferguson, Sheila 119, 131
Fetherston, Dr Guy 9, 16, 80
Fetherston, Sarah (née Harvey) 16, 17
Fields, Gracie 142
Fischer, Anne 274
Flack, Alice Mowbray 55, 56, 69, 77
Flett, Doris 258, 258, 259, 260, 261, 264, 266
Flower, Ivy 119, 155, 165, 166, 166, 167, 186, 190, 216
food/mealtimes, for nurses 55, 72, 86, 90, 115, 118, 130, 155, 157, 165, 165, 167, 170, 200, 216, 239; for patients 51, 125–6, 141–2, 157, 164, 165, 165, 170, 198, 200, 206, 208, 209, 210
fomentations 26
Ford, Anna 17
Forster, Lady 97
Forster, Dr Wilfred 147

Forsyth, Pam 303
Fowler, Blanche 60
Fowler, Robert 300
Fox, Mona 180
Frankston Orthopaedic Hospital 81, 111, 126, 127, 130, 133, 133, 134, 134–5, 135, 136, 136–9, 139, 140, 140, 141, 141–2, 142, 143, 144, 144, 145, 150, 151, 153, 157–8, 160, 171, 174, 186, 191, 209, 218, 227, 237, 238, 240, 241, 251, 276, 286, 305, 306
Fraser, Lillias Sharpe 41
Fraunfelder, Jo 309
Frizon, Josie 215
Furnell, Nancy (née Heane) 161–2

Galbraith, Dr Douglas 130, 140, 143
Gardner, Irene 175
Garson, Miss 18
gastroenteritis 7, 8, 126, 180, 198
Gendle, Joan M. 129, 130, 154, 223, 227, 228, 229, 230, 232, 236–7, 238, 241, 242, 247, 300
Gibson, Karen 312
Gifford-Burgess, Elizabeth 203
Gillespie, Sally 188
Goddard, Eleanor 43
Gooderham, Nance 227
Gordon, Anne 156, 159
Gosling, Vivien 283
Goudge, Jan 304
Goulding, Phillip 304, 312
graduation 188, 212, 215, 217, 228, 239, 283, 284, 288
Grant, Audrey (née Laugher) 199, 250
Gray, Nancy 221
Great Ormond Street Hospital (London) ix, 9, 17, 18, 24, 128, 247, 275
Greenwood, Mavis 283
Grey, Helene 221
Grieg, Dr Janet 82
Grieve, Dr John W. (Jock) 112, 115, 162
Grieve, Patricia 212
Grimwade, Mrs 233
Guaran, Christina 283
Gunn, Kelly 156
Gunter, George 205
Guthrie, Mary 73, 86, 87, 117

haemophilia 300
Halford, Professor George 13, 23
Hall, Mrs 106
Hall, Jennifer 212
Hampson, Barbara 189
Hampton Convalescent Cottage ix, 126, 133, 134, 136, 144, 145, 145, 146,

INDEX

147–9, 150, 157, 158, 160, 185, 191, 207, 222
Harden, Kate 202, 203, *230*, 267
Hardham, Anne (née Coventry) 242, 273–4, 274, *282*, 283
Hardham, Jean 94, 115, 119, 123, 171, *171*, 172, 283
Hardy, Ida 54
Hardy, Nancy (née Hurst) 204, 204, 205, 236
Harswell, Joan *253*
Harvey, Emily 16
Harvey, Marian 16–17, 18
Harvey, Sarah *see* Fetherston, Sarah
Hatswell, Joan *189*
Head Nurses 17, 18, 25–6, 36, 38, 40, 42–3, 57, 59, 68 (*see also* Home Sisters, Sisters, Staff Nurses)
Healy, Ellen 26
Heath, Alfred 57
Heley, Judith *155*
heliotherapy and exposure therapy 126, 129, 135, 137, 138, *140*, 144, 160
Hennessy, Dr Raymond 180, 214
Herald (newspaper) 96, 97, 147
Heriot, Bev *187*, *188*
Higgins, Mrs 76, 82, 150
Hines, Frances (Fanny) Emma 52, *53*, 53
Hoadley, Jean *156*
Hocking, Elizabeth (née Strickland) *187*, *188*, 203, 204
Hodge, Isabel 281
Hogan, Karen 306
Hogan, Meryl *215*
Holcombe (née Heley), Noel 154
Holder, Nurse 117
Holland, Jennifer *212*
Hollow, Fay *135*
Home Sisters 69, 77, 103, 115, 118, 119, 125, 155, 161, 163, *190*, 285
Homeopathic Hospital *see* Prince Henry's Hospital
Honey, Mavis 208
Hooper, Reginald 207, 246
Hopetoun, Lady 51
Hôpital des Enfants Malades (Paris) 9
Hosking, Marjorie (née Tomlinson) *156*, 171, 180
Hospital in the Home 298
Hospitals and Charities Commission 147, 221
Howard, Paula *271*
Howard, Russell 195, 205
Howse, Neville 80
Hughes, Lee *293*
Hulls, Betty *187*, *188*
Hunt, Nan *187*
Hunter, Dr Charles 16, 23
Huntingfield, Lady 150

Hurst, Dr John 303
Hurst, Nancy *see* Hardy, Nancy
Huxley, Clara 17
hydrocephalus 207, 237, 300

illnesses and nurses 33, 35, 38, 39, 50, 53, 60, 69, 71, 72, 76, 86, 89, 96, 97, 115, 117, 130, 138, 145, 162, 195 (*see also* Sick Nurses' Ward)
industrial issues 69, 100, 102, 105, 285, 286, 288
infantile fever 16
infectious diseases nursing 28–9, 29, 30–1 94, 95 (*see also* diphtheria, poliomyelitis, tuberculosis, typhoid, typhus, Isolation Pavilion, Medical Flat)
initiative, and nurses 197, 213–14, 244
injections, for babies 179, 199, 203
Ingpen, Enid 203
Inspector of Charities, Report of (1892) 58
instrument trays, set-up of 169, 178, 269
Intensive Care Unit (ICU) 234, 237, 247, 251, 253, 254, *254*, 255–7, *258*, 258–62, *263*, *264*, 264, 265–6, *277*, 278, 292
interviews for prospective trainees 112, 117, 274
invalid cookery 18, 25, 56, 56, *130*, 164
Isolation Pavilion *29*, 29–30, 31, 82, *85*, 121 (*see also* Medical Flat)

Jackson, Chevalier 254
Jackson, Elizabeth 223
Jackson, Janet *188*
Jacobs, Nancy 216
Jaffray, Elizabeth 229, *230*, 231, *254*, 255, 257, 258, 259, 265, 266, 283
James, Dr Edwin 23
James, Elizabeth *212*
Jarrett, Trixie 115, 118, 155
Jarvis, Jenni 312
Jenkins, Dawn *212*
Jenkins, Elizabeth *209*
Jennings, Mrs 4
Jergamanis, Hilda 270
Jess, Sheila *215*
Jewell, Anne 172
Johnson, Paula 300

Kelly, Justin 300
Kelly, Paul 270
Kelsey, Dr Helen 82
Kendall, Anne *188*
Kenny, Elizabeth 112, 126, 147, 148, 149
Keogh, Dr Julian 234, 235
Kerr, Mona 55

kidney disease 122, 198, 200
(Annie Stirling) Kindergarten 231
kindergarten work, and nurses 123
King, Christine *283*
Kinney, Sharon 288
Kirschner, Thekla 250
Knox, Mrs J. 156
Krysz, Sheila (née Mackenzie) *176*, 178

La Trobe University 250, 293
Lady Bowen Ward *19*, 32
Lady Superintendents *see* Matrons
Lady Talbot Milk Institute 105, *107*
Laidlaw, Ina Annie 81, 86, 106, 143, 144, *144*, 171, 286
Lancaster, Francine *283*
Lane, Lucy (née Mackenzie) 106, *176*, 177
Lanyon, Judith 178, 179
Lark, Valerie *155*
Latham, Lady Ella 138, 150, 153, 154, 156, 158, 160, 189
laundry 28, 31, *32*, *33*, 69, 86, 97
League of Former Trainees (LOFT) x, 52, 98, 105–7, 127, 173, 174, 178, *239* (*see also* awards/prizes)
Leckie, Janet (née Menzies) *176*, *249*
Lee, Kim 271
leeches 28
Lempriere, Janie McRobie 52, *53*, 53, 56, 80
Lewis, Muriel *106*, 250
Liddicut, Lillian 122
Lindell, John 221
Lindsay, Hilda 87–8, 89, 90, 96
Lister, Joseph 10
Loch, Lady Elizabeth 32, 38
Loch, Lord 32
Logan, Sister 170
Long, Margaret *212*
Longstaff, Patience *165*
Lord Somers League 136
Love, Robert J. (Jim) 95
lumbar punctures 88, 169, 202
Lyall, Doreen 125–6, 157, 165, 170, 208
Lying-in Hospital *see* Royal Women's Hospital

Macauley, Wilma *187*
MacDonald, Dr Bill 180
MacEachern, Malcolm 129
Macfarlane, Miss 25
Mackenzie, Catherine *176*, 177, *177*, 178

Mackenzie, Dr Helen *176*, 177
Mackenzie, Lucy *see* Lane, Lucy
Mackenzie, Sheila *see* Krysz, Sheila
Mackinnon School of Nursing 288, 293, 312
Mackinnon, Emily 90, 117, 135
Mackinnon, Dame Patricia 190, 233, 276, *280*, 285, *307*
Mackintosh, Gwen (née Easton) 250
Macleod, Diane *188*
Macnamara, Dr Jean 145, 147
Magnus, Ruth 300
Mair, Margaret *187*, *188*
Marles, Fay 287
Martelli, Alice 40, 42–3, 55, 59
Martin Committee 242
Massey, Pearl *187*
Massie, Cathleen 55
Matrons/Lady Superintendents/ Directors of Nursing 16–17, 18, 25, 34–5, 36, 38, 51, 57, 67, *68*, 68, 72, 76, 77, 81, 82–3, 86, 90, 94, 95, 97, 99, 100, 102, 106, 107, 114, 121, 124–5, *125*, 126–7, 143, 144, *144*, 151, *151*, 156, 157, 160, 161, 163, 164, 167, 169, 171, 178, 185, 186–8, *188*, *189*, 189–90, *190*, 191, 196, 197, 213, 217, 218, 221, 222, 223, 227, *228*, 229, *230*, 231, 232, 236–7, *238*, 241, 242, 247, *266*, 268, 273–5, *275*, 276–7, 278, *280*, 283–4, 286, *286*, 287, 289, 312; use of 'Lady Superintendent' title 34–5, 67, 227, *288*, 288, 300, 303; use of 'Director of Nursing' (DON) title 34–5, 227
Matthews, Dr Rae 203
McCallum, Mary *188*
McCausland, Irene *249*
McClelland, Dr Margaret 257
McComas, Dr Elizabeth 144
McCoy, Julia *304*
McCredie, Rhonda *155*
McDonald, Ian 257, 261
McDonald, Jean *187*
McDonnell, Geraldine 267, 268
McElhinney, Helen *212*
McEwan, Janette 292, *292*, 293
McFarland, Mary 118
McGeachin, Neil 235, *283*
McGowan, Mary 299, *299*, 300

McKay, Dr 51, 52
McKay, Noreen 255, 258, 270
McKenzie, Ian 235
McKinley, Di 288
McLaren, Robyn see Smith, Robyn
McMeekin, Helen 156
McMurtrie, Amanda 283
McNaught, Kaye 300
McNeill, Ella Grace (née Robinson) 103
(Emily) McPherson College of Domestic Science 25, 56, 222
McPherson, Mrs 4
McPherson, Sir William 25
McVilly, C. L. 158
Medical Flat(s) 87–8, 89, 89, 91, 96
Medical Society (Melbourne) 9
Medical Ward(s) 32, 46, 68, 82, 85, 122, 165, 192, 197, 198–204, 209, 236–7, 251, 299, 304 (see also specialty areas)
Mee, Roger 269, 293
Meehan, Michelle 304
Mekking, Esselina 283
Melbourne Hospital see Royal Melbourne Hospital
Melbourne School of Nursing 221
Melbourne University x, 148, 288, 293, 312
Memishi, Adele 283
Menadue, Win 234
meningitis and related illnesses 87–8, 161, 163, 180, 198, 202, 210–11, 262
Menzies, Kate (née Carew) 118, 175–6, 176, 249
Menzies, Kathleen (née Gardner)
Meredith, M. 160
migrant children 199, 207, 211–12, 269
Milburn, Ann 103, 150, 151, 151, 160
Miles, Maggie 197–8
Millard, Nola 283
Miller, Celeste 283
Miller, P.A. 278
Milliken, Doris 203, 267, 267
Minogue, Christine 312
Mitchell, Margaret 203
Moline, Mrs 4
Morey, Yvonne 165
Morgan, Fred 136
morphine 122, 206
Morris, Agnes 115, 118, 121, 127, 154, 155, 161, 178, 186
Morris, Barbara see Brian, Barbara
Morrison, Jessie 125, 154
Morrison, Margaret 283
Morton, Eileen 259

Morton, Trish 305
Moss, Eleanor (née Peck) 146, 147, 149
Mothercraft nursing 123, 197, 208, 241
Motherwell, Dr James 13, 23
Munnerley, Leanne 283
Murdoch, Lady (later Dame) Elisabeth 150, 186, 230, 233
Murphy, Sarah 17
Murray, Constance Mary 61
Murray, Lois 259
Myers, Dr Nathaniel 195, 205, 311

Nason, Joan (née Joynes) 282, 284
nasotracheal intubation 259–61
Neild, Dr James 23
Neilson, Sue 239
Neilson, Wendy 297
neonatal nursing 199, 202, 203, 236, 260, 261, 262, 267–8, 288
neuroscience nursing 236, 237, 246, 257, 296, 296, 297–8, 305
Newing, Gertrude 222
Newman Morris, Lady Sheila (née Brown) 174–5, 280
Ng, Oi Yuet 212
Nicholas, Alfred ('Aspro') 158
Nicholas, Isabel 150, 151, 158
Nicholas, Jennifer 187
Nightingale, Florence ix, 9, 10
Nightingale nursing 9, 11, 16, 21, 25, 34, 35, 55, 125 see also St Thomas' Hospital
Nixon Esme (née McCormack) 167, 179, 180, 181
Noble, Emily 164
Norris, Dr Kingsley 91
Nott, Helen 283
Nunn, Debra 283
Nurse Educators 265, 274, 277, 278, 287, 288, 310, 313
nurse–doctor relations 21, 23, 29, 34, 35, 36, 57, 76, 82, 170, 174, 236–7, 269, 276–7, 287, 293, 296
nurses/nursing, private 9, 16, 43, 57, 61, 102, 103
nurses/nursing, public perception of 10–11, 16, 114, 115, 117, 178
(Student) Nurses' Council 194, 196–7
Nurses' Homes 43, 58, 77, 84, 90, 114, 115, 116, 117, 118, 119–20, 134, 135, 136, 151, 154, 156,

157, 158, 160–1, 162, 163, 165, 168–9, 179, 186, 190, 193, 196, 198, 214, 216–18, 229, 238, 239, 240–2, 284: at Frankston 134, 135, 136, 241; at Sherbrooke ('Marybrooke') 151, 157, 158, 160; for Sisters 120, 196, 198, 242; for Matrons 120, 190, 191
Nurses' Registration Act 1924 (Vic.) and amendments 76, 102, 106, 128
Nurses' Registration Board of Victoria 106, 126, 127, 130, 154, 171, 221
nursing aides 186, 221, 238, 241
Nursing Aide School (Hawthorn) 227, 283, 284
Nursing School at RCH 24–5, 36, 43, 46, 48, 48, 55, 56–7, 61, 71, 74, 75, 75, 76, 81, 83, 86, 89, 100, 127–8, 288 (see also Preliminary Training School, RVTNA)
nursing, as women's work 10–11, 12, 76; as men's work also 235, 270, 283

O'Callahan, Janice 283
O'Connell, Rev J. H. 84
O'Donnell, Aileen 303
O'Dwyer, Joseph 254
Oberklaid, Dr Frank 303
Occupational Therapy Section 231
Officer, Dr 57
Oliver, Nan 258
operating theatres 71, 72, 90, 95, 100, 121, 125, 161, 168, 174, 180, 191, 195, 201, 205, 235, 246, 247, 254, 255, 255–6, 268–9, 269, 270, 271
Orford, Peg 143, 163–4, 167, 168, 181
Orr, Elaine 217, 268, 273–5, 275, 276–7, 278, 280, 283–4, 286, 300, 303
Orr, Dr R. Graham 198
Osburn, Lucy 9, 25, 35
osteomyelitis 111, 137, 144, 161, 202
Out-patients Department ix, 17, 22, 23, 31, 34, 52, 59, 68, 72, 73, 73–4, 74, 83, 94, 100, 120, 121, 129, 156, 167–9, 170, 180, 195, 286, 291, 301, 303, 306
Oxnam, Cathy 309, 309

Packham, Alma 43
pain control 208, 235, 269, 310
Palmer, Jan 283
parents' (and wider family's) involvement in

child treatment ix, 73, 88–9, 111, 120, 121, 138, 139–40, 178–9, 198, 199, 200, 205, 206, 207, 209–10, 211–12, 232, 236, 242, 265–6, 267, 269, 270, 271, 285, 293, 294, 295, 297–8, 299–300, 303, 304, 306, 308, 309, 310–11
Parkes, (Sir) Henry 9
Pasteur, Louis 10
patient care, and nurses 4, 14, 16, 17, 21, 21, 22, 23, 26, 27, 28, 29–31, 38, 40, 41, 45, 46, 47, 49, 54, 65, 65, 66, 72, 75, 79, 85, 88, 89, 95, 97, 100, 111, 111, 120, 121–3, 124, 128, 130, 133, 134–6, 137, 138–9, 140, 141, 141–2, 143, 144, 147–8, 149, 149, 150, 153, 161, 162–3, 164, 166, 167, 168, 178–80, 195, 198–201, 201, 202–3, 204, 204–8, 210–12, 213, 216, 219, 220, 227, 227, 231, 231–5, 242, 244, 251, 253, 253, 254–5, 259–61, 276, 280, 285, 291, 296, 297, 298, 299, 300, 301, 303, 305–6, 308–310
patients: average length of stays 111, 136, 169, 185, 218, 291, 295, 309; in-patient numbers ix, 3, 13, 18, 31, 32, 51, 81, 129, 133, 204, 229, 291; out-patient numbers ix, 13, 81, 204, 291, 301; schooling for long-termers 139, 140; segregation of girls and boys 13, 32, 139, 139, 140, 140 (see also food, rules)
Patten, Mary 242, 266, 286, 286, 287, 288, 288, 289, 300, 312
Patterson, Mrs 20
Payne, Gwenda 215
Peck, Eleanor 161, 181
Peck, Muriel Anna 103, 104, 105, 107
penicillin 179–80, 181, 202, 203
Penn, Edith 156
Perry, Bishop Charles 5, 9, 12
Perry, Frances 12
Peter MacCallum Clinic 297
Peters, Olive see Raymond, Olive
Pex, Patricia 217
pharmacy at RCH 57
Philpott, Sue 288
Pierce, Evelyn 169
Pilkington, Isabel 112, 113, 125, 127, 128, 153, 154, 155, 156, 169–70, 173–4

378

INDEX

Pink disease 198
Playfair, Margaret 220, 283
Player, Hilda 55, 66–7, *68*, 68, 69, 70, 76, 77, 82, 83, 86, 89, 90, 96, 97, 106, 107, 284
pneumonia 122, 126, 163, 180, 233
Pohlman, Robert Williams 4, 5
poisonings 210, 211, 247, 291
poliomyelitis (infantile paralysis) 72, 87, 91, 112, 120, 126, 133, 134, 137, 140, 144, 145, *146*, 160, 161, 185, 306
Pollard, Christine *283*
Pollard, Dianne *283*
Pollock, Jeanette *230*, 278
post-basic/postgraduate education 130, 221, 222, 248, *250*, 251, 264–5, *266*, 277, 278, 280, 287, 288, 293, 300, 311, 312 (*see also* tertiary)
Potts, Francis 286
poultices 26
Powell, Dr Mostyn 197, 236
Preece, Helen 277
Preliminary Training School (PTS) 112, 115, 116, 118, 128, 130, 154–5, *155*, 164, 169–70, 178, *187*, 189, *193*, 196, 213–14, 221, 222, 227, 240, 244, 245, 273, *274*, 275, 285, 288
premature babies 162, 181, 198, 310
Presbyterian Babies' Home 129
Price, Dr Eric 147
Price, Margaret 43
Priest, Susan *283*
Prince Henry's Hospital 14, 76, 96, 128, 137
Princess May Pavilion 66, 67, 73, 82, 84, 120, 203
Prowse, Rosemary *283*
Proy, Silvio 303
psychiatric conditions 305
public health education 23–4, 66, 97, 105, 170, 291, 292, 309
Puckle, Mrs 4
Pullar, Sue 310
Purcell, Kathy 244

(RCH) qualifications, portability of 61, 75, 128, 275, 277
Queen Elizabeth II, visit of 229, *230*
Queen Victoria Hospital (Melbourne) 221
Quiney, Helen 286
Quiney, Mary *156*, 208

radiotherapy 297
Ragg, Dr Philip 235

Ramsey, Diana (née Harrison) 191
Rank, Benjamin 205
Raymond, Olive (née Peters) *164*, 164, 167–8
Recovery Room 254, 257, *263*, 270
recreation, and nurses 69, 98, 100, 114–15, 117, 118, 119, 130, 135, 136, 155, 161, 217, *240*
Red Cross 90, 98 (*see also* awards/prizes)
Reddihough, Dr Dinah 306
Rees, Catherine *283*
registration, and nurses 76, 112, *126*, 128 (*see also* Nurses' Registration Board of Victoria)
remote area nursing 102, 103, *106* (*see also* Cottage Bush Nursing Hospitals)
rheumatic fever 8, 160, 198, 233
Richards, Gwenneth *156*
Richmond Dispensary 9
Rintel, Mrs 4
Risby, William Andrew 8
Robertson, Janet *215*
Robinson, Andrew 310
Robinson, Gwendoline *283*
Rodda, Libby *228*
Rogers, Grace 208, *209*
Rogers, Margaret (née Stockwell) 163, 175, *175*
Roman Catholic patients, and priestly visits 84, 162
Ronald McDonald House 299, 311
Ross, Rev David 117
Ross, Isabella Younger 82, 103
Ross, Norma *188*
Rossiter, J. F. 281
Rouse, Mrs 196
Royal Alexandra Hospital for Children (Sydney) 67
Royal Australian Armed Forces Nursing Service (RAAFNS) 177
Royal Australian Navy Nursing Service (RANNS) 144, 171
Royal Australian Nursing Federation (RANF) 242–3, 276, 286
Royal Children's Hospital, Melbourne (RCH) (formerly Free Hospital for Sick Children): Annual Reports of 7, 16, 18, 48, 58, 81, 129, 133, 204, 213, 291; Committee of 4, *5*, 5, 11–13, 14, 17, 18, 23, 31, 34, 35, 36, 38, 40, 42, 48, 51, 54–5, 56, 58, 60, 67, 68, 69, 70, 72, 75, 77, 80, 82, 83, 84, 87, 90, 96, 97, 98, 99, 100, 102, 117, 121, 126, 128, 138, 145, 150, 156, 157, 158, 161, 167, 169, 186, 189, 190, 196, 197, 221, 222, 223, 229, *230*, 232, 241, 274, 276, 284; centenary celebrations of 278, *280*, 280; founding purpose of 4, 13, 77; fundraising/donations for 60, 86, 90, 91, 96–7, 117, 136, 141, 150, *189*; locations/expansions of 3, 3–4, 6, 13, 14, *15*, 18, *19*, 21, 31, 32, *33*, 38, 43, 60, 66, *67*, 72, *73*, 76, 77, 82, 90, 90, 97, 133, *134*, *145*, 145, *148*, *157*, 168, 185, 186, *192*, 222, 227, *228*, *230*, 238, *239*, 251; nurse numbers at 76, 96, 100, 102, 133, 218, 238; Royal Charter of 218
Royal Commission on Charitable Institutions (1890–91, Report 1892) 35, 43, 59
Royal Melbourne Hospital (RMH) 5, 67, 70, 74, 75, 76, 91, 96, 100, 102, 112, 130, 137, 167, 179, 180, 214, 216, 221, 222, 235, 240, 258, 286
Royal Victorian College of Nursing 98, 221
Royal Victorian Trained Nurses' Association (RVTNA) 61, 65, 67, 74–5, 98, 100, *101*, 102, 106, 130 (*see also* College of Nursing, UNA)
Royal Women's Hospital (formerly Lying-in Hospital) 8, 16, 76, 86, 91, 128, 137, 221, 235, 236, 250, 312
rules, and nurses 40, 48, 54, 65, 68, 72, 76, 83, 100, *111*, 114, 118, 119, 163, 205, 213, 218, 240–2, 244, 268; and patients 17, 34, *111*; and visitors 199, 209–10
Russell, Robert Hamilton 71, *71*
Ryan, Charles 70, *70*
Ryan, Julia 86

Sadlier, Elizabeth *see* Chalmers, Elizabeth
Sage, Annie M. 170
St Thomas' Hospital (London), Nightingale School at ix
St Vincent's Hospital 216, 242, 245, 297
Salter, Elaine 270
Salter, Gillian *212*
Saunders, Dorothy 191, 223, *255*, 256, 268
Savage, Ellen 173

'Save the Babies' Appeal 96–7
Sawrey, Dr Cliff 162, 164
Sax Committee Report 285
Scantlebury (Brown), Dr Vera 82, 105
Schapper, Barbara *155*
Schilov, Andre and Alexandre 199
scholarships 222
scoliosis 308, 309
Sechiari De Neeve (née Walmsley), Lucy 178, 186–8, *188*, *189*, 189–90, *190*, 191, 196, 213, 218, 221, 222, 223, 227, 229, 231, 241, 286
Semmens, Margot *187*
Sexton, Dr Helen 82
Shannon, Beryl 250
Sheehan, Marie *212*
Sheldon, Mrs 14
Shepherd, Joan *187*
Sherbrooke Convalescent Cottage ix, 103, 112, 133, 134, *148*, *149*, 149–51, *151*, 154, *157*, 157–8, *159*, 160, 185, 191, 209
Shergold, Dr Una 303
Shine, May 86
Shipp, Anne 294
Sick Nurses' Ward 121, 145, 162, 204
Simpson, Paula 288
Singleton, Dr John 4, *5*, 5, 9, 12, 17
Sisters 68, 77, 81, 82, 83, 95, 100, 103, 115, 117, 119, 121, *129*, *129*, 130, 143, 154, 155, 160, 161, 162, 165, 166, *166*, 167, 170, 178, 180, 181, 185, 191, *194*, 195, 197–8, 202, 203, *204*, 206, 208, *209*, 210, 211, 212, 216, 217, *219*, 222, 223, 229, *230*, *231*, 231, 233, 234, 241, 244, 245, 248, *249*, *250*, 255, *255*, *258*, 258, 259, 262, *263*, 264, 267, 270, 271, 276, 278, *279*, 281, *282*, 285, 289, *302*, 303 (*see also* Nurse Educators, Home Sisters, Staff Nurses, Tutor Sisters)
skin care treatments 169
Slater, Pat *156*, 242
Sloan, Dr Lionel (L. E. G.) 203, 251
Smith, Barbara (née Catto) *155*, *189*
Smith, Cecily *209*
Smith, Durham 246, 300
Smith, Elsie 106
Smith, Dr Gordon Keys 238, 306
Smith, Iris 100
Smith, Judith 269
Smith, Marg *239*
Smith, Meryl *155*

Smith, Robert Murray 59
Smith, Robyn (née McLaren) *273*, 305
Smith, Dr William 4, *5*, 5, 14, 17; Mrs Smith 86
Snowball, Dr William ix, 17–18, 23, 24–5, *25*, 31, 36, 43, 56, 70, 76
Snowball Ward 85
Social Work Department 281
Solomon, Dr John 234
Southby, Dr Robert 94, 121
Spanish influenza 77, 91, 93, 95–6
Spargo, Dr 76
Sparks, Beryl 162
Spencer, Sean 312
spina bifida 238, 300, 306, 309
Squibbs, Amy E. A. 169
Staff Nurses 68, 81, 82, 83, 103, 129, 161, 166, 180, 227, 236, 241, 245, 264, 285
Stafford, Mrs 4
Stainsby, Jill Harris 153
State Registered Nurses 221
State Enrolled Nurses 284
Stawell, Dr 52
Stawell, Sir William 5
Stephens, Dr Douglas 164, 300, 301
Stephenson and Turner (architects) 156, 229
sterilisation techniques 10, 31, *256*, 269
Stewart, Nurse 36
Stocks, Dr John 257, 259, 260, 261
Stokes, Lola (née Cumber) 284
Street, Annette 310
Street, Debra *283*
Street, Faith *215*
Strickland, Elizabeth *see* Hocking, Elizabeth
stringency measures 84, 90–1, 97, 118, 155, 167, 170, 198
Stuart, Rev 162
study block training 130, 214, 221, 222, 243
study leave 222–3, 278
sulphonamide drugs 163, 203
Sumner Ward 32, *46*
Surgical Ward(s) 32, 33, 65, 68, 82, *120*, 121, *204*, 204–8, 209, 214, 235, 236, 238, 246, 255, 300–1, *301* (*see also* Edward Wilson Surgical Pavilion and specialty areas)
Sutherland, D'arcy 293
Sutton, Anne *283*
Sutton, Lesla 248
Swift, Wendy *279*, 294, *295*, 295

Teasdale, Anne Maree 311
Teasdale, James *291*, 311
Telfer, Heather 203, 260, *264*, 264, 265, 266, 278, 288
Terry, Joan *155*
tertiary education 242, 285, 287, 288, 293
Testar, Elizabeth 13, 35, 38
tetanus 203–4
textbooks and course notes 18, 21, 57, 125, 169, 170, 197–8, 208, 280–1
theatre technicians 262
Thomas, Maria 34, *68*, 77, 90, 100, 106
Thomas, Phil (née Richey) 211–12
Thomas, Thyra (née Watson) *146*, 147, 148, 149
Thompson, Elizabeth *188*
Thompson, Judy *188*
Thomson, Marge *187*, 235–6, 296
Thorburn, Patricia 114
Thorne, Bev *see* Touzel, Bev
Tiballs, Dr Jim 235, *264*
Tomlinson, Marjorie *see* Hosking, Marjorie
tonsillitis 168, 195, 201, *201*, 270
Tonzing, John 270
Toohey, Deborah *283*
Topp, Nurse 57
Touzel, Bev (née Thorne) 306, *307*, 308, *308*, 309
tracheo(s)tomy 8, 82, 161, 179, 202, *253*, 254, 255–6, 259
Trained Nurses' Guild 100, 102 (*see also* College of Nursing)
(nurse) trainees and probationers 10–11, 16, 18, 26, 36, 43, 46, 48, 50–1, 55–7, 58–9, 61, 65–6, 69–70, 71, 76, 82, 83, 84, 85–6, 87–8, 89, 90, 94–5, 100, 111–12, 114–16, *116*, 117–19, 121–4, 125, 127–8, 131, 134, *135*, 136, 137, 143, 147–8, 149, 151, 154–5, *155*, 156, 160–3, *164*, 164–5, 167–8, 178–80, 186, *187*, *194*, 196–7, 198, 199, 200, 203, 204, 205, 206, 208, *209*, 213–14, 216–18, 221, 222, 234, 238, 240, *240*, 241–5, 269–70, 273–4, *274*, 275, 276, 277, 278, 285, 286 (*see also* awards/prizes, certification, graduation, Preliminary Training School, Nursing School)
tuberculosis and related illnesses 5, 8, 52, 111, 126, 134, 137, 139, 144, 185, 195, 200, 306

Tucakic, Marina 288
Turnbull, Hilda 80
Turner, Dr Elizabeth 162, 180, *181*, 181, 197, 203, 267
Turriff, Haldane 35
Tutor Sisters 99, 112, *113*, 118, 125, 127, 128, 130, 131, 153, 154, *155*, *156*, 160, 169–70, *187*, 213, 221, 227, 236, *243*, 243, *250*, 251 (*see also* Nurse Educators)
typhoid 4, 5, 8, 16, 28, 30–1, 35, 38, 39, 52, 60, 76, 80, 162, 169
typhus 8

UNA (Journal of (R)VTNA) 67, 98, 105
Uncle Bobs Club 278, 306
uniforms 18, 36, *37*, *42*, 43, 83, 115, 116, 117, 118, 136, 150, 179, 185, 196, 197, 213, 241, 242, 243, 245, 258, 284
Upton, Mr 155
urine testing 122–3
urological nursing 300, 301

vaccinations 185
Van Leewin, Mary *201*
Van Valen, Jo 245, *246*, 246–8, 270
Vance, Marjorie *135*
Vaughan, Rose 21
Venables, Dr Alex 233, 236
venereal diseases nursing 16, 93–5, 102, 200, 203
Venereal Diseases Act 1915–16 (Vic.) 91, 94
Vernon, Esther Dorothea Harcourt 43
Victorian Infant Asylum an Foundling Hospital 65
Victorian Nursing Council 245, 286
Victorian Trained Nurses' Association (VTNA) *see* RVTNA
Vietnam, nurses in 245, *246*, 246–7, 248
Vintiadis, Anne *287*, 288

Waddington, Brendan 233
Wakefield, Alan 205–6
Wall, Cathy *215*
Walsh, Hilda 94, 106, 107, 112, 115, 116, 117, 118, 124–5, *125*, 126–7, 156, 157, 161, 163, 164, 165, 167, 169, 171, 186
ward (nurse) assistants ('Pinkies') 161, 186, 200, 205, 238, 261
Warr, Margaret 137, 151, 155
Waterhouse, Jill *188*
Waters, Joan 250
Watson, Beatrice Middleton 81
Webster, Katherine (Kit) 115, 116, *116*, 119, 121, 155, 161, 162, 163, *190*
Webster, Dr Reginald 89, 96, 121
Were, J. B. 31
West, Charles ix, 18
Westlake, George 233, 246
Westland, Betty (née Jeffrey) 170–1
Whitbourne, Graham 277
White, Beryl (née Letcher) 118
White, Mrs F. *239*
Whittaker, Dr J. G. 141
Whitfield, Doris *129*
Wigg, Dr Henry 17, 23
Wilkins, Leanne *283*
Williams, Dr Howard 124, 156, 157, 160, 170, 195, 197
Williams, Jacquie 288
Williams, Leanne *283*
Williams, Dr Stanley 197
Willis, Roslyn 300, 301, *301*
Wilson, Beatrice *135*
Wilson, Charles 149
Wilson, Grace Margaret 34, 77, 97–8, *98*, 99, *99*, 100, 102, 105, 124, 170
Wilson, Judith *215*
Wilson, Kathleen (Kate) *129*, 130, 131, 160, 170, 186, 221–2, 227, 236
Wilson (née Alderson), Mary 69, 85–6
Winstanley, Bon 134
Wiseman, Lorraine *283*
Wishart, Una 117, 143, *156*, *159*, 160, 163, 164, 171, *194*
Women's and Children's Health Care Network 312
Women's Hospital *see* Royal Women's Hospital
Wood, Dr Arthur Jeffreys 35, 60, 61, 66, 70, 72, 74, 88, 94, 103, 105, *106*, 254 (*see also* awards/prizes)
Wood, W. Atkinson 74, 103
World War One, and nurses 53, 76, 77, 80–91
World War Two, and RCH 126, 131, 144, 150–1, 153–4, 156–7, *157*, 158, *159*, 160, 162, *164*, 167, 170–1, *171*, 172, *173*, 173–5, *175*, 176, *176*, 177, 181
Wright, Professor 148
Wright, Verna *215*

X-ray Department 82, 120, 129

Youl, Dr 8
Young, Dr Simon 304
Younger, Dr Isabella *see* Ross, Dr Isabella